The Psychiatric Treatment
of Adolescents

THE PSYCHIATRIC TREATMENT OF ADOLESCENTS

Edited by

Aaron H. Esman, M.D.

International Universities Press, Inc.

New York

Library of Congress Cataloging in Publication Data

Main entry under title:

The Psychiatric treatment of adolescents.

  Bibliography: p.
  Includes index.
  1. Adolescent psychotherapy. I. Esman, Aaron H.
[DNLM: 1. Mental disorders—In adolescence. 2. Mental disorders—Therapy.WS 463 P974]
RJ503.P73 1982   616.89′14′088055   83-208
ISBN 0-8236-5595-4

Manufactured in the United States of America

Contents

PART IV: GROUP THERAPY

PART V: BEHAVIOR THERAPY

PART VI: PSYCHOPHARMACOLOGY

Acknowledgments

My thanks and appreciation are due to:

—the authors and publishers of the papers printed herein, for their generosity in permitting the publication and republication of their work;

—Mrs. Phyllis Rubinton, Librarian, and Miss Mary Mylenki, Assistant Librarian, of the Department of Psychiatry, Cornell University Medical College, for their gracious assistance with the arduous business of locating material for this book;

—Mrs. Sandra Schneiderman, for her unfailingly cheerful and efficient work in the preparation of the manuscript;

—Dr. John Sours, for his catalytic suggestion at a strategic moment;

—my wife, whose support and encouragement are eternally helpful.

Introduction

The psychiatric treatment of adolescents has a relatively brief and somewhat checkered history. Indeed, the recognition—some would say the designation—of adolescence as a unique developmental phase was a late occurrence in human history (see Ariès, 1962). Until the last century adolescents in trouble tended, with certain exceptions, to be dealt with by society in the same manner as adults, with little or no concern for their special characteristics and phase-related needs.

The modern approach to the psychological treatment of adolescents derives from two major historical channels. The first, of course, is psychoanalysis, beginning with Freud's (1905a) report of his analysis of the patient he called "Dora." Although he gave little explicit consideration to Dora's adolescent status, it is clear, as Blos (1979b) and Glenn (1978) demonstrate, that adolescent issues were paramount in the structure of her neurosis, in the complex family entanglements that helped to shape it, and in the unresolved transference issues on which the analysis foundered. In any case, Freud's (1905b) conceptualizations of adolescent development and his general views on the role of transference and resistance led to the pioneering contributions of Aichhorn (1925) and his followers to the treatment and education of troubled youths. Anna Freud's explication (1936, 1958) of the adolescent's defense structure led to further clarification of the nature of conflict and its modes of maladaptive resolution during this developmental phase.

The second major factor in the development of the modern approach was the evolution of the juvenile court system. Now fallen under serious criticism for its alleged failure to provide adequate rehabilitative measures for the more aggressive adolescent, the juvenile court represented, at least in its conception, a major effort to humanize the care of young offenders and to provide an institutional framework for a treatment approach based on the recognition of the adolescent's special circumstances. It was in 1899 that Illinois established the first statewide system of juvenile courts, and the other states followed rapidly in the early years of this century, applying the ancient principle of *parens patriae* whereby the state or ruler assumed responsibility for the protection of infants in the realm (see Malmquist, 1978, pp. 735-737). A network of guidance clinics and residential treatment centers, many of them using the new ideas of psychoanalytic psychology, grew up in conjunction with the juvenile justice system and its corollary, the child welfare system—all struggling to find new ways of helping troubled adolescents and of reducing the burden they place on society.

It was thus the socially troublesome adolescent who was the beneficiary—or target—of the earliest treatment efforts. Only later, as ideas about prevention began to gain currency, did professionals begin to apply their methods and extend their interest to other groups of adolescents in difficulty—the neurotic, the sexually confused, the psychophysiologically afflicted, and the psychotically withdrawn. At first, enthusiastic students of psychoanalysis sought, as far as possible, to use classical treatment techniques. Given the complexities of adolescent psychology, however—the shifting defenses, the intolerance of frustration, the pressure toward action—it was "not surprising," said Anna Freud (1958), "that besides analytic therapy many alternative forms of treatment for adolescents have been evolved and practiced . . . " (p. 263). As Zellermayer (1975) has pointed out, however, the difficulties may rest as often with the therapist, whose own unresolved adolescent conflicts may be stirred up by his work with the patient and compromise his status as an effective adult.

Most of the newer therapies—group therapy, residential treatment, family therapy, brief or specially focused psychotherapies—have drawn their basic concepts and some of their treatment strategies from psychoanalysis. Behavior therapy, in contrast, has developed independently of—even perhaps in reaction against—psychoanalysis, deriving its principles from learning theory and conditioning techniques. Most recently, new developments in psychopharmacology have also been applied to the treatment of adolescent patients.

This book aims to provide the reader with a survey of the range of therapies currently available for adolescents and, where possible, the historical background from which they have sprung. In selecting the papers to be included, I have sought to present as fairly as possible a variety of points of view and theoretical perspectives. It will not be lost on the reader, however, that for me a basic framework of psychoanalytic developmental psychology is the optimal structure on which to build rational therapeutic efforts. Indeed, a number of non-analytic treatment approaches appear to flow from this primary source and others to derive nourishment from it. I hope that, similarly, this volume will provide intellectual nutriment for those who are devoted to the clinical and educational care of young people who are, as Winnicott (1965) put it, "struggling through the doldrums."

Aaron H. Esman

PART I

*Psychoanalysis
and Psychoanalytic
Psychotherapy*

1

INTRODUCTION

The Transference, by August Aichhorn

August Aichhorn (1878-1951) was the pioneer in the development of efforts to apply psychoanalytic concepts to the treatment of troubled youth. A teacher by training, he early became interested in work with the abandoned and the delinquent, and found in psychoanalysis the instrument that served him, as had no other, in his efforts to understand and influence the young people who came into his charge in the residential center he founded in Vienna after World War I. The distillation of his highly original, idiosyncratic, empathic approach to delinquent youths and their families appeared in 1925 as his enormously influential little volume, *Verwahrlösten Jugend,* translated as *Wayward Youth.*

Aichhorn served as inspiration and model to a generation of gifted child therapists and child analysts such as Anna Freud, Fritz Redl, Erik Erikson, and Peter Blos, all of whom, like Aichhorn, came to psychoanalysis through education. His mastery of the use of the clinical interview as a psychotherapeutic tool was unrivaled; as Kurt Eissler (1949) put it: "He has forged an exquisite therapeutic tool out of a procedure which is usually a matter of routine. . . . a single interview [has] a significant effect on the family equilibrium, an effect which persist[s] years after the interview had taken place" (p. xii).

3

In this excerpt from *Wayward Youth*, Aichhorn demonstrates both his understanding of Freud's concept of "transference" and his unique way of exploiting it to establish what
would now be called a "working relationship" or "therapeutic
alliance" in his clinical work with delinquents. Aichhorn had
no illusions about the efficacy of the "blank screen" therapist
in such cases, and was by no means adverse to using his own
authoritative bearing and position as therapeutic agents. Different times and social attitudes may by now have diminished
the power of such devices, but it is still worth being reminded
by a master of their occasional utility, even within the framework of psychoanalytically inspired therapy.

1

The Transference

August Aichhorn

We have used the term "transference" several times, and in the last case we attributed the therapeutic results to the transference without further definition of the word. We shall now consider more closely the emotional relationship which is thus designated. During a psychoanalytic treatment, the patient allows the analyst to play a predominating role in his emotional life. This is of great importance in the analytic process. After the treatment is over, this situation is changed. The patient builds up feelings of affection for and resistance to his analyst which, in their ebb and flow, so exceed the normal degree of feeling that the phenomenon has long attracted the theoretical interest of the analyst. Freud studied this phenomenon thoroughly, explained it, and gave it the name "transference." We shall understand later why he chose exactly this term.

I cannot reproduce for you all of Freud's research about the transference, but must limit myself to essentials. When we speak of the transference in connection with social re-education, we mean the emotional response of the pupil toward the educator or counselor or therapist, as the case may be, without meaning that it takes place in exactly the same way as in an analysis. The "countertransference" is the emotional attitude of the teacher toward the pupil, the counselor toward his charge, the therapist toward the patient. The feeling which the child develops for the mentor is conditioned by a much earlier relationship to someone else. We must take cognizance of this fact in order to understand these relationships. The tender relationships which go to make up the child's love life are no longer strange to us. Many of these have already been touched upon in the foregoing chapters. We have learned how the small boy takes the father and mother as love objects. We have followed the strivings which arise out of this relationship, the Oedipus situation; we have seen how this runs its course and terminates in an identification with the parents. We have also had opportunity to consider the relationships between brothers and sisters, how their original rivalry is transformed into affection through the pressure of their feeling for the parents. We know that the boy at puberty must give up his first love objects within the family and transfer his libido to individuals outside the family.

Our present purpose is to consider the effects of these first experiences from a certain angle. The child's attachment to the family, the continuance and the subsequent dissolution of these love relationships within the family not only leave a deep effect on the child through the resulting identification; they determine at the same time the actual form of his love relationships in the future. Freud compares these forms, without implying too great a rigidity, to copper plates for engraving. He has shown that in the emotional relationships of our later life we can do nothing but make an imprint from one or another of these patterns which we have established in early childhood.

Why Freud chose the term "transference" for the emotional relationship between patient and analyst is easy to understand. The feelings which arose long ago in another situation are transferred to the analyst. To the counselor of the child, the knowledge of the transference mechanism is indispensable. In order to influence the dissocial behavior, he must bring his charge into the transference situation. The study of the transference in the dissocial child shows regularly a love life that has been disturbed in early childhood by a lack of affection or an undue amount of affection. A satisfactory social adjustment depends on certain conditions, among them an adequate constitutional endowment and early love relationships which have been confined within certain limits. Society determines these limits just as definitely as the later love life of an individual is determined by the early form of his libidinal development. The child develops normally and assumes his proper place in society if he can cultivate in the nursery such relationships as can favorably be carried over into the school and from there into the ever-broadening world around him. His attitude toward his parents must be such that it can be carried over to the teacher, and that toward his brothers and sisters must be transferred to his schoolmates. Every new contact, according to the degree of authority or maturity which the person represents, repeats a previous relationship with very little deviation. People whose early adjustments follow such a normal course have no difficulties in their emotional relationships with others; they are able to form new ties, to deepen them, or to break them off without conflict when the situation demands it.

We can easily see why an attempt to change the present order of society always meets with resistance and where the radical reformer will have to use the greatest leverage. Our attitude to society and its members has a certain standard form. It gets its imprint from the structure of the family and

the emotional relationships set up within the family. Therefore the parents, especially the father, assume overwhelming
responsibility for the social orientation of the child. The persistent, ineradicable libidinal relationships carried over from
childhood are facts with which social reformers must reckon.
If the family represents the best preparation for the present
social order, which seems to be the case, then the introduction
of a new order means that the family must be uprooted and
replaced by a different personal world for the child. It is
beyond our scope to attempt a solution of this question, which
concerns those who strive to build up a new order of society.
We are remedial educators and must recognize these socio-
logical relationships. We can ally ourselves with whatever
social system we will, but we have the path of our present
activity well marked out for us, to bring dissocial youth into
line with present-day society.

If the child is harmed through too great disappointment
or too great indulgence in his early love life, he builds up
reaction patterns which are damaged, incomplete, or too
delicate to support the wear and tear of life. He is incapable
of forming libidinal object relationships which are considered
normal by society. His unpreparedness for life, his inability
to regulate his conscious and unconscious libidinal strivings
and to confine his libidinal expectations within normal
bounds, creates an insecurity in relation to his fellow men
and constitutes one of the first and most important conditions
for the development of delinquency. Following this point of
view, we look for the primary causes of dissocial behavior in
early childhood, where the abnormal libidinal ties are established. The word "delinquency" is an expression used to describe a relationship to people and things which is at variance
with what society approves in the individual.

It is not immediately clear from the particular form of the
delinquency just what libidinal disturbance in childhood has

given rise to the dissocial expression. Until we have a psychoanalytically constructed scheme for the diagnosis of delinquency, we may content ourselves by separating these forms into two groups: (1) borderline neurotic cases with dissocial symptoms, and (2) dissocial cases in which that part of the ego giving rise to the dissocial behavior shows no trace of neurosis. In the first type, the individual finds himself in an inner conflict because of the nature of his love relationships; a part of his own personality forbids the indulgence of libidinal desires and strivings. The dissocial behavior results from this conflict. In the second type, the individual finds himself in open conflict with his environment, because the outer world has frustrated his childish libidinal desires.

The differences in the forms of dissocial behavior are important for many reasons. At present, they are significant to us because of the various ways in which the transference is established in these two types. We know that with a normal child the transference takes place of itself through the kindly efforts of the responsible adult. The teacher in his attitude repeats the situations long familiar to the child, and thereby evokes a parental relationship. He does not maintain this relationship at the same level, but continually deepens it as long as he is the parental substitute.

When a neurotic child with symptoms of delinquency comes into the institution, the tendency to transfer his attitude toward his parents to the persons in authority is immediately noticeable. The worker will adopt the same attitude toward the dissocial child as to the normal child, and bring him into a positive transference, if he acts toward him in such a way as to prevent a repetition with the worker of the situation with the parents which led to the conflict. In psychoanalysis, on the other hand, it is of greatest importance to let this situation repeat itself. In a sense, the worker becomes the father or the mother but still not wholly so; he represents their claims, but in the right moment he must let the dissocial child know that he has insight into his difficulties and that he will not interpret the behavior in the same way as do the parents. He will respond to the child's feeling of a need for punishment, but he will not completely satisfy it.

He will conduct himself entirely differently in the case of the child who is in open conflict with society. In this instance he must take the child's part, be in agreement with his behavior, and in the severest cases even give the child to understand that in his place he would behave just the same way. The guilt feelings found so clearly in the neurotic cases with dissocial behavior are present in these cases also. These feelings do not arise, however, from the dissocial ego, but have another source.

Why does the educator conduct himself differently in dealing with this second type? These children, too, he must draw into a positive transference to him, but what is applicable and appropriate for a normal or a neurotic child would here achieve the opposite result. Otherwise the worker would bring onto himself all the hate and aggression which the child bears toward society, thus leading the child into a negative instead of a positive transference, and creating a situation in which the child is not amenable to training.

What I have said about psychoanalytic theory is only a bare outline. A much deeper study of the transference is necessary to anyone interested in re-educational work from the psychoanalytic point of view. The practical application of this theory is not easy, since we deal mostly with mixed types. The attitude of the counselor cannot be as uniform as I have pictured it for you. We do not have enough description of individual forms of dissocial behavior to enable us to offer detailed instructions about how to deal with them. At present our psychoanalytic knowledge is such that a correct procedure cannot be stated specifically for each and every dissocial individual.

The necessity for bringing the child into a good relationship to his mentor is of prime importance. The worker cannot leave this to chance; he must deliberately achieve it and he must face the fact that no effective work is possible without it. It is important for him to grasp the psychic situation of the dissocial child in the very first contact he makes with him, because only thus can he know what attitude to adopt. There is a further difficulty in that the dissocial child takes pains to hide his real nature; he misrepresents himself and lies. This is to be taken for granted; it should not surprise or upset us. Dissocial children do not come to us of their own free will but are brought to us, very often with the threat, "You'll soon find out what's going to happen to you." Generally parents resort to our help only after every other means, including corporal punishment, has failed. To the child, we are only another form of punishment, an enemy against whom he must be on his guard, not a source of help to him. There is a great difference between this and the psychoanalytic situation, where the patient comes voluntarily for help. To the dissocial child, we are a menace because we represent society, with which he is in conflict. He must protect himself against this terrible danger and be careful what he says in order not to give himself away. It is hard to make some of these delinquent children talk; they remain unresponsive and stubborn. One thing they all have in common: they do not tell the truth. Some lie stupidly, pitiably; others, especially the older ones, show great skill and sophistication. The extremely submissive child, the "dandy," the very jovial, or the exaggeratedly sincere are especially hard to reach. This behavior is so much to be expected that we are not surprised or disarmed by it. The inexperienced teacher or advisor is easily irritated, especially when the lies are transparent, but

he must not let the child be aware of this. He must deal with
the situation immediately without telling the child that he
sees through his behavior.

There is nothing remarkable in the behavior of the dissocial; it differs only quantitatively from normal behavior.
We all hide our real selves and use a great deal of psychic
energy to mislead our neighbors. We masquerade more or
less, according to necessity. Most of us learn in the nursery
the necessity of presenting ourselves in accordance with the
environmental demands, and thus we consciously or unconsciously build up a shell around ourselves. Anyone who has
had experience with young children must have noticed how
they immediately begin to dissimulate when a grown-up
comes into the room. Most children succeed in behaving in
the manner which they think is expected of them. Thus they
lessen the danger to themselves and at the same time they
are casting the permanent molds of their mannerisms and
their behavior. How many parents really bother themselves
about the inner life of their children? Is this mask a necessity
for life? I do not know, but it often seems that the person
on whom childhood experiences have forced the cleverest
mask is best able to cope with reality. It is not surprising that
the dissocial individual masquerades to a greater extent, and
more consciously, than the normal. He is only drawing logical
deductions from his unfortunate experiences. Why should
he be sincere with those people who represent disagreeable
authority? This is an unfair demand!

We must look further into the differences between the
situation of social retraining and the analytic situation. The
analyst expects to meet in his patient unconscious resistances
which prevent him from being honest or make him silent;
but the treatment is in vain when the patient lies persistently.
Those who work with dissocial children expect to be lied to.
To send the child away because he lies is only giving in to

him. We must wait and hope to penetrate the mask which covers the real psychic situation. In the institution it does not matter if this is not achieved immediately; it means merely that the establishment of the transference is postponed. In the clinic, however, we must work more quickly. Talking with the patient does not always suffice; we must introduce other remedial measures. Generally we see the delinquent child only a few times; we are forced to take some steps after the first few interviews, to formulate some tentative conception of the difficulty and to establish a positive transference as quickly as possible. This means we must get at least a peep behind the mask. If the child is not put in an institution, he remains in the old situation under the same influences which caused the trouble. In such cases we wish to establish the transference as quickly as possible, to intensify the child's positive feelings for us that are aroused while the child is with us, and to bring them rapidly to such a pitch that they can no longer be easily disturbed by the old influences. To carry on such work successfully presupposes a long experience.

Let us interrupt our theoretical considerations here and see how the worker tries to grasp the situation, to establish the transference, and to lift the mask. How others work, I do not know; I can only try to show you what I usually do. A youth comes into the consulting room. At first glance he seems to be the bully type. If we take a stern tone with him, he rejects us immediately and we can never get a transference established. If we are cordial and friendly, he becomes distrustful and rejects us or he takes this for weakness on our part and reacts with increased roughness. If we approach a boy who is intellectually superior with a severe air, he feels himself immediately on sure ground and master of the situation because he meets that attitude often in life. He looks with suspicion on people who are nice to him and is more than ever on his guard. The timid ones, who come in frightened, are easily reduced to tears by a stern demeanor and fall into a state which may be confused with sulkiness. How shall we conduct ourselves in order to establish a good contact with the child? I usually begin with a friendly look or attitude; sometimes I say, "How do you do," or I may only shake hands in silence. I say that there is nothing here to be afraid of, that this is neither a police station nor a court. Sometimes I tell a joke by way of introduction. This gives me an opportunity to size up the situation. We sit down opposite each other. Just how I proceed toward the establishment of the transference in an individual case depends on the impression I have of the youth as he first enters the room.

I consider this first moment of our coming together of the utmost importance. It is more than a "feeling out" of the situation; it must have the appearance of certainty and sureness and must be put through as quickly as possible because in most cases it forms the foundation for our later relationship. The adolescent does the same thing when he comes into contact with me. He wants to know right away what kind of person he is dealing with. Children usually try to orient themselves quickly, but for the most part they are not clever about it. The adolescent, however, often develops an amazing ability at this. We can observe a momentary gleam in the eye, a hardly perceptible movement of the lips, an involuntary gesture, a "watchful waiting" attitude, although he may be in a state of conflict. The older he is, the harder it is to know whether he will prove stubborn, or openly scornful and resistant. It is especially difficult when he assumes an air of sincerity or unctuous submissiveness. If I accept this as genuine, he immediately feels superior although he may sense that I have the upper hand.

After this sizing up of each other is over, a struggle begins for the mastery of the situation. This may be brief or it may be prolonged, and I must confess that I do not always come out victorious. You must not think of this struggle, however, as a mutual show of conscious strength. There are many unconscious factors in it; we feel rather than know what actually takes place. My attitude from the very beginning lets the boy feel that I have a power over him. He is justified when he senses this as a danger. He does not feel this as an entirely new situation; he has experienced it often before. I am thus no different from his mother, father, or teacher. If he is a borderline case of neurosis with dissocial features, or a mixed form where the dissocial features are predominant, I remain in the position of the parents but, as our association progresses, I act somewhat differently. If the child is in open conflict and expecting an attack, he is disappointed. I do not ask him what he has done, I do not press him to tell me what has happened, and, in contrast to the police or juvenile court, I do not try to pry out of him information which he is unwilling to give. In many cases where I feel the child wants to be questioned so that he can come into opposition to me, I say that he may hold back whatever information he wishes, that I understand that one does not want to tell everything to a person he has met for the first time. When I add that I would do likewise, he is usually willing to fall into conversation with me about something remote from his difficulties but in line with his interests. To describe my attitude from the moment when I let the boy feel some activity in me, I would say that I become progressively passive the more he expects an attack from me. This astonishes him, he feels uncertain, he does not know where he stands. He feels, rather than understands, that I am not an authority with whom he must fight, but an understanding ally. I avoid the word "friend" intentionally since he has no friends; he allies himself with others only because he needs them to achieve some end.

In a natural fashion, I begin to speak of things which interest most boys but are in no way connected with their dissocial behavior. Eight out of ten are interested in football. One must know the teams, the best players, the last match, the scores, etc. Less often one finds a contact through books, mostly through adventure and detective stories. It is often easy to talk about movies and in this way make the child lose his caution.

With little girls I talk about fairy tales and games. Often one does not need to go far afield. A remark about the clothes or jewelry they wear may start the ball rolling. I let the half-grown girls tell me about styles in clothes, in haircuts, or the price of toilet articles. I ask the youngest children who are afraid to talk what they like to eat; we discuss desserts and candies. Thus I reach topics which the child carries on in the conversation. Sometimes it is difficult, sometimes easy, but as a rule it is possible to arrive unobtrusively at what I wish to know. In the first interview I usually get the positive transference well enough underway to secure some explanations and to gain some influence.

It is also necessary to get some idea of the child's relationship to the members of the family and other people in the environment. Adolescent children usually answer such questions directly; with younger children this is more difficult. Either they do not answer questions at all or they answer in a way which is worthless for our purpose. We must learn their attitudes through various makeshifts, such as talking about games and stories.

I asked a 10-year-old girl if she liked to read. When she said, "Yes," I asked what she liked best.

"Fairy tales."

"Without stopping to think, tell me the name of a fairy tale you like."

"Snow White."

"What part in it?"

"Where the old witch sold Snow White the poisoned apple."

"Were there pictures in your book?"

"Yes."

"One of the witch, too?"

"Yes."

"Describe the witch for me, not exactly as she is in the picture, but how you think of her."

She described the witch in detail, her size, her hair, her facial expression, mouth, teeth, and clothes. When I asked where she got these various characteristics, it turned out that they were a collection from people whom the child disliked. This does not always turn out so propitiously. Sometimes the figure described does not fit the disliked people in the environment.

Another little girl told me that she liked to play with dolls. I asked her to describe in detail a doll she would like to have. This again resulted in a composite figure, but this time it had the features of the people she loved.

A 12-year-old girl once sat opposite me giving no sign through her facial expression, movement, or speech what kind of emotional situation she was in. I asked what color she liked best.

"Red."

I continued, "When I think of a color, I always think of something which has that color. On what do you see red?"

"On the front car of the grotto-train in the amusement park."

"Now tell me what color you like least."

"Black."

"Where do you see black?"

"Your shoes and tie."

"But surely something else black occurs to you, too?"

"The hole where the grotto-train goes in is black, too."

What all this may symbolize need not concern us at the moment. We need only consider how the anxiety connected with the ride in the grotto-train has been displaced onto me. She sat in front of me in the same anxious tension that she sat in the train in the amusement park. Perhaps she wanted to ask, "What's coming next?" How do we know this? My shoes and my cravat (which was really gray) had for the child the same color as the grotto which she did not like. You can see how we get material from which we draw conclusions about the psychological situation of the child. I certainly would not have received a satisfactory answer to a direct question, for even if she had been ready to tell the truth she would not have known how to describe how she felt.

In such a tense situation we can accomplish nothing. I let her tell me about the trip through the grotto. Brightly lighted pictures appeared suddenly in the dark, devils roasting poor souls on hellish fires, dwarfs digging in the bowels of the earth for treasure, and such things. Something uncanny was always appearing and nothing cheerful or happy ever happened. We went from this to the shooting galleries, from one stand to another, and to the merry-go-round. Then laughing, she told me about a funny fortune-teller who could tell what was going to happen to you. When I asked what amusing experiences she could remember, she told of another trip to the amusement park at the time she was confirmed. With this her mood changed completely, making it possible for the transference to begin. She was now accessible to questions which came to the point. I do not need to mention the fact that the child had no conception of my intention.

Sometimes a deep distrust shows itself. Perhaps I have acted clumsily, perhaps I am dealing with a special type of personality. Then I must resort to some other method. I will report such a case where in a brief time I succeeded not only in overcoming the distrust but also in discovering how it arose.

A 16-year-old girl, who had been suspected of being a prostitute because of her behavior and appearance, had suddenly shown a complete change. Her bold manner had disappeared and in her dress and behavior she had become a conventional, respectable girl. The social worker wanted to know what had happened. Naturally I did not know, but asked to see the girl. We sat down together and she showed very evident distrust of me. I asked how things were at home but got no answer. Did she like to read? What did she think about? No answer. Would she tell me a dream? Continued silence. Thereupon I laughed and said, "You think it's dangerous to talk to me. I can understand that, but certainly it can't be dangerous to tell me a story of a movie you've seen." She laughed and started to tell about a circus acrobat who had to dive from a high place through a burning ring. Two girls were in love with him. One of the girls, out of jealousy, cut the wire and made him fall into the fire-ring. The second girl saved him but sacrificed her life to do so. As you can guess from this summary, the story did not tally exactly with what she had seen, but showed her own version of it. I asked her what pleased her best in it and got the answer I expected, namely, that the girl sacrificed herself for her lover. I then asked if she could remember how the hero looked. When she answered in the affirmative, I asked her to describe what he must look like to please her. She described him as a strong, young, slender, dark-haired, clean-shaven man with bright eyes. Now I said, "Tell me, what does Franz look like?" She understood immediately that I meant her boyfriend, was a little embarrassed, and then described him to look just like the movie hero. She went on without further effort on my part to say that he was studying chemistry but her mother refused to let her go with him. It was clear that the change in the girl was to be ascribed to her affection for the man. By attacking her distrust, I soon succeeded in overcoming her resistance.

I shall now present a case to show you how the transference can help one to find the deeper-lying causes of dissocial behavior.

A city school reported that for several months a 13-year-old boy had been absent on Tuesdays and Fridays. The history stated that instead of going to school he went to the horse market, not out of any special interest or because of the tips he may have got for small chores, but only to be in the neighborhood of the horse dealers. I do not regard every unusual bit of behavior as springing from some obscure motive, but try first to find a simple explanation. Since I have always found that, after the transference is established, the child will go to school regularly if I show him that it pleases me, I tried it in this case. We must realize that in many cases no one troubles himself about a child's going to school and that he therefore has no incentive to endure the unpleasantness of school life. In such truancy cases, I have the boy come to me first every week, then every two weeks, and later less often. When he knows that I am interested in all the pleasant and unpleasant happenings in the previous school week, he enters into the school life, and the truancy subsides. With this boy who went to the horse market, the transference was established in the first interview. He came for the next two weeks and reported that he had been in school. The third week the mother came to say that he was going to school regularly, but twice a week he did not come home until late in the evening and she thought from the way he smelled that he must have been in the horse market again.

We see in this case how the transference blocked the outlet for a symptom. The force behind the symptom, however, was still effective and produced a new symptom. The boy could not stay away from school because of his feeling for me. Now we see that this was not a case of ordinary truancy. Something attracted him to the horses and it was only a coincidence that the time for school and the horses was the same. Through the transference, I could see that we were dealing with a deeper mechanism. One needs psychoanalytic methods in the treatment of such a case. I do not want you to conclude from what I have said that I have any hard and fast rules which enable me to establish the transference in all cases. I only want to protect you from making the crudest mistakes in your practice by giving you some hints from my own experiences.

When the child comes to us in the institution, we do not feel obliged to hurry the establishment of the transference. Unless it is a case of neurosis with dissocial features, we are friendly, but show no extraordinary interest in him or his fate and do not force ourselves upon him. We ignore his distrust, his secret or open opposition, his condescension, scorn, or whatever he may show against us. The preparation for the transference he gets from his companions. He usually makes quick contacts with the other boys not because he shows his real self to them or because he needs friendship, but because he must have an audience to whom he can relate an exaggerated account of his adventures, for whom he even improvises new escapades when reality offers nothing impressive enough. According to his custom, he begins to collect information about the details of the organization and the people with whom he comes in contact. Is the counselor a "good fellow," can he be annoyed or teased, and how? He hears a great deal from the boys who are about ready to leave the institution. He learns the characteristics of the people on the staff, what the real life of the institution is like. Through this contact with the other boys, he saves himself from the disillusionment which often follows first impressions, and comes in touch with an authority from which he does not need to turn distrustfully away, or which he tolerates, with clenched teeth, until such time as he attains his freedom and attempts a revenge.

If the *milieu* has done its part, the transference begins to develop as the counselor gradually lets himself be drawn out of his passive role and responds to the newcomer in a neutral but friendly manner. Sometimes he pays more attention to the boy, sometimes less. This fluctuation of interest is not a matter of indifference to the youth. If he is distrustful because the counselor seems to pay undue attention to him today, tomorrow he will be reassured if no notice is taken of him. He betrays a definite excitement the next day, however, if he thinks the counselor has observed his unpolished shoes with displeasure. The shoes will be more highly polished or dirtier according to the positive or negative feeling aroused in him, or they will remain the same if no transference is underway. In this case we must wait. What I have said about the shoes is true for a host of other small details which the educator must be quick to recognize and to evaluate. He must sense the ambivalence or changes from affection to distrust in the relationship of his charge to him. There are no general directions for this. We must observe at first hand how the experienced counselor directs these waves of feeling and strives deliberately to raise the crests to a higher point. It is easy to recognize when the positive relationship reaches a climax. Often the feelings of affection break out with such vehemence and strength that the child waits in great tension for his counselor to appear, does something to attract his attention, runs after him, or finds something to do which brings him into his counselor's vicinity. The unskilled worker will not recognize the importance of this moment, will be on the defensive and not realize that the affection of the boy can thus be changed into hate. On the contrary, when the hate reaction sets in, he will flatter himself that he has always seen through the hypocrite. If we try to show him how he mis-interprets the situation, he turns a deaf ear. He does not understand that he is interpreting as cause what is really effect.

I would like to show you how hard it often is to establish a transference with individuals of the highly narcissistic type—that is, those who are in love with themselves. I cite the case of a 17-year-old boy who had gambled and specu-lated on the stock exchange and had made a lot of money. He had begun at 15 as a cashier for a street moneychanger, who entrusted him with orders on the exchange and made it possible for him to speculate on his own. He accumulated a small fortune for a boy, and made himself independent. He travelled to other countries and imported things which he sold as a bootlegger. This business paid well. He led a free and easy life in night clubs, gambled, and associated with the demimonde. When his money gave out, he began pawning his mother's clothes. His mother, who had been left a widow after an unhappy marriage, had repeatedly tried to reform the boy. Since she could do nothing with him, she appealed for help to a social agency which brought him to us.

He was one of those boys who gave no apparent trouble in an institution. Such youths are polite and obliging, handy and useful in simple office work. They know how to get along with others and soon achieve the role of gang leader. When one works more intensively with them, one learns to see their difficulties. Inwardly demoralized but outwardly as smooth as glass, they offer no point of attack. Their behavior is a mask, but a very good one. They show no interest in the personnel, and ward off every attempt to establish a real relationship to them. Thus the transference, which must of necessity be very strongly positive if one is to accomplish anything with them educationally, is almost impossible to establish. In the institution they give the impression of being cured very speedily but when at large again they revert to their old behavior. We must use the greatest caution with them.

Our man of the world knew how to withdraw from every effort to influence him. He was with us several months without any transference having been established in the psychoanalytic sense. We could see, however, that he had been influenced by the environment. I thought it a good idea to get him away from it for a time so that he could compare the discomforts of another environment with the comforts he enjoyed with us, feeling that this realization might make him accessible to therapy. For this purpose, however, he must not be sent away; he must go of his own accord. I had to avoid letting him know of my intention. The best way to achieve my purpose was to influence his feeling about the institution. Occasionally, running away from the institution takes place as the result of a sudden emotional state or because of a dream, and then it is hard to prevent. In most cases, however, it requires long preparation and should not escape the sharp eye of the counselor. Aside from our position against punishment in general in a reform school, we regard it as a complete lack of understanding to punish returned runaways. The running away takes place only when the "outside" is a more attractive place than the "inside." If we can induce the boy to talk to us while he is in this conflict, we can often make the "inside" seem more attractive without mentioning his intention of running away. We can accomplish the opposite effect if we recall the outer world to his memory as more attractive than the life in the institution.

A short talk was sufficient to put our gambler in the right mood. A half hour after he left me, I got the report that he had run away. The first part of my treatment had worked. The counselor did not know that I had provoked this. I confide such things to the personnel only when I need their cooperation, since it is extremely difficult when one lives among the boys to conceal such things. If such a plan does not succeed, it gives rise to unending differences of opinion. With our gambler, this successful provocation to run away was a prologue to the establishment of the transference. I expected his return on the second day. When he had not turned up after a week, I feared that I had make a mistake.

At nine o'clock in the evening 10 days later, someone knocked on my door. It was the runaway. He was so exhausted physically and under such psychological tension that I felt I could accomplish much more with him than I had planned. I did not reproach him for going away, as he evidently expected. I only looked at him seriously and said, "How long has it been since you had something to eat?" "Yesterday evening." I took him into the dining room of my apartment where my family was at supper and had a place set for him. This boy, who was usually the complete master of a situation, was so upset that he could not eat. Although I was quite aware of this, I said, "Why don't you eat?" "I can't. Couldn't I eat outside?" "Yes, go into the kitchen." His plate was refilled until he was satisfied. When he finished eating, it was 10 o'clock. I went out and said to him, "It's too late for you to go into your group tonight. You can sleep here." A bed was fixed for him in the hall. I patted him on the head and said goodnight to him.

The next morning the transference was in effect. How strongly positive it was I learned from a mistake which I made later. Without realizing it I gave him grounds for jealousy, in that I let one of his comrades check up on his bookkeeping, in which he often made errors. The counselor to whom he was entrusted succeeded, however, in making good the mistake in this especially difficult case. Soon after this he was allowed to bring the supplies from the city. He never let himself be led astray after that. He left the institution to become a salesman and for years has had a satisfactory record as a clerk in a business establishment.

The establishment of the transference seldom necessitates such an artifice. Generally the ordinary course of events is enough. I reported this case merely to show you how impossible it is to lay down general rules.

2

INTRODUCTION

*Notes on Problems of Technique in the
Psychoanalytic Treatment of Adolescents:
With Some Remarks on Perversions*, by K.
R. Eissler

Aichhorn's technical approach to the treatment of delinquents involved, among other things, active efforts by the
therapist to arouse the patient's interest, curiosity, and respect. Kurt Eissler is a compatriot of Aichhorn, reared in the
fertile atmosphere of between-the-wars Vienna that saw the
flowering of psychoanalysis and its application to a wide
range of problems. Though primarily an analyst of adults,
he has had a special interest in the propagation of Aichhorn's
ideas (Eissler, 1949), and during World War II had the opportunity to test them in the treatment of psychiatric cas-
ualties in the United States Army. It was Eissler who
formulated the concept of technical "parameters" (1953)—i.e.,
modifications of classical analytic technique in response to
the specific requirements of patients who do not conform to
the classical neurotic model. It is precisely the elaboration of
such parameters that he describes here, in setting forth a
model based on the special developmentally determined
characteristics of adolescent patients. Indeed, Eissler pro-
poses an approach based on an extraordinary degree of flexi-

bility, with the therapist attuning himself to what at times may be moment-to-moment shifts in ego organization and defense structure.

Eissler is a true psychoanalytic polymath and in the course of this essay offers characteristically scholarly reflections on a wide range of issues from artistic creativity to the psycho-biological function of the orgasm. His observations about the central role of masturbation and masturbation fantasy in adolescent development have been reaffirmed and elaborated in recent work by Borowitz (1973) and Laufer (1978), among others.

As he acknowledges, the technical prescriptions set forth here are idealized and paradigmatic, unlikely to be fully realized in practice by an actual therapist. They do, however, demonstrate the way in which informed psychodynamic and structural assessment of the patient's mental state can and should serve to direct the form and content of the therapist's intervention.

2

Notes on Problems of Technique in the Psychoanalytic Treatment of Adolescents: With Some Remarks on Perversions

K. R. Eissler, M.D.

This paper undertakes to outline an ideal technique for the treatment of adolescent patients. I have not actually used the projected technique, nor do I claim to have mastered it, and offer only a construct built on chance observation and applied theory.

Even on this limited basis it may be worthy of consideration because the psychoanalytic treatment of adolescents is an area of continuing controversy (Gitelson, 1948). Even analysts who agree on other areas of technique hold widely divergent views on this subject. Some analysts do not undertake treatment of adolescents on the grounds that psychoanalysis cannot be used for this age group and advise only psychotherapeutic, supportive, or educational measures. Those who have used psychoanalysis for adolescents have reported occasional good therapeutic results with modified techniques; but also the

Reprinted by permission from *The Psychoanalytic Study of the Child*, 13:233-254, 1958. New York: International Universities Press.

painful surprise of unforeseen failures or severe aggravation of the patient's condition. These analysts believe that the crux of the clinical problem lies in the proper selection of adolescent patients for therapy. There is also a small group which maintains an optimistic view of the psychoanalytic treatment of adolescents.

The controversy encountered in this area of psychoanalysis is reminiscent of the situation in child analysis (A. Freud, 1945). The limitation of age as a criterion for treatment potential was raised early in the history of psychoanalytic technique. It was clear that the process of aging diminished the flexibility necessary for psychoanalytic therapy and eventually a point was reached where it becomes impossible to effect even minor reorganizational processes.[1]

In general we expect greater, that is to say, more profound clinical success with younger patients than older ones. In 1904 Freud regarded patients close to or over 50 no longer amenable to psychoanalytic treatment, while prepubescent patients (depending on special circumstances) were thought to be promising subjects (p. 264). It can be learned from Freud's *Studies on Hysteria* (Breuer and Freud, 1893-1895) and *The Interpretation of Dreams* (1900) that he did not hesitate to subject adolescent patients to the cathartic method. "Elasticity of mental processes" and educability apparently determined the eligibility of patients (Freud, 1904). Elasticity and educability are indeed two prominent features of adolescence, yet grave doubts exist regarding the treatability of patients at that stage of their growth.

Although it is easy to define puberty in terms of biological

[1]Here one may recall Freud's clinical impression that women of about 30, in contrast to men of the same age, frequently show signs of such "psychical rigidity and unchangeability" as to leave "no paths open . . . to further development" (1933, pp. 134-135). However, diminished transformability is generally noticeable from the third to the fourth decade.

maturation, it is difficult to reach equally acceptable definitions of the psychology and personality development of adolescence. Whereas the biological processes are identical (with the possible exception of the time of onset) in all races and social groups, the psychology of this developmental period differs widely. Bernfeld (1923) has made this the focus of his research. Indeed, the syndromes may embrace extremes, and it seems almost impossible to find a common denominator in their bewildering variety. Bernfeld's thesis (1929) of the social *topos* and its influence on forms of psychopathology may be usefully applied to clinical research on adolescence.

Adolescence may pass without conflict when no inner objection is raised against heterosexual intercourse, and instinctual gratifications are assured by favorable external circumstances. Or, this period may end in suicide if the resistances to and the fear of impulses and fantasies concerning heterosexual or substitute gratifications are so strong that the ego cannot cope with the new demands upon the psychic apparatus. Although puberty may take many courses, we think predominantly of stormy and unpredictable behavior marked by mood swings between elation and melancholy (Bernfeld, 1938). We assume the adolescent will be subjected to great inner suffering and be a source of worry to those who feel responsibility for his welfare. Indeed, storminess to some degree can be considered normal during this period, and its origins are easy to trace, no matter how it is manifested. In most instances the personality of the pubescent undergoes a process of reorganization which subjects the psychic apparatus to great strain. Parts of the personality which had solidified are loosened and new structures must be formed (A. Freud, 1936). The outcome depends to a certain extent on imponderables, and the feeling of doom or the tortured preoccupation with the uncertainty of the future reported by some adolescents reflects an objective feature of this period of life.

I wish to emphasize here one of the many aspects of this process of reorganization. It seems well proven that the basic conflicts or the interplay of basic psychic forces are determined in almost all persons in the period between one of the pregenital phases and the oedipal phase, or the latter and some point in the latency period. These basic conflicts probably do not undergo subsequent alteration, but the clinical *form* in which they will be manifest in the adult often appears to be decided only during adolescence. The principal forms in which psychopathology may make its appearance are neurosis, perversion, delinquency, and psychosis, and their equivalent character syndromes.

Of course, this statement needs to be qualified. There are instances where specific psychopathology has been firmly established before puberty and sometimes even before prepuberty and where consistent uniformity of pathology is encountered between the years of infancy and adulthood. Thus the history of an adult's neurosis may start in childhood with a severe phobia that changes to a compulsive neurosis during latency and becomes a neurosis of mixed type during adolescence, essentially unchanging in its clinical form in subsequent years. It is not difficult to trace a similar course for psychopathological forms such as delinquency and perversions. Thus the development may continue from the pregenital phase without a change in clinical form during puberty. But there are many instances in which the persistent psychopathology is formed only during adolescence, beginning, as the case may be, with the early manifestations of prepuberty. This is important to a discussion of technique in the analysis of adolescents.

When an adolescent enters treatment with a solidified form of psychopathology—a severe neurosis, or schizophrenia, full-blown delinquency or a perversion in which he indulges to the exclusion of any other sexual gratification—then psychoanalytic treatment involves no particular technical problem essentially different from its adult counterpart. However, with adolescent patients whose need of treatment is evident but whose psychopathology is still in flux, we encounter a technical problem specific to puberty. In many instances psychopathology switches from one form to another, sometimes in the course of weeks or months, but often also from one day to another and even within one and the same psychoanalytic hour. The symptoms manifested by such patients may be neurotic at one time and almost psychotic at another. Then sudden acts of delinquency may occur, only to be followed by a phase of perverted sexual activity. Thus, correlated with the psychobiological particulars of this developmental phase, the patient may exhibit a variety of psychopathological forms in quick succession. One would have to study the conditions (internal and external) under which self-observation becomes so much exaggerated that it renders the adolescent a *Heauton Timoroumenos* and those conditions under which these functions are checkmated by ungovernable passions, in order to select a random example. Parallel to this delineation of extremes it would be necessary to specify the technical measures to counter these extreme clinical manifestations. The frequency of symptomatic changes manifested by many adolescent patients makes it evident that no one technique can fulfill the requirements for the treatment of adolescents. Therefore, I shall digress now and outline the techniques evolved to treat a variety of disorders and then discuss the feasibility of their application to the treatment of adolescent patients.

A technique which aims at inducing a change of personality depends mainly on three factors: (1) how material is obtained from which conclusions about the unconscious parts of the patient's personality are drawn; (2) how the resistances are dealt with; (3) the structure of the patient's transference and how it is to be handled.

The best-known and most studied technique is that with which the common neuroses are treated, the classical method developed by Freud. Here no particular effort is necessary for the recovery of material. The subjective material can be obtained with relative ease mainly because:

1. The discomfort the patient suffers from the neurotic disorder impels him to meet the requirements of treatment.
2. The capacity for self-observation is uninjured in neurotic disorders. In the neurotic patient a firm separation is maintained between representations of the external and the internal reality. Despite temporary confusion of the two, observable in neurotic projections and displacements, enough capacity for self-observation and self-criticism remains potentially to enable him to separate one from the other.
3. In a neurosis the conflict is internalized and the disorder does not subside with changes in external conditions. That is to say, wish fulfillments do not remove symptoms. Fulfillment of unconscious wishes may even aggravate the symptoms since such gratifications arouse anxiety and, in general, unconscious feelings of guilt.

Consequently, internalization of the conflict draws the patient's attention toward his inner life; his capacity for self-observation enables him to discern internal processes, and the pain inherent to his disorder induces compliance with the analyst's demand to verbalize his observations.

The whole process is greatly supported and even rests mainly upon the buoyancy of the repressed, which emits derivatives into the conscious part of the patient's mind, particularly in the supine treatment position which excludes distraction by external stimuli and makes possible full attention to whatever crosses his field of consciousness.

Under these conditions the analyst is in a position to study all provinces of the patient's personality, particularly the resistances and defenses which the patient institutes against the emergence of the repressed and, therefore, also against the therapeutic process. The principal tool used in this technique is interpretation. Interpretation of the repressed and of the unconscious part of ego and superego provides the patient with insight and permits reconstruction of his history.

Among the patient's numerous associations, those referring directly or indirectly to the therapist are of particular interest. They illuminate the patient's transference in which significant conflicts and unconscious memories make their—usually distorted—appearance. In ideal instances, the transference absorbs the whole disorder and becomes the battlefield on which the dissolution of the neurosis takes place. In neurosis the transference is spontaneous and does not need stimulation or manipulation (Freud, 1937, p. 233). Interpretation remains the exclusive tool of operation.

Insight into the structure of his personality and into his history provides the patient with freedom of choice within the limits set by reality and by his own endowment. His personality is now enabled to meet frustrations without renewal of symptoms.

The next best-studied psychoanalytic technique is that of child analysis. The structure of the child's personality requires basic changes from the technique outlined above. Anna Freud has devoted extensive study to the derivation of the technique of child analysis and to the structure of the child's personality.[2] Since the time of her study, knowledge about both child and adult personality has grown and the technique of child analysis has changed.[3]

Many salient points in the technique of child analysis seem to have derived from the absence of a fully developed, self-observatory function in the child and his relative inability to distinguish between what is inside and outside of his personality. Here I am concerned mainly with the child at the peak of the Oedipus conflict. The extent of self-observation, its various forms, and its integration at particular age levels deserves separate investigation and will not be pursued here. Suffice it to say that the child's capacity for self-observation is not sufficiently developed to permit the use of the classical technique. Material has to be obtained, therefore, in a different way, through daydreams, play, games, storytelling, or from any situation which facilitates expressive verbalization on the child's own level.

The child produces fantasies and tells stories with relative ease and, owing to his comparative closeness to the primary process, he usually reveals more of the repressed than an adult. But the child's quick susceptibility to anxiety arouses correspondingly quick mobilization of the defenses. Usually, then, what is revealed of the unconscious cannot be interpreted in a way the child could accept. Thus, the unconscious

[2]See Anna Freud's *Introduction to the Technique of Child Analysis* (1926). This book could be called the first text on comparative psychoanalytic technique since the author consistently compares the technique of psychoanalysis for adults with that necessary and adequate for children. Comparative technique is a fruitful area, but neglected in the literature of psychoanalysis.

[3]For an admirable report of a child analysis, see Bornstein (1949). Since I am not a child analyst, the outline that follows is based on the literature and on discussions with colleagues. At present it is difficult to abstract a general scheme of the technique of child analysis and my presentation may be inadequate.

may be projected onto outer reality and be readily understood by the analyst in terms of the repressed, but it may be impossible to demonstrate to the child the meaning of the projection for he will remain fully convinced of the outer reality of his projections.

The transference problems in child analysis are important. To a child the analyst is another adult who shares this status with all other adults in his environment. The analyst therefore does not possess that unique and exclusive place he holds with adult patients, and is more than the focus for transference (A. Freud, 1927). To the child, the adult (and the analyst) is the source of authority, of assistance, of knowledge and affection. Since he has not yet repressed his oedipal strivings, not all reactions and behavior patterns in the child's relationship to the analyst can be viewed as displacements of elements originating in his relationship to the parents.

Furthermore, the superego of the child is not yet functionally reliable. At most this province of the personality is only slightly developed. His ego, unassisted by the superego and lacking its later power to synthesize, still tolerates contradictions. Moreover, regressions are easily precipitated and the child's ego may not be adequate to deal with the new situation except by indulging in the pleasures of regressed activities or to recoil in horror from them. As Anna Freud (1927) has also pointed out, analytic interpretations may have quite different effects on the child than on the adult. Depending on the developmental stage and individual factors, the child may infer, from the analyst's benevolent neutrality and abstention from prohibitions, implicit permission to carry out repressed impulses. Whereas, in the adult, an internal structure, the superego, is the main source of prohibition, in the child it is usually fear of punishment or of loss of love that impels him to abstain. Therefore the role of the child analyst is to be also that of pedagogue, a role the analyst strictly avoids when treating adult patients (A. Freud, 1927).

Thus, interpretation of transference in child analysis is very different from its interpretation to adults. The whole technique must acknowledge the necessity for the child to evolve additional structure in the course of his analysis.

The technique of child analysis is contingent upon the characteristics of a developmental period. In other situations it may be the nature of the disorder which makes the classical technique inapplicable. Principally, there are two groups of disorders which require special therapeutic techniques in treatment. These are the delinquencies and the schizophrenias. In outlining the models of technique appropriate to many instances in these two groups, I will refer to the structure of the ego wherein the respective symptoms reside. A psychoanalytic technique makes sense only in reference to ego structure and can rarely be derived from symptomatology (Loewenstein, 1958, p. 202).[4]

I shall turn now to a third psychoanalytic technique which has been fairly well systematized, mainly through the efforts of August Aichhorn (1925). The technical difficulty in treating a delinquent arises from his total lack of desire to change. His symptoms are painful not to him but to others in his environment.[5] He has no need or motive to reveal to the analyst what is going on in him. Furthermore, he sees the analyst as a representative of that society against which his aggressions are directed and therefore meets him with distrust or fear. Yet, even if the delinquent wanted to confide

[4]A symptom such as stealing, which unquestionably constitutes an act of delinquency, may be based on neurosis or appear in a schizophrenic patient. Yet, stealing may also be symptomatic of an ego structure characteristic of the delinquencies.

[5]This is also often true of the symptoms that the child develops. See Anna Freud (1945).

in the analyst, he would verbalize almost nothing but the content of his unfulfilled desires and his plans for gratification since, in accordance with the structural defects of his superego, his capacity for self-observation has scarcely been developed or has been badly damaged.

Thus, even under the optimal conditions, never obtained in practice, a structural change would first have to be effected in the delinquent before one could learn about the interplay of forces and his development. If, during the initial phase, a typical delinquent were put on the analytic couch for the purpose of free association, he would either fall asleep or report that nothing comes to mind. Although bearing the marks of resistance, such behavior reflects even more the consequences of a structural defect. Therefore, the first phase of treatment consists in making the delinquent analyzable, that is to say, neurotic. Once this is achieved, society is safe from his aggressions and he will cooperate with the analyst and be amenable to the classical technique.

But how can one transform the delinquent into a neurotic? By instituting those processes we know lead to the formation of superego structure. The analyst, by forcing the patient into a strong emotional dependency and exposing him to frustration, compels the patient to undergo the process he defied during the oedipal phase, namely, identification with an authoritative person. Once this is established, the delinquent will be unable to gratify his asocial impulses. First he will learn to keep them in suspense without ensuing discharge; and then, in accordance with basic laws, his unfulfilled desires will be subjected to repression.

Clinical experience demonstrates that, in such instances, repression is not complete and the warded-off impulses return in the form of neurotic symptoms, making the patient amenable to the classical technique. This can be achieved when the analyst consistently behaves so as to offer an ego ideal that is acceptable to the delinquent patient. Discussion of the variety of measures necessary for this exceeds the confines of this paper. Suffice it to say that the analyst may afford partial wish fulfillment to the delinquent in a way that does not draw the latter further into impulsive behavior; he may demonstrate repeatedly to the patient that the analyst's knowledge of ways and means to gratify delinquent impulses are vastly superior to the patient's. The analyst has also to relieve the delinquent's archaic feelings of guilt and provide healthier safeguards against archaic impulses. Setting prohibitions which do not transgress the patient's current level of tolerance is, of course, an integral part of the treatment.

Technique in this phase is further characterized by a minimal use of interpretation, since defenses must not be broken down but raised against archaic impulses. What then is the dynamic equivalent of interpretation as used in the classical technique? The experienced analyst is capable of using seemingly trivial details as clues to the delinquent's recent misdeeds and his plans for future misbehavior. By verbalizing the delinquent's secret thoughts the analyst creates an illusion of omniscience which greatly contributes to the development of a positive transference in the patient.[6] This induces the delinquent to accept the analyst as a superego figure concomitant with the occurrence of anxiety and the aforementioned symptomatic change. When this is achieved, the second phase begins.

[6]"In the neurotic the secret is hidden from his own consciousness; in the criminal it is hidden only from you. In the former there is genuine ignorance, though not an ignorance in every sense, while in the latter there is nothing but a pretence of ignorance. Connected with this is another difference, which is in practice of importance. In psycho-analysis the patient assists with his conscious efforts to combat his resistance, because he expects to gain something from the investigation, namely, his recovery. The criminal, on the other hand, does not work with you; if he did, he would be working against his whole ego" (Freud, 1906, pp. 111-112).

The schizophrenic personality has a different structure; consequently the therapeutic technique must differ. We observe in the schizophrenic disorders, too, a victory of the pleasure principle over the reality principle. But this is achieved by a dysfunction of perception and thinking. The barrier between the ego and the instincts is weakened and permits the wishes stored in the repressed to impinge upon the functions of thought and perception which cooperate with the id far more than is compatible with the reality principle.

To understand the requirements for the psychoanalysis of schizophrenia it may be useful to elucidate some differences between the delinquent and the schizophrenic. In the delinquent the functions of thought and perception are intact, but the volitional system, abetted by the patient's intelligence and observational power, is put into the service of the pleasure principle unchecked by the restraint of an adequately developed superego. All the delinquent's energy is directed toward immediate wish fulfillment. Thus the delinquent and the schizophrenic fail to curb or conquer the pleasure principle. However, with the delinquent, his wishes are well circumscribed and can be potentially fulfilled. Dissatisfaction for the delinquent lies in sectors of reality which in his estimation withhold pleasure. If, for example, he had all the money and all the girls he desires, he would not commit his asocial acts. His aggressions are carried out with basic ego functions intact.[7]

The schizophrenic, too, lives in an unacceptable reality. But his conflict with reality is eliminated by falsification of perceptions and thoughts. The faulty action which results from his disorder is the secondary effect of faulty perception

[7]This is an oversimplification which does not consider the effect of superego pathology on the rest of the delinquent's ego, his inclinations toward perversions and homosexuality.

and thought. Thus a schizophrenic may commit murder because a hallucinated voice commands him to do so. The different effects of the fixation upon the pleasure principle can best be characterized by the autoplastic nature of the schizophrenias versus the alloplastic nature of the delinquencies.

In discussing the treatment technique for schizophrenia, two phases of the treatment are to be considered: (1) the acute stage in which the whole personality is overpowered and the patient's objectivation of the symptom becomes impossible; (2) a phase in which the acute disease process has subsided and a foothold can be found in the patient's personality from which he can maintain some distance from his symptoms. The technique required in each of the two phases differs.

The latter phase, in a surprising number of instances, permits a technique with a surface resemblance to the classical. The patient can recline on a couch and pursue the trend of his associations. However, the content of the interpretations, their sequence, the way the transference is handled differ essentially from the classical technique. These differences do not concern us here. Only the procedure which may help a patient out of the acute phase is of interest in this context.

Here the problem is how to approach a patient who has withdrawn from reality because it has taken a turn that is unbearable to him. A variety of techniques have been suggested, one of which I will present briefly since it is applicable to critical phases in the treatment of the adolescent patient.

The disappointment that forces the patient to withdraw always involves a conflict with another person. Even when the precipitating factor is a particular event, such as a financial setback or an impending graduation, one regularly finds behind it a temporary (sometimes perhaps a permanent and therefore incurable) incapacity to trust or love a human being. The world from which the nonschizophrenic expects love and kindness, or hatred and unfriendliness, as the case may be, becomes for the schizophrenic patient a world from which *only* hatred and unfriendliness can be expected.[8]

The initial technique to break through the barrier created by the schizophrenic's withdrawal must eliminate whatever tends to confirm the patient's expectations and then expose the patient to stimuli which will disprove the primary equation he has established or which has been imposed on him. The manner in which this is to be brought about varies, of course, from patient to patient, and has to be found out anew in each individual case. Since the patient misinterprets reality, that is to say, he draws incorrect inferences from various environmental conditions, it is no easy task to eliminate everything that may have an aggressive meaning to him. If the quality of the therapist's tone evokes in the patient a memory of his father's stern voice, the therapist will lose his chance to allay the acute crisis. Indeed, the schizophrenic may sense aggression which, though present, would be imperceptible to a normal person (Freud, 1922), for example, if the therapist perhaps unconsciously is impatient and his voice takes on a rasping note. Clinical experience demonstrates in many instances that when all stimuli which the patient can interpret as aggressive are eliminated, and a sustained variety of stimuli which the patient interprets as affectionate is proffered, the acute conflict subsides. The patient turns toward the world again, though still in a pathological way. The relationship to the therapist becomes the point of crystallization around which other friendly channels are organized. Once this state is reliably established, the second phase of treatment, of less interest in this context, can set in.

[8]See Kogerer (1934). I owe thanks to Dr. Laci Fessler for calling my attention to Dr. Kogerer's work. Dr. Kogerer has coined the term "crisis of trust" ("*Vertrauenskrise*") that excellently characterizes the state I have in mind.

Thus we see that in the therapeutic setup for the acute phase transference and resistance analysis are radically different from the classical technique. The schizophrenic is in the grip of his unconscious and information about the acute conflict usually is easy to obtain. The report of the patient's environment locates more frequently than not the external sources of his current plight. Resistances are not to be analyzed since this would only stimulate more intense breakthrough from the unconscious into the patient's ego, and result in further regressions. Positive transference must be actively induced, and the therapeutic task centers on the removal, not of intersystemic barriers, but of those that interpose between the patient and external reality.

In accordance with my initial diagram, I should now set forth the psychoanalytic technique for the treatment of perversions. Unfortunately, no such technique has been developed. Nevertheless, I will permit myself a few general remarks about perversions that may be justified in view of the fact that manifest perversions so frequently have a direct connection with adolescence.

Initially, perversions were put into a clinically well-delineated group by Freud (1905b) who called them the negative of the neuroses, thereby emphasizing a characteristic contrast between the dynamics of the two disease entities. However, Freud's decisive paper on perversions (1919), which to a certain extent became paradigmatic for psychoanalytic research, was based upon knowledge obtained from perverted fantasies of neurotic patients. This is easily understandable. In almost every psychoanalysis of a neurotic patient one encounters a considerable number of sexual fantasies that express impulses toward sexual deviation. The bulk of our information concerning the origin and development of perversions is derived from the analysis of this material. But the structure of the personality that wards off perverted impulses by the formation of neurotic symptoms differs from the personality structures of actual deviants. Furthermore, the psychoanalyst has an opportunity to investigate the psychology of manifest perversions only in patients in whom the disturbance arouses (usually severe) feelings of guilt. Otherwise the patient would not seek treatment at all. Yet, this feeling of guilt is again indicative of a neurotic personality. Why, in the case of a neurosis, frustration sometimes leads exclusively to bona fide neurotic symptoms and in other instances aside from neurotic symptoms also to manifest perversions accompanied by feelings of guilt has not yet been sufficiently explained (Freud, 1937). Be that as it may, perversions in predominantly neurotic personalities do not require a modification of the classical technique, but respond to this technique like neurotic symptoms. Also, the perversions encountered in schizophrenic patients, if at all treatable, do not require a technique different from that used with other schizophrenic symptoms.[9]

From the point of view of psychoanalytic technique, the perversions proper (in the narrower sense of the word) are of primary interest. In this syndrome we find a more or less "normal," unneurotic ego disturbed only by the insistence that adequate sexual gratification can be achieved solely by one or several variations from an almost unlimited choice of deviant patterns. The impulsion does not cause the patient anxiety or guilt. Being ego-syntonic and well integrated, the deviation is not accessible to the classical technique. The patient has no reason to seek treatment, and even if forced to do so by court order, he would have no motivation toward an internal change and therefore would be incapable of compliance with the basic rule of free association.

[9]A perversion in a schizophrenic is often a safety valve on which the functioning of his ego depends and the therapeutic effort should then not extend to the sexual dysfunction.

In order to analyze this type of patient (and only here can one study the technique specifically adjusted to the treatment of perversions), it is necessary first to make his symptom ego alien; that is, to create a conflict between him and his urge for sexual gratification through his perversion. To achieve this, a technique quite different from the classical one would have to be applied. When the patient's transference has reached a level of sufficient intensity, some analysts forbid further indulgence in the perversion. I do not think that this technique can suffice when there has been full integration of the perversion. Moreover, prohibition may precipitate unbearable anxiety, but I assume this occurs mainly in the neurotic pervert (Loewenstein, 1958, p. 202).

There is much to be said about the structure of perversions, concerning which there is a dire lack of enlightenment. I am convinced that research in this field is hampered by our ignorance about the psychology of orgasm. The phenomenon of genitality is fairly well investigated in biological terms and man's intense longing for the orgastic experience is easily understood because of the pleasure it affords and the awareness of deprivation in its absence. But biological knowledge has little value when it is observed that the pleasure premium is unconditionally tied to a rigid individual pattern. Notwithstanding the limited range of foods the average person is capable of eating without disgust, a hungry man can be gratified by almost any edibles, and almost under any conditions. Yet, even if tradition and ethics are set aside, most people are capable of gratifying the sexual drive in only one particular way; a substantial percentage of the rest may have two means at their disposal; but three different ways become exceptional.

The group of truly perverted patients is even more remarkable since all possibilities of sexual gratification are rejected except one, although it may endanger their social status and career. Despite many other available channels for gratification, the physical demand remains ungratified, even for long periods of time if reality withholds the particular conditions they require. This finding surprisingly demonstrates that orgasm (aside from the biological aspect) when viewed in its relationship to the ego must contain a meaning and function beyond the attainment of physical pleasure and the reduction of tension. To repeat the argument from a slightly different viewpoint: The clinical fact that, in general, satisfactory orgasm can be obtained by a person in one exclusive form (which is contrary to general biological principles) presumes a significance in orgasm which cannot be resolved into mere psychobiological processes.

Before presenting a hypothesis regarding this significance I wish to interpolate a few remarks that may at first appear unrelated to the point in question. Man accepts something as true from two diametrically opposed criteria. One is the requirement of logical and scientific thought culminating in the incontrovertible propositions of mathematics. In its application to reality, mathematics safeguards scientific statements from falsification which may be brought about either by shortcomings of ratiocination or by the interference of emotions and illusions. In the form of mathematics the human mind has evolved a kind of watchdog that almost completely precludes error.

The opposite criterion is emotional conviction, a good example of which is belief in the Bible. Scriptural content is believed in with a conviction more intense if possible than that of the scientist in his mathematical formulae. Yet, scriptural content does not live up to the requirements of logic. Its various statements about the same things are contradictory. Its terms are either undefined or ill defined and are open to more or less arbitrary interpretation.

Psychological inquiry into such belief suggests that any attempt to cleanse the text of its contradictions or to reconcile it halfway with the requirements of logical or scientific thinking loosens its grip on the human mind. Thus it can be summarily stated that the illogic in the text is a prerequisite for its hypnotic effect. To avert misunderstanding, I must add that by no means do I identify illogic with hypnotic suasion. Contradiction is only one among a number of elements in religious texts which impress the human mind with incontrovertible truth. No text has yet been created to satisfy the demands of mathematical and scientific thought that is comparable to the Bible in its effect on the human mind. Whereas the effect of mathematical-scientific texts is unaffected by a change of form (the symbols can be changed arbitrarily if the structure of the definitions is preserved), the effect of religious texts is weakened once their form is tampered with.

Evidently the conviction of absolute truth, independent of the probability or improbability of the correctness of its content, results from the arousal of certain feelings. The actual correlations in this sequence are open to dispute. Is the primary factor the text that creates conviction, which in turn evokes a certain set of emotions; or is there an emotional demand which requires satisfaction and under whose sway an external configuration is raised to the level of absolute truth? Both sequences are feasible and, I think, will be encountered clinically, depending on circumstances and individual bent. Returning for a moment to my confrontation of the mathematical-scientific text with the Bible, it is obvious that the former is correlated with the secondary process and the latter with the primary. The application of mathematics to science is the maximum abstraction to be reached by the secondary process. It is not probable that the human mind will ever reach a higher level. Yet, despite the prevalence of the primary process in the origin of religious texts and in the relationship of the believer to his creed, it must be remembered that here we are not dealing with primary process in its bare form. After all, in rationalization the human mind has an efficient mechanism at its disposal with which it makes the result of primary process acceptable to reason. Therefore, it becomes reasonable to assume that there are still other even more archaic forms which provide man with the conviction of truth. Descartes' famous *cogito, ergo sum* which was the starting point or end result, as the case may be, of his quest for incontrovertible truth, is after all the genetic product of a long development. The infant, if it had the power to verbalize, would never base incontrovertible truth on such flimsy evidence. Rather, it would say: "I experience pleasure, hence I exist." Since the greatest pleasure available to the human organism is orgasm, I hypothesize that one of the ego functions of orgasm is to ascertain an incontrovertible truth. If the ego has to resort to such archaic tools to make sure that something is true, then this truth must be even more irrational than that which is ascribed to religious texts.

In perversions, where the selectivity of orgastic conditions comes so conspicuously to attention, my hypothesis has an area for validation. From my limited experience in the study of fetishism, I have gained the impression that a principle, or general view, underlies this form of perversion. In contrast to Freud (1927), I have not found that the fetishist denies that women have no penis, that in terms of the unconscious they are castrated. It was my clinical impression that the fetishist is ready to acknowledge that some human beings have no penis, but with the reservation that this condition is reversible. His denial concerns only the immutability of female anatomy. In his concept the penis is an organ, or perhaps an object, which can be put on or removed rather than an integral part of the organism. Where hair is the fetish this is particularly evident. But it can also be found in the idol worship from which the term fetish is derived. An idol that does not give satisfactory service is cast off by the worshiper and a new one is set up in its place. In the primitive mind the idol is replaceable—a thought alien to Occidental religiosity. The fetishist, therefore, modifies one reality element and declares the penis to be only an accessory appendage.

Only about one other perversion, male masochism, am I able to hypothesize the underlying principle. The male masochist, I believe, "proves" that despite castration orgasm can be experienced. The masochist's intense castration fear is well known. In his dealings with reality he is overaware of anything that may imply castration. Yet, in the perverted act, he exposes himself to conditions that have the meaning of castration represented either symbolically or in pregenital form. In the frequent fantasy of inducing orgasm by hanging, the castrative feature is particularly clear, the whole body assumes the role of the threatened phallus.[10] In the moment of sexual release the masochist, in my opinion, reaffirms that, despite castration, he can preserve the penis and/or the orgastic capacity. One of the many factors responsible for the difficulty of curing masochism is the contradiction inherent in the perversion—the attempt to prove the simultaneous existence of two mutually exclusive facts, namely that an event takes place and simultaneously does not take place. It is as if the masochist wanted to say, "I am castrated and I have a penis."[11] This is the maximum reassurance a person suffering from strong castration anxiety can obtain and at the same time the maximum of spiteful triumph over an aggressor (Freud, 1927).

[10]Masochism is sometimes explained as a defense against or denial of castration since the masochist submits to all kinds of procedures except those containing any threat to the penis. See Wilhelm Reich (1932).

[11]Cf. Nunberg's interpretation of a patient's reaction to circumcision. It seemed as if the patient tried to say: "Even castration cannot deprive me of my masculinity" (Nunberg, 1947, p. 16).

My main point is the hypothetical connection evidenced in the pervert between a special conviction about a reality factor and orgasm. According to my hypothesis, the pervert obtains the maximum of unconscious conviction man can achieve about a reality factor. Yet what is the nature of the reality factor about which he needs such archaic and convincing evidence? It seems that it is regularly related to some detail of the sexual situation. I presume that each type of perversion is related to a different detail of the basic situation of human intercourse. In the fetishist it is the accessory character of the penis; in the male masochist it is the orgastic function of the penis. By achieving orgasm in a reality consistent with his view, the pervert confirms, solidifies, and obtains over and over again the conviction that reality is actually as he needs it to be.

Among the many points in my hypothesis liable to objection, I will elaborate only on two concerning this function of orgasm.

Where does orgasm derive its power to create or confirm conviction? I think the roots of this mechanism go far back to early stages of development, namely, to a period in which pleasure is equated with reality. Freud speaks of the estrangement (*Entfremdung*)[12] between the subjective and the objective that occurs in the course of installing the reality principle, particularly with the development of reality-adequate thinking. The conscious part of the ego is forced to perceive and, if possible, to acknowledge as true certain conditions that disprove what is represented as true in the unconscious. The ego is then, depending on quantitative factors, endangered by the necessity of accepting either reality as it is represented in the unconscious (which would lead to a

[12]See Freud (1925a, p. 238) where the term is translated as "differentiation." Cf. Freud (1925b, p. 6).

psychosis), or to accept reality as it exists, which could entail intolerable anxiety. If, in the state of orgasm, the ego succeeds in giving reality a structure that conforms to the unconscious representation, it escapes both alternatives.

In orgasm the estrangement between the subjective and objective is temporarily abolished. The self has to accept as true the meaning of external reality at the time when orgasm is experienced, since in that moment the maximum pleasure available to the psychobiological person occurs. Metapsychologically we are dealing here with a modality of the infantile pleasure ego that "wants to introject into itself everything that is good and to eject from itself everything that is bad" (Freud, 1925a, p. 237). When the external and internal worlds are fused, as happens in the moment of orgasm, the unconscious representation of reality and the specific external setup meet and become one. The pervert gives a structure to reality that coincides with its conscious representation and thus the ego, in an archaic way, obtains an incontrovertible confirmation that reality is what is claimed by the unconscious.[13]

What does orgasm mean to the person who is free of perversions? The question is most difficult to answer since a subject in whom sexual behavior coincides with the requirements of biological and social reality will not permit analysis to penetrate to the depths of the unconscious where the answer might be found. I can only suggest that possibly Ferenczi (1924, p. 379) is right to attribute to male intercourse the meaning of a return to the mother's womb. It is feasible that

[13]To a certain extent I am doing no more than spelling out certain implications inherent in Freud's concept of the sexual overvaluation of the love object. See Freud (1905b, pp. 150f.). If the prerequisites and consequences of sexual overvaluation are carefully considered the inherent delusional elements will be recognized. Freud speaks of the weakness of judgment in the infatuated person (1905b, p. 150).

under normal circumstances orgasm might affirm that the very first frustration man has suffered, the greatest grievance he has to complain of, namely, his separation from the maternal organism, has never occurred. (Cf. also Nunberg, 1947, p. 17, and Freud, 1923, p. 144, n. 2, 145.)

In my opinion, orgasm is the strongest affirmation possible to man. Its antipode is sleep which, though life-necessary, is the strongest negation of life and reality. Possibly, at this point the objection will be raised that by assigning to orgasm the function of an affirmation I try to reduce it to a defense whose form is an affirmative sentence. This, however, I did not have in mind. Orgasm is a wish fulfillment and its function of affirmation occurs probably in most instances on the preverbal level. The truth that is affirmed by orgasm is not represented by words and not necessarily by explicit fantasies. Thus the reality situation that is fused with the orgasm becomes indisputably true; if orgasm occurred under different circumstances, this would deny reality to the particular and necessary configuration which constitutes to the pervert a sine qua non. Why this reassurance is indispensable to the pervert is a question that need not occupy us here. The main point, however, is that orgasm is endowed with the power to confirm, create, and affirm conviction. It is this point which makes the psychoanalytic therapy of adolescents more crucial and responsible than the psychoanalysis of any other phase.

It is during adolescence that the convictions which ultimately become associated with orgasm are decided. It is during puberty when the first orgasm occurs and later in adolescence when orgasm has obtained a permanent place in the patient's life that the decision is made as to the permanent form his sexual life will take.[14] I believe the conditions

[14]However, see Freud (1905b, p. 146) in a footnote added in 1915: "A person's final sexual attitude is not decided until after puberty."

under which the first orgasm occurs may have an effect as fateful as early traumata in infancy.

Still another point is to be considered. A fully integrated perversion shares an important feature with a psychosis. In the moment of orgasm a world that may be delusional is affirmed. This is reminiscent of the temporary, short-lasting dream psychosis (Freud, 1938, p. 202). As a matter of fact, when force of circumstance (internal or external) prevents the pervert from gratifying his sexual urge, he may be pushed to the border of a psychosis. This factor must be considered in the treatment of adolescents, yet with it we encounter a technical problem almost impossible to solve.

Clinical experience has demonstrated that a delayed onset of masturbation or even its total absence (unless there is an early onset of heterosexual intercourse) during adolescence is generally a bad prognostic sign. Therefore, masturbation is an indispensable part of healthy adolescence. However, adolescent maturbation favors the evolution and integration of perverted fantasies.[15] Thus the analyst has to remove restraints that may prevent the adolescent from masturbating and at the same time forestall the growth of perverted fantasies and promote internal conditions that will channel the adolescent's fantasy life toward heterosexual intercourse.

In his therapeutic dealings with the adolescent the analyst has the following techniques at his disposal. With the classical technique he can undo the damage of inhibition or neurotic symptoms evoked by a reality that has imposed too great a restraint on the instincts; by the technique used with delinquents he is able to close the gaps or lacunae in the adolescent's superego and curb his antisocial impulses; with the technique evolved for the treatment of the acute phase of

[15]See, however, Freud (1912, p. 252) where he agrees with Stekel that through the compromise obtained in masturbation strong perverse inclinations are rendered innocuous.

schizophrenia he is enabled to reconcile the adolescent patient with his total environment when it becomes so intol-
erably painful that he withdraws and surrenders to the id
with a minimum of defense. By instigating a conflict between
the ego and perverted impulses the analyst seeks to safeguard
in the unconscious the cathexis of adequate heterosexual
objects and of the genital function.

The ultimate and most difficult task in the treatment of
adolescents is to synthesize these four techniques. Unless the
psychopathology of the adolescent has solidified and he enters treatment with symptomatology that makes him a "reliable" member of one of the four major groups, the
technique of treatment has to be correlated with the respective phase in which the patient's symptomatology moves for
it can change so drastically that if the analyst persists in a
technique bound to the initial clinical impression, the risk of
failure is great. I surmise that the widespread pessimism regarding the success of psychoanalysis in adolescence stems
from rigid adherence to one technique throughout the course
of treatment. To demonstrate the clinical relevance of a flexible technique I will present a hypothetical situation.

A boy of 15 goes into psychoanalysis because of headaches,
a neurotic symptom. The classical technique is instituted;
quickly an intense transference is established and he responds
favorably to the treatment. He becomes aware that the unconscious conflict which caused his head to ache was the
repression of aggressive impulses toward his father. But as
the headaches disappear they are replaced by increasing anxiety. His need for punishment being no longer satisfied by
painful physical symptoms, he manifests castration anxiety,
fearing retaliation for his aggression. As this fear is analyzed
and greatly reduced, the patient begins to release aggression.
He becomes argumentative and unruly at home, associates
with delinquent boys, and participates in minor acts of de-

linquency. Thus, the reduction of restraining forces interacting with the defense against an increase of passive wishes,
which are partly due to the positive transference, results in
a pseudomasculinity expressed through aggressive behavior.
If, in accordance with the technique of the treatment of neuroses, analysis of his passive wishes is carried out, the patient
is necessarily driven deeper into this delinquent behavior
since his passive wishes are dangerous and unacceptable.
Their analysis only weakens defenses, increases the intensity
of fear-arousing wishes, and almost forces the patient toward
compensatory acting out.

An equilibrated treatment situation is restored, however,
as soon as the therapist establishes himself as a temporary,
friendly superego figure with whom the patient can gratify
his passive wishes in a narcissistic, sublimated way. At this
point the therapeutic situation is so structured as to permit
appropriate prohibitions to reduce the patient's feelings of
guilt. The technique has thus been switched to that of the
therapy of delinquents. Let us assume that under its beneficial effect the delinquent behavior subsides since the passive
homosexual desires are now made acceptable by their investment in a superego representative. Furthermore, reacting to the analyst's interpretations, the patient falls in love
with a girl, initiates heterosexual activity, starts necking and
is greatly stimulated sexually. He feels successful and ani-
mated.

Then the girl deserts him and he is terribly disappointed.
Having stopped masturbating while he was involved with the
girl, he recoils from regressing to his former means of gratification. He becomes sexually tense. The fact that his sweetheart deserted him for an older boy stimulates homosexual
fears and rivalry. Again he becomes provocative at home; his
parents berate him; his schoolwork suffers and his grades
decline; he misses a few appointments with the therapist. He

is in conflict with the representative of his superego, feeling that his ego ideal (the analyst) has failed to protect him against unbearable frustration. When he returns to the analyst's office, he appears depressed, complains of symptoms that imply feelings of depersonalization, and shows signs of hypochondriasis. He spends most of his time daydreaming and is almost incapable of participating in social activities.

If the therapist continues the technique which was appropriate to the delinquent phase, the disequilibrium which has extended to the therapeutic situation will increase and the patient will progressively withdraw. Reality is filled with unendurable frustrations and the patient's conflict with reality is similar in structure to that observed in schizophrenic psychoses. Concomitantly, the ensuing symptomatology is reminiscent of that in psychosis: depersonalization, hypochondriasis, seclusiveness, etc. Should the psychoanalyst still try to function as the patient's superego, the therapeutic situation will have frustrating implications for the patient, reminiscent of the way the rest of the world appears to him, and the therapeutic situation itself will founder in the process of withdrawal.

Nor will a return to the classical technique be successful. The patient's positive transference has sunk far below the optimal level, and any reference to an unconscious content will bring about feelings of revulsion in the patient.

This serious threat to the patient's safety and to his therapy can be met by a new change of technique. The therapist must offer the patient gratification that will stimulate his interest in the world, beginning with the therapeutic situation. However, no specific suggestion can be made here since the practical measure depends entirely upon the patient's needs which have become familiar to the analyst from his previous observations. Sessions may be filled with storytelling, a meal may be served or small talk may fill the therapeutic hour.

Whatever occurs during the session should be pleasurable to the patient without arousing feelings of guilt. It should persuade the patient that he is still accepted and liked by the therapist. The first indication that the withdrawal process has come to a standstill will be the patient's readiness to come for treatment and the pleasure he obtains from spending time with the therapist. Next, announcing that the process of withdrawal has been reversed, the patient will find sexual pleasure in the release of masturbation.

Yet, even after harmonious relations with his environment are restored, the patient may evince a symptom that bears definite earmarks of the past regressive phase. The traumatic disappointment of his sweetheart's desertion and the ensuing regression left their mark in the form of an internal estrangement from the other sex. Consequently, his sexual fantasies, those accompanying masturbation as well as those occurring independently, show pregenital elements focused mainly on his own sex. Their content centers in an oral-sadistic tendency; the adolescent has entered a phase of perversion. It is evident that continued use of a technique which has its fulcrum in the fulfillment of the patient's wishes and avoids the arousal of guilt feelings will risk fixating the patient in a perversion.

In most instances analysis of the defensive functions, the underlying repressed childhood conflicts and castration fear may suffice to end this phase. However, if the pleasure derived from perverted fantasies or practices is so great that a purely interpretative technique will not avail, then a temporary wedge must be driven between ego and id; a conflict must be created. The ego has to be alienated from a set of fantasies it is inclined to integrate. A powerful weapon with which the ego exerts influence upon the id is anxiety, and it may become necessary to institute a technique that will increase the patient's anxiety. In other words, if a perversion is on the verge of being integrated, it has to be changed into a neurotic symptom. Yet when this is achieved, the point of departure is reached and the patient again is in a neurotic phase. Possibly this time his symptom will not be somatic, but one of a well-delineated neurosis so that reinstating the classical technique perhaps will not lead to the complications previously noted.

This hypothetical case may have no exact parallel in clinical practice. Phases are not as distinctly separate as I have postulated. What is important, and probably most difficult to achieve, is the correct timing of a change in technique. In the instance outlined above, the symptoms of delinquency would not have appeared if the classical technique had been changed to fit the needs of delinquency at the very first hint that neurotic symptomatology was on the verge of transformation. If the approach of a new phase could always be recognized in time, it is feasible that a technique could be devised which might limit dramatic symptom change to the treatment situation, leaving almost untouched the adolescent patient's behavior in his social world.

The suggested changes of technique may have to occur not only in broad phaseal changes of the patient's disorder, but sometimes within the same treatment hour. An adolescent may start a session under the sway of neurotic fears that give way to outright delinquent tendencies. If only one technique is used to cope with the varieties of psychopathology that may be encountered in the treatment of an adolescent, resistances are necessarily increased or reduced below the optimal level, as the case may be, or symptoms may become dangerously aggravated.

There is a fifth form of psychopathology that I have not mentioned up to now. In its purest form it appears in the genius, and attempts to classify it under the heading of almost any known psychopathology have been in vain.[16] It has not escaped attention that most intelligent adolescents go through a phase in which they strike the observer as a potential genius. This phase is the repetition of an earlier one when an intelligent child discovers the world and makes those frequently reported bewitching remarks that portray a surprising power of original observation. Through his discovery of new values and his contemplation of the world in a new light, the gifted adolescent is stimulated to an onrush of original thoughts and interests. This process is highly instinctualized and results in the outward appearance we expect and sometimes actually encounter in genius, particularly in the arts. But even if adolescence does not lead to such an attractive efflorescence, something similar can be observed unless the particularly alarming prognostic signs of dullness and uneventfulness characterize the period.

I introduce the problem of genius in the belief that if we had insight into its psychology, we would be better able to protect, safeguard, and encourage mental development and creativity in the adolescent. Just as the final decision as to the form of adult sexuality occurs during adolescence, the potential and momentum of his manifest intelligence and creativity is decided during the same developmental stage. I am not certain that Jokl (1950) is right in his conclusion that creativity can never be endangered or impaired by analysis. Jokl cites a letter by Freud in which he declared that "a real talent could not be damaged by analysis, which would only rid the patient of her difficulties."[17] To be sure, an excep-

---

[16]I cannot set forth here the reasons for calling genius a special form of psychopathology in its own right. I have justified and believe to have demonstrated the constructiveness of this approach in an unpublished manuscript on Goethe.

[17]I wonder when this letter was written. Does it remain true in view of the vast expansion of ego analysis in the last three decades?

tional mind may successfully resist all environmental influence that may constrain or injure a less exceptional one; but in the psychoanalysis of adolescents we almost never deal with such a favorable clinical situation. Moreover, I surmise Freud had in mind psychoanalysis properly applied, for Jokl reports that Freud assigned to him a patient endowed with unusual creative ability with the request "to be particularly careful."[18] In adolescence, when creativity has not yet been integrated, unless we adhere to a primitive belief in inheritance and deny the bearing of environmental factors, the problem of creativity involves exceedingly great therapeutic responsibility. To measure the scope of this problem in this context one must consider that we do not yet have a circumscribed technique for the treatment of adolescents, and the therapist is hardly ever in a position to deal with a subject in which the creative potential is genius-like and therefore invulnerable to external vicissitudes. Finally, it must be the therapist's task not only to protect the adolescent's creativity from stunting influences, but also to activate its potential toward maximum fulfillment.

Although the optimal conditions for creativity have not yet been ascertained, it can be safely assumed that among many variables conflict is a necessary one. But it is totally unknown what intensity or structure of conflict is most conducive to the development of creativity. If, from this lack of knowledge, it is concluded that psychotherapy or psychoanalysis may injure the creative potential of an adolescent and therefore should be avoided, this would be misplaced caution. True, we have not yet obtained sufficient knowledge about a therapeutic milieu optimal for the growth of creativity, but we

[18]It strikes me as generally meaningful that Freud limited his therapeutic activity to psychotherapy when he was consulted by Gustav Mahler and Bruno Walter. For the latter, see Walter (1947) and Sterba (1951).

know that if left to chance, social reality and inner conflicts destroy the seed of creativity in the adolescent whereas there is the possibility that careful analysis may avert this. It is my impression that an enormous psychic tension is often built up during adolescence which functions as a fulcrum for many years to come. However, we also notice in other cases that conflicts presenting a similar clinical appearance prove devastating and the adolescent becomes an adult completely lacking in creativity. Can psychoanalysis influence the direction adolescent conflicts will take, namely, their constructive or damaging effects? Goethe, who for a variety of reasons can be considered the model of creative man, had a particularly stormy adolescence culminating in two, short-lasting psychotic episodes in whose wake a particular artistic function was released. I am not saying that adolescence, so to speak, made Goethe a genius; it is reasonable to assume that without the two psychotic episodes, his creativity would still have been distinguished. But it is significant that a function of by no means subordinate importance arose out of the turmoil attached to these two episodes; and possibly a general conclusion can be drawn therefrom.

The question arises concerning a functional connection between the conflicts and solutions of the oedipal phase and those of adolescence. Jones (1922) has devoted a study to this question and emphasized the parallel between them. I do not doubt that such parallels exist. I would even go a step further and emphasize here as one extreme those life histories from which it is evident that the patient's fate was sealed shortly after the peak of the oedipal conflict. These, as I said before, are patients who usually develop distinct psychopathology at an early age which continues during latency to a varying degree, and who enter adolescence with a fixed pattern that is maintained throughout life. One can observe this developmental course with particular clarity in patients who are homosexually seduced at three or four and continue their sexual deviation uninterrupted until adolescence. If a patient of this type is treated during adolescence, the problem of technique is simplified, for the chance of his psychopathology veering from one form to another is lessened, though not entirely absent. Yet it is my impression that the other course of adolescence characterized by reorganizational processes is more frequent. Oddly enough, both types of development are also observed in the genius. Mozart is the outstanding example of the former. His musical endowment, discovered at four, had an uninterrupted growth. He was already a master when he entered adolescence. I regard such person-alities as inappropriate for a study of the functions of ado-lescence. Goethe is a representative of the other type. Despite early signs of creativity, I doubt whether its fabulous extent could have been predicted before the end of his adolescence.

Adolescence appears to afford the individual a second chance; it is a kind of lease permitting revision of the solutions found during latency which had been formed in direct re-action to the oedipal conflict. Some structure of the earlier personality seems to dissolve in the course of adolescence. Perhaps a comparison with a process of liquefaction is more appropriate. Regressive features are certain to appear, but I prefer to emphasize the release of forces that were bound in the structure and the ensuing reorganization through new identifications and the cathexis of new objects. If there are processes of liquefaction combined with restructuralization, the course of adolescence will be stormy. With or without psychoanalysis, swings are to be expected in the adolescent; and depending on the inner constellations of forces and frus-trations, temptations and gratifications in external reality, there may be sudden acts of delinquency, bursts of creativity, or times of a general withdrawal.

To take such sequences out of the realm of the fortuitous

and to prevent damaging effect from conflicts that otherwise have a constructive function, a stormy adolescence ought to be subjected to psychoanalytic therapy. Yet even under optimal conditions therapy will hardly succeed in settling the patient's psychopathology forever, just as child analysis is not to be expected to do more than strengthen the child's ego and enable him to respond with less intense psychopathology to later demands. The final determination of psychopathology can occur only during adult years. But analysis in adolescence can and should prevent the formation of a fixated reaction to conflict in the ego. It is so frequently observed as to be considered statistically normal that at the end of adolescence the individual has evolved a rigid pattern for solving conflicts; only one way of reacting is at his disposal when stress exceeds the optimal level of tolerance for him.

When the personality leaves adolescence with its ego structure capable of varied reactions instead of being fixated on one, the general prognosis seems to me far better. The suffering that is to be expected is greatly reduced and the flexibility of adjustive processes is much greater. Besides, there is under such circumstances the chance that the individual will preserve the capacity to re-experience phases of adolescence.

Goethe said to Eckermann (March 11, 1828) that geniuses "experience a repeated puberty whereas other people are young only once" ("*Geniale Naturen . . . erleben eine wiederholte Pubertät, während andere Leute nur einmal jung sind*") (Eckermann [1836, p. 538]), and he referred to such a period in his own life which occurred when he was 65 years old. Of course, this was not the only adolescent episode during his adult years. The constructive effect of such adolescent resurgences is immense. Is it only the genius who can enjoy them? Or is this privilege bound to a special psychobiological constitution? Perhaps it depends too on the manner in which a person went through his physical puberty, on the extent of fear, on the tribulations and dangers he experienced at that time, or on the exhaustion of forces in that period which may deplete the energic abundance which is necessary for such a period and which must remain if periods of adolescence are to recur.

In discussing the technique of child analysis I have referred to the position held by the analyst in the child's life as necessarily trespassing beyond a purely therapeutic relationship. I wonder whether the analyst's obligation to empower maximum creativity in the adolescent necessitates a similar step beyond the realm of therapy as defined by psychoanalysis. The patient's later creativity, I believe, depends also on the unconscious evolution and integration of creative goals during adolescence. During that period a mental horizon which future action should strive toward is unconsciously constructed. Although this aspiration does not develop independently of the oedipal phase, the function of the psychoanalyst is perhaps not only to clear the way for it, but also to facilitate its expansion.

Be that as it may, the clinical reality of the psychoanalysis of adolescence appears quite different from what may be expected from the foregoing, and I wish to add a few arbitrarily selected clinical problems.

(1) In the majority of instances, the analyst is consulted only in cases of such severe psychopathology that the psychoanalytic procedure can scarcely be instituted at all. What should be done under such not infrequent extreme conditions? I recall a severely troubled youngster of sixteen who could not tolerate the slightest recognition of any of his problems. To any reference to his troubles no matter how circumspectly formulated, he responded with immediate resentment. It was clear that renewed attempts would precipitate an open break between therapist and patient. Dis-

continuance of the therapeutic relationship seemed advisable, but regular contact was maintained for two more years although it did not lead to more than ordinary small talk. I felt that lighthearted contact unburdened by any external limitation, combined with an absence of ambivalence in my reaction to his antics and provocative behavior, would have a wholesome effect on this patient's devastated ego, enabling him to effect at least a minimum of adjustment. The therapeutic relationship was a kind of crystallization point around which some ego functioning could be preserved or regressions averted. Three years after leaving this quasi therapy the patient spontaneously asked for psychoanalytic treatment. I doubt that he would have sought therapy if I had previously dismissed him as untreatable, or if I had tried to force therapy on him.

(2) In another case I have observed the deplorable effects brought about in a patient who was coerced by his parents into psychoanalysis during adolescence, and I do not recommend such a procedure.

(3) As Dr. Sidney Kahr pointed out in a discussion, psychotherapy during adolescence frequently keeps the patient from entering psychoanalysis later. I could observe this in a severely disturbed adolescent patient whom I met once a week for about two and a half years and whom I helped successfully through the many crises which beset his adolescence. The therapeutic measures were taken with a plan to institute a bona fide psychoanalysis as soon as the patient entered a phase of less acute problems and conflicts. But when he reached this point, he rejected my suggestion, although in an earlier state of severe suffering he had asked for full analysis. Now that the assistance he had received made it possible for him to maintain a semblance of adequate adjustment, he refused to enter analysis. It would have been better for this patient had I given him less help during the

acute adolescent crisis, or had risked a full analytic course at that time.

In view of our present knowledge of adolescent patients I am inclined to plead in favor of regular psychoanalysis rather than for substitute measures in case of doubt.

I hope this construct of an ideal model of technique for the treatment of adolescents will not be taken as a deterrent to the psychoanalytic treatment of adolescents, but as an outline of the many areas for positive action as well as the range of problems inherent in the quest for a reliable psychoanalytic technique appropriate for this development phase.

3

INTRODUCTION

Intensive Psychotherapy in Relation to the Various Phases of the Adolescent Period, by Peter Blos

Our knowledge of adolescent psychological development and, in particular, our understanding of its subphase variations derive very largely from the work of Peter Blos. Blos has devoted a richly productive lifetime to the psychoanalytic study of adolescence and has provided us with a detailed map of the territory which has served as an invaluable guide to a generation of fellow explorers. His major works (1962, 1979a) are landmarks in psychoanalytic developmental psychology.

The idea of subphases is fairly generally accepted; although there may be some differences as to their precise number and specific characteristics (e.g., Miller, 1974), most workers agree that there are significant structural and cognitive changes from puberty to late adolescence that dictate different strategies and techniques of intervention. In this paper Blos sketches his conception of five definable subphases and suggests some of its implications for differential psychotherapeutic technique. More detailed clinical descriptions can be found in his casebook *The Young Adolescent* (1970).

3

Intensive Psychotherapy in Relation to the Various Phases of the Adolescent Period

Peter Blos, Ph.D.

The application of intensive psychotherapy during the adolescent period has been questioned over the years as often as it has been affirmed with regard to its appropriateness and effectiveness. The negative opinion was based on the notion that intensive therapy tends to undo repressions, to weaken defenses, in short, to flood the adolescent mind with unconscious fantasies and urges which easily overtax its integrative potential. Psychoanalysis seemed therefore an especially inappropriate method for this age. Supportive, reassuring, manipulative, and relationship therapy, that is, ego-building and ego-strengthening techniques, were consequently considered the more appropriate interventions during adolescence. Therapists in favor of intensive therapy of adolescents saw no intrinsic danger in the analytic method

Reprinted by permission from the *American Journal of Orthopsychiatry*, 32:901-910, 1962. Copyright © the American Orthopsychiatric Association, Inc. Reproduced by permission of Peter Blos, Ph.D., and the American Orthopsychiatric Association.

because the ego's integrative capacity is kept under constant scrutiny during analytic therapy.

The relative weakness of the ego vis-à-vis the powerful drives is considered typical for the pubescent individual. Consequently, the need for proper dosage and timing of the instinct interpretations became generally accepted as an intrinsic aspect of adolescent therapy. Ego interpretations take the center of the stage for long stretches of time. The fear that the adolescent ego will be overwhelmed by the instincts if we weaken the defensive system by ill-timed interpretations and consequently invite a state of panic, even if only transient, seems to me to be true for any age. The reluctance to use intensive therapy with adolescents is based on cases which at no age would be considered promising candidates for intensive therapy. No generalization can be based on these adolescent cases of borderline functioning with reference to adolescence in its typical form. We often mistake preconscious as unconscious material, and project our own apprehensions onto the adolescent. The controversy resolves itself to the question: What do we mean by intensive therapy?

In answering this question let us first rule out as criteria such formalities as frequency of sessions and the supine position on the couch. We would come closer to a dynamic formulation by saying that intensive therapy makes resistance (defenses) and transference the object of systematic investigation or interpretation. This focus necessarily leads to reconstruction with the help of memories or dreams. In a broader sense we might say that intensive therapy restores a lost or disrupted continuity in ego experience. Such a restorative achievement has far-reaching consequences: It promotes the process of individuation, it establishes firm ego boundaries, it stabilizes the distinction between self and object, and it enhances the faculty of reality testing. I shall be content for the moment with this definition of intensive psychotherapy and proceed to ask a question of a more practical bent.

When we talk about adolescents we refer to male and female individuals between the ages—roughly speaking—of 10 and 20. The representatives of such heterogeneous developmental stages cannot possibly be lumped together with the hope of establishing overall congruities and similarities which render their behavior intelligible. What the various adolescent stages have in common is the simple fact that all through the second decade a process of personality differentiation takes place which transforms the child into an adult. Regarding the treatment situation, the adolescent shares with the child the fact that an outside agency initiates his therapy; with the adult he shares the privilege that others, especially the parents, are excluded from his therapeutic privacy. What started as an act initiated by the environment must become a totally self-motivated endeavor.

The two facts—namely that the personality at adolescence is in flux and that therapy is called upon to serve various interests of the environment, both characteristic of adolescent therapy—suggest that a planned and explicit preparatory phase in adolescent treatment is indicated. This is more true for some cases than for others. However, such a preparatory phase seems desirable in order to put the therapeutic work on firm ground. The time needed for this preparatory work varies from case to case. We can often observe that a too vehement initial eagerness by the therapist evokes in the adolescent a negative reaction. In general terms the preparatory phase aims at establishing a therapeutic alliance by eliciting in the adolescent the trust and conviction that the therapist's actions and interferences are in the interest of the adolescent's progressive development. By siding with the adolescent's ego or, rather, with that part of his ego which desires change through therapy, the therapist will necessarily arouse recurrent waves of frustration which will always threaten to disrupt the therapeutic alliance. The preparatory phase is instituted to acquaint the adolescent with the therapeutic situation, with technique and role designations. To say it differently, the preparatory phase deals, superficially perhaps, with the most obstructive and disturbing fantasies, fears, and hopes with which the adolescent approaches treatment. If these adverse forces are not dealt with at the outset, they threaten to disrupt treatment before it can begin.

It often happens that the parents' divided and contradictory attitudes toward treatment render the therapeutic situation the battleground for mutual ambivalence conflicts between parent and child. If this displacement is allowed to persist, the adolescent uses the treatment situation as such to act out his positive and negative attitudes toward his parents or theirs toward him. The displacement of an ambivalence conflict to the therapeutic situation is often mistaken as a transference problem. This clinical picture presented itself to me in the case of an 18-year-old girl with social inhibitions, temper outbursts, and hysterical symptoms. The mother had made all the arrangements for treatment while the father was ignored by both mother and daughter. During the first weeks the girl complained repeatedly that she was afraid the expenses of treatment might kill her hardworking father. In her family nobody told anything to anybody. While she was most cooperative and eager for therapy, she could not see how she could possibly have three sessions weekly; her father could not afford them. This was confirmed by the mother, who was eager for the treatment of her daughter.

I insisted on seeing the father and did so with the full endorsement of the patient. When I finally talked with him I realized that the therapeutic situation had been used to act out a pathological family constellation in which the daughter had reluctantly sided with the mother. The father, presumably antagonistic to treatment, showed in a forthright manner his appreciation for my insistence on talking with him. He wanted his daughter to have the number of sessions she needed, and he added that it was up to him to make them financially possible. Safeguards against similar exploitations of the therapeutic situation as such must be established early in therapy; only then will the conflictual problem become accessible to therapy instead of remaining extraneous to it through acting out. Dealings with parents should take place at the very beginning of treatment because later on such interferences only tend to complicate the therapeutic situation.

In this connection it should be mentioned that the passivity of the therapist, often considered an obligatory hallmark of intensive therapy, can have a most detrimental influence on the therapeutic situation at adolescence. The adolescent tends to experience his own feelings and thoughts as originating outside himself. He has a tendency to project. Prolonged silences in therapy are contraindicated in most adolescent cases. The "screen therapist" has no place at this age, certainly not at the onset of treatment. Here one has to consider the adolescent state of increased narcissism, which has to be counteracted by outside stimuli. Prolonged silences in therapy mobilize projective mechanisms with the result that the patient's ego boundaries become blurred and anxiety drives the adolescent into acting out, withdrawal, or negativism. It is necessary in adolescent therapy constantly to keep in mind the disorganizing influence of silences. The therapist's activity must remain always tuned to the adolescent's threshold of tolerance in relation to noncommunicated internal stimuli.

The fact that the adolescent personality is in constant flux requires a constant change of therapeutic technique or emphasis. It is hardly ever possible to concentrate the therapeutic endeavor on a given problem for long. Instinctual problems tend to intermingle with problems of ego integration. Because of the adolescent condition, namely, because of the psychic restructuring taking place at this period, the ego is threatened not only by the pubescent drives, but in equal measure by the threat of losing contact with reality. The narcissistic defenses in particular weaken reality contact and as such have to be counteracted by the therapist. This might require his engaging actively, often dramatizingly, in the therapeutic interchange. Therapy must be stimulating and interesting to the adolescent in order for him to tolerate it. Adolescent acting out is often nothing more than a frantic attempt to keep in touch with reality and to ward off a surrender to infantile greed and dependency.

The goal of therapy during adolescence is to restore progressive development, i.e., to counteract regression or adolescent fixation. This therapeutic approach requires first of all an orientation in the adolescent process and in its distinctive developmental phases. These phases must be characterized by their typical drive and ego organizations and in terms of phase-specific tasks involved. Only then are we in a position to select from the multitude of data in a given case those aspects which are relevant to a specific developmental impasse or to a given clinical picture.

I shall not be able in the following to present the whole adolescent period in the orderly sequence of its developmental phases because time does not permit such an expansive presentation. I shall, however, illustrate the practical relevancy of phase definition for the conduct of therapy in one phase, namely, preadolescence. Before I turn to this phase, I must make clear that some essential achievements of the latency period constitute a prerequisite for the entrance into adolescence. Otherwise the pubescent drive increase results only in the intensification of infantile sexuality with nothing typically adolescent appearing on the mental scene. Some adolescent disturbances are erroneously treated as adolescent problems simply because of the age or of the sexual connotations involved. If the latency period has not made its distinctive contribution to personality formation, the quasi-adolescent behavior is misleading as to its nature. I classify such cases as "simulated adolescence." In them therapy has to deal first with the developmental deficit. This shows up in a deficit as to tension tolerance, resistivity of ego functions to regression, formation of the self-critical ego, capacity for verbal expression in isolation from motor activity, capacity of "postponement" and "anticipation." We must keep in mind that adolescence, a psychological process, does not necessarily run parallel to the biological process of puberty.

Let us now turn to preadolescence in its typical form. What strikes us first is the different picture in boy and girl. The boy reacts to the advent of puberty—which is physiologically active before it is physically apparent—with a regression to pregenitality. Witness his diffuse motility, his oral greediness, his sadistic and anal propensities as expressed in coprophilic pleasures, dirty language, his disregard for cleanliness, his fascination with odors, and his phallic-exhibitionistic play. A 14-year-old boy made an astute observation about himself at 11 and at 14. He said: "At 11 my mind was only on filth, now it is on sex. There is a great difference." In addition, the preadolescent boy behaves hostilely to girls, he belittles them, in fact, he is afraid of them. The castration anxiety which brought the oedipal phase to its decline reappears and forces the boy into the exclusive company of his own sex. The boy's typical preadolescent conflict can be defined as one of fear and envy of the female. Both are dealt with by denial and overcompensation. The castration anxiety is not experienced in relation to the father but rather to the archaic phallic mother, the witch of folklore. The danger of this phase lies in the boy's identification with the phallic woman. A fixation on the preadolescent phase in terms of the ego organization becomes apparent in diffuse, scattered, and unstable interests, with no one ever capturing a lasting position of supremacy. Ego autonomy is easily surrendered in exchange for comfort and safety; an undercurrent of magical thinking never ceases to operate; a fascination with gadgeteering takes the place of orderly activity; primitive science fiction adventures represent the collective fantasy of this stage.

The girl offers a picture totally different. She is either a tomboy or a young aggressive female. To the young preadolescent boy she appears as Diana, the young Goddess of Hunting who displays her physical charms while roaming through the woods with a pack of hounds. The girl at this stage can by no stretch of the imagination be called feminine. She is the aggressor and seducer in the game of pseudolove. She turns to the opposite sex as a defense against the regressive pull to the preoedipal mother. The regression which is open to the boy without interference with his normal development is closed to the girl. We discern the reasons for this difference in the fact that regression throws her back to a stage of object love, the nurturing mother, which in the pubescent girl would open the door to homosexuality. What often appears in the young adolescent girl as heterosexual preoccupation represents on closer inspection a defense against the regressive pull as just described. This condition is characteristic for female delinquency.

From these sketchy delineations of the preadolescent male and female conflict, we can deduce the phase-specific tasks of boy and girl respectively. In essence, the boy has to overcome hostility and fear in relation to the female and advance to the stage of heterosexual orientation, while the girl has to resist regression to the active archaic mother and advance to an identification with the oedipal mother. These formulations provide guideposts of sequential patterns in development. As such they bring some order into clinical observations, offer reference criteria to determine to which midway station of the adolescent process a certain disturbance belongs, and, last but not least, provide a rationale for therapeutic strategy. It needs to be emphasized again that chronological age is the most unreliable indicator for determining the developmental or psychological position. Some component parts of the personality might be precociously developed while others are abnormally retarded.

I will now illustrate with some case excerpts the formulation of the preadolescent phase which I have advanced. The first case is that of a girl of 16. She came to therapy because she acted out sexually and had failed in school. It was clear to me that her acting out was a revenge on the mother for whose love she yearned in a childish way by making unreasonable demands on her, by wishing that the interests of mother and child should merge and be one and the same. One day she reported one of the many scenes with the mother, whom she accused of not understanding her needs; she ended the tale by saying that she had walked out on her mother, angrily slamming the door. I remarked that I knew what she had thought of at that moment. Her curiosity was aroused and I told her that she had decided at that very moment to sleep with her boyfriend. This proved to be correct. The surprise and shock quality of this interpretation made it more effective than previous generalities or discussions. The girl suddenly realized that her love for her boyfriend was not love at all but was motivated by revenge on the mother whose love she could not obtain; it served as an anchor on the level of pseudoheterosexuality, as a defense against the regressive pull to early dependency. This interpretive tour de force marked the end of the girl's sexual acting out and opened the door to a new phase in therapy in which the recognition of internal conflicts replaced the effort to resolve them through interaction with the environment. When this girl came for therapy she was fixated on the preadolescent phase: The task of this phase had to be fulfilled before progressive development could be resumed.

The second illustration concerns a boy of 12 who showed passive feminine tendencies and suffered from a learning disability. His play-acting and overcompensatory manliness made him feel at home with girls; he secretly envied them since they were spared the dreadful competition with boys. The defensive nature of his pseudomasculinity was apparent; it remained the task of therapy to reach the preadolescent conflict because only then could genuine masculinity assert itself. We knew what the theme of this conflict generally is and paid therapeutic attention to it whenever it appeared in one of countless derivative manifestations. The fear of the castrating female was contained in a fantasy which the boy revealed before going to a mixed party of his peers. In order to appear manly he felt compelled to kiss the girls on the mouth in case a kissing game should take place. This prospect evoked anxiety which derived from his conviction that "girls are diseased." He feared to get sick from the kiss. Again, the seemingly heterosexual interest masked the preadolescent conflict as outlined above. Phase-specific anxiety had temporarily brought progressive development to a standstill, thus initiating a deviate, i.e., a pathological, development.

On the basis of clinical experience I have become especially interested in adolescent research to investigate the dissimilarities between male and female, and to draw up separate schemata of adolescent drive and ego development characteristic for either boy or girl.

I have described the preadolescent phase of development in detail in order to present to you a model of phase definition

and its relatedness to intensive therapy. The adolescent process is composed of several phases which have to be understood in their epigenetic sequence and order. It is misleading
to view adolescence only as a repetition on a higher level of
early childhood development. The therapist of the adolescent
has to be oriented with equal interest toward the goal of
psychic transformations as toward the resuscitation of the
past. What appears as a defense in adolescence can turn into
an adaptive process and contribute essentially to the formation of character. This change of a defense into an adaptive mechanism is enhanced whenever ego functions become
isolated from object relations or, to say it differently, whenever the desexualization of ego functions is achieved. This
will protect ego functions from being drawn into the life of
the instinct and thus contribute to the extension of ego autonomy. What appears, for instance, as intellectualization or
as an exhibitionistic defense can turn into an autonomous
ego activity in the form of scholarship or showmanship, provided an innate endowment for such endeavors exists.

In summary, we might say that intensive psychotherapy is
guided by three coordinates: biological givens, genetic determinants, and adaptive norms. The last can be defined
during periods of growth such as adolescence only by phase-
specific requirements in terms of psychic restructuring. In
any given adolescent disturbance we therefore attempt to
relate the adolescent impasse in progressive development to
an adolescent fixation point, to genetic antecedents, and to
constitutional factors. Each of the various phases of the adolescent process, as exemplified by preadolescence, is characterized by a dominant theme, by a typical conflict, by a
personal crisis, and by an idiosyncratic adaptive solution.

It is not the purpose of this paper to recount the adolescent
process in terms of its various phases. It must suffice here

to point out the need for such a schema because it brings order into the perplexing phenomenology of adolescence.

I will now introduce a concept about adolescent conflict resolution which has a bearing on the understanding of adolescent personality formation and, indirectly, on psychotherapy with this age group. From my work with adolescents I have arrived at the conclusion that adolescence does not aim at conflict resolution per se, nor would the accomplishment of such a task be desirable. One should rather consider that during the terminal period of adolescence certain conflictual themes or complexes acquire an ego-syntonic nature. They become integrated into the ego and thus give rise to persistent life tasks. Following these lines of thought, the termination of *adolescence proper*, or *middle adolescence*, would be in evidence with the delineation of an idiosyncratic conflict and drive constellation which, during *late adolescence*, is transformed into a unified whole that forms an integral part of the ego. *Adolescence proper* has elaborated a core of internal strife that has resisted adolescent transformation. During this phase, conflicts and disequilibrizing forces have moved into sharp focus, but only *late adolescence* will bring about a final settlement by rendering conflictual residues ego syntonic. This is subjectively felt as having found "one's way of life," or "being in harmony with oneself."

The terminal stage of adolescence confronts the individual with the renunciation of a host of expectations and wishes. Up to this stage many kinds of lives seemed possible; approaching adulthood requires the pursuit of limited goals and the commitment to selective values. The magnitude of this task is usually underrated. To let go of the megalomania of childhood can easily upset the narcissistic balance of a predisposed individual and consolidate the syndrome which I have described as "prolonged adolescence."

The adolescent's need for the relinquishment of childhood

megalomania pushes the therapist into a most precarious position: In siding with the adolescent's megalomanic self-expectations he makes himself indispensable to the adolescent but in so doing he forestalls his growth. Siding with reality, on the other hand, means whittling down the inflated adolescent self-image to proportions which are in consonance with his mental resources and factual accomplishments; in so doing the therapist easily becomes an irritating bore or a nagging frustrater. Yet the therapist has to play his part on both sides of the dilemma. In practical terms this means that the therapist has to offer himself first as a person who provides narcissistic gratification: This might run the gamut from mutual daydreaming to the show of strength. Eventually, it is hoped that through the formation of the ego ideal an internal agency becomes the regulator of the narcissistic balance. In this process the therapist makes himself indispensable to the adolescent because the need for objective or real achievements that are in harmony with the ego ideal becomes increasingly more urgent for the maintenance of self-esteem. Toward this goal he needs the therapist's help.

A question not often disputed in the discussion of adolescent therapy concerns the sex of the therapist. It has been my experience that by and large the adolescent alterations of psychic structure occur through identification and polarization equally well, which is to say that they will proceed with a therapist of either sex. Transference reactions are not intrinsically determined by the sex of the therapist, who becomes the target, for example, of mother and father transference reactions. The therapist's own inflexible self-image often stands in the way of perceiving the shifting roles into which the adolescent places him.

An exception to this general rule is to be found in the case of the preadolescent girl. I had occasion to continue the analysis of a girl at 20 whom I had seen in child analysis at the

age of 11. I learned from this girl that as an 11-year-old she
was in constant fear when alone with me that she would be
raped. Wish and fear made her a dependent but a guarded
patient. The same rape fantasy was confirmed in other preadolescent girl patients of mine, some of whom I referred
successfully to a woman therapist. The interpretation of the
resistance usually aggravates the situation. The girl's consent
in the transfer to a woman and her acknowledgment that
conscious fantasies blocked verbal communication were an
indirect admission of the fact that being alone with a man
was too stimulating and disturbing for therapy ever to become fruitful. An equivalent situation concerning the boy
does not ordinarily exist. The dissimilarity is rooted in the
resolution of the oedipal conflict, which, in the case of the
girl, is not accomplished until adolescence while, in contrast,
it is forcefully repressed in the boy before he enters the
latency period.

One more word about the therapist and the proverbial
difficulties which the treatment of adolescents entails. I refer
to the countertransference. From supervision I have become
convinced that the adolescent presents a peculiar threat to
the therapist. Some embers of his or her own adolescence
usually still continue to glow, or, as it happens not infrequently, the adolescent conflicts of the therapist have been
inadequately analyzed. We must not forget that the reconstruction of adolescence as an intrinsic part of an analysis has
received wider acceptance only during the last decade. One
of the major obstacles to adolescent therapy is to be sought
in the vicissitudes of the countertransference.

In order to present a balanced view of the factors which
complicate intensive therapy with adolescents, I must now
introduce a condition which is inherent in the adolescent
process and which will always work against the therapeutic
endeavor. It is well known that two paradigmatic situations

in the affective life deprive therapy of its effectiveness; I refer to being in love and to the state of mourning. These two affective states epitomize the adolescent tasks of object relinquishment and object finding; both these states make themselves felt in varying intensity throughout adolescence. Of course, these states are the normal affective accomplishment of the adolescent process: They tend, however, to leave the therapist and what he stands for outside the patient's interest. Professional narcissism often makes it difficult to accept such banishment gracefully. Changes in the adolescent's attitude toward therapy that are due to the affective states mentioned are often treated as resistance; this only adds insult to injury.

Everybody who has treated adolescents has had occasion to witness the increasing meaninglessness of therapy when an adolescent falls in love. This occurs mainly during the terminal phase of adolescence, when love assumes a quality quite different from previous attachments and infatuations which we relegate to the stage of affection and sexual experimentation. The ensuing disinterest can lead to the total abandonment of therapy, which might, however, be resumed after a love relationship has acquired permanency. It is often extremely difficult to differentiate between "acting out" and "falling in love." As a rule only the stage of "falling in love" will drain therapy entirely of meaning and purpose, while transient and experimental attachments result only in fluctuations of attitude and interest.

The work of mourning is more silent. The withdrawal of cathexis from inner objects, the internalized parents and siblings, has to be effected before object libido can again be turned outward. This process is comparable to mourning; it represents a permanent detachment from infantile love objects. The self-absorption and the regressive states which constitute typical aspects of the mourning process leave the outside world temporarily without interest and the future without concern or attractiveness. The mood swings of adolescence are partly reflections of the mourning process or object relinquishment. At such times, the adolescent expects the therapist to stand ready with the appropriate attitude once his turn to the object world signals the awakened interest in the business of living.

The turn to the object world is always fraught with the repetition of prototypical experiences. Their display offers therapy again all the chances to render to the growing individual the unique service of relating the present to the past and the future. Establishing an essential continuity in ego experience is thus enhanced; the formation of the self in its final structure has come within reach. We might say that with the formation of the self in its definitive and stable form adolescence has fulfilled its developmental task. In moving toward this level of personality integration, the goal of the adolescent process and the goal of therapy have become one and the same.

4

INTRODUCTION

On Some Problems of Technique in the Analysis of Early Adolescents, by Marjorie Harley

It has often been pointed out (e.g., A. Freud, 1958) that the very developmental position of the early adolescent conflicts with fundamental aspects of the psychoanalytic situation. His need to modify or attenuate his attachment to parental figures tends to impede the establishment of the working alliance and skews the transference; rising drive pressures propel him to action rather than reflection; and the fragility of his self-esteem disposes him to tenacious externalization rather than self-observation.

Nevertheless, profitable analytic work with young adolescents—those, at least, who experience significant subjective discomfort—has been and can be done, and Harley describes here with unusual candor her struggles in attempting to do so. Her discussion is of particular interest for its consideration of special nuances of the transference and the subtleties of interpretation required to allow for insight while preserving the adolescent's delicate narcissistic balance. Further, she suggests ways in which the analyst can gain access to some of the more rigidly protected aspects of the young adolescent's mental life—his maturbation fantasies and their ramifications in his daily living.

It is likely that, despite her sensitivity to preoedipal issues, some of Harley's clinical formulations might be challenged by those who would see, for instance, her patient's early compulsive masturbation as a sign of affective deprivation rather than of sexual overstimulation. But in any case her sensitive technical suggestions, couched in the language of classical metapsychology, merit attentive consideration.

4

On Some Problems of Technique in the Analysis of Early Adolescents

Marjorie Harley, Ph.D.

The aim of this paper is to discuss a few of the technical difficulties which have cumbered my way in the analyses of early adolescents. First, however, I shall briefly review, as I see them, some of the metapsychological aspects of the subphase *early adolescence*. Since the views of child analysts on the distinction between preadolescence and adolescence are somewhat diversified, such an introduction may be a necessary prelude to the clinical material which I shall include in my discussion of technique.

I have thought it somewhat misleading to characterize preadolescence by the quantitative changes in the drives *in contradistinction to* the qualitative changes which occur in early adolescence. It is, of course, incontestable that in preadolescence there is an indiscriminate instinctual arousal from

Reprinted by permission from *The Psychoanalytic Study of the Child*, 25:99-121, 1970. New York: International Universities Press.

Originally read at the Fifth Annual Meeting of The American Association for Child Psychoanalysis, April 1970, at Hershey, Pennsylvania. This paper was designed to provide a point of departure for an associated workshop discussion of technical problems in the analysis of early adolescents.

all developmental levels (A. Freud, 1936); and it is equally incontestable that in early adolescence the biological processes of puberty work toward a qualitative shift in drive organization. But these processes also further augment the quantitative factor, and it is this quantitative factor that largely accounts for the now relative weakness of the ego vis-à-vis the drives. In addition, it is the quantitative as well as the qualitative factor which results in the recathexis of the oedipal strivings with a renewed vigor. As these strivings press toward the surface, the concomitant conflicts may constitute a potentially powerful impediment to the ego's acceptance of genitality and hence a potentially disturbing influence on "the later development of the ego after puberty" (Freud, 1938, p. 191).

From the foregoing, it follows that I do not question the existence, in early adolescence, of the interplay of forces associated with the Oedipus complex and the attendant structural conflicts. It is my impression, however, that the recathexis of the oedipal strivings is as yet a contributing rather than the dominating factor in the early adolescent's initial attempts to loosen his infantile object ties; and that these endeavors are motivated at least as much by the ego's need to repudiate preoedipal protection and comfort, and to move toward self-reliance and self-direction, as by the need to relinquish the incestuous (oedipal) bonds. In this sense, they reflect the first steps on the long road toward the final attainment of adult maturity. I would further add that they are closely bound up with the maturation of the ego apparatuses and that they draw upon ego as well as id energies.

In the ego-superego conflicts of early adolescence, the incestuous strivings obviously play their role, particularly as manifested in the frequently observed sexualization and resultant externalization of the superego. Here, nonetheless, in this early subphase of adolescence, I would again see the ego's strenuous endeavors to negate parental standards as springing in no small measure from the conflictual wishes to establish independence. Further (and in contrast to the older adolescent), the early adolescent is as yet relatively undiscriminating in his quest for new values and standards: Instead, self-consciously and protestingly, he is primarily driven to adopt behavior which is in direct opposition to parental dictates. Underneath, however, his state of mind generally runs counter to his overt behavior; and his unconscious anxiety and guilt, arising from his furtively or truculently aggressive methods of self-assertiveness, are often easily detectable.

The object relations of early adolescence also may be said to have their own peculiar characteristics. In contrast to the (homosexual) peer relationships of preadolescence, where it is not so much the objects that are sexualized as those mutual activities of exploration of the physical selves and exchanges of sexual knowledge and theories, the bisexual (Blos, 1962) relationships of early adolescence are often highly libidinized. On the one hand, they provide a displaced medium through which to enact the various facets of the positive and negative oedipal triangles; on the other hand, they serve as narcissistic buttresses for acquiring and establishing a new and different status, and as experimental maneuvers for demonstrating one's appropriate sexual role. In any event, these relationships lack those dimensions of emotional richness and depth which mark the ardent friendships and love affairs of later adolescence; and there are as yet, as I have implied, no efforts toward object removal (A. Katan, 1937) contingent on the finding of new (heterosexual) love objects.

I am inclined to conceive of early adolescence, then, within a framework which takes into account a rather wide view of ego development and which also allows for failures in meeting the new ego and drive demands. It has seemed to me that those pubertal or early postpubertal girls, and those somewhat older boys who are in an analogous maturational stage, whom I would speak of as early adolescents, are in many ways different beings, confronted with a different situation, than the children whom I would regard as still being in the preadolescent phase. To be more explicit, the individual whom I conceive of as an early adolescent has by now, as a rule, attained a more complex level of (autonomous) ego functioning; and he is now faced with a different set of demands, both internal and external. In respect to the internal, there will be new ego tasks among which, of course, the demands to deal with the awakening genital urgencies, to integrate a changing body image into the self-representation, and to loosen the infantile object ties are foremost. From the external, there will be demands to meet new standards that come from two directions: from the peer group and from the adult world, so that, in addition, these new standards often will clash. If, however, the individual is burdened with pregenital and preoedipal fixations, or in other ways is ill-equipped to meet the maturational demands for a shift in drive organization and for new modalities of ego adaptation,[1] I would still consider him an early adolescent—albeit one very much in need of treatment. I realize that there may be those who feel that, in speaking of early adolescence, I am not free of discrepancies and contradictions; and that there may be others who feel I have placed undue emphasis on the assumption that an individual who is faced with certain phase-specific problems which he is unable to solve, and who retreats to or maintains earlier positions, in many respects

[1]In my introductory summary of some of the metapsychological aspects of early adolescence, I deliberately excluded the adaptive factor. I am quite in accord with K. Eissler's (1969) statement that neither adaptation nor genetic processes "can be the stuff of special metapsychological categories" (p. 465). I further agree that the topographical factor is indispensable to a complete understanding of mental processes.

is not comparable to the individual for whom the same positions are still phase appropriate.

Against this background I shall discuss a few of the technical problems which I have encountered in the analysis of early adolescents. These problems, which admittedly have occurred to me in a haphazard fashion, have nonetheless tended to organize themselves into three groups: (1) problems relating to the initial contact with the early adolescent, that is, to the consultation period; (2) problems pertaining to the early adolescent's transference manifestations; and (3) problems dealing with the handling of perverse masturbation practices and passive homosexual problems in the early adolescent boy.

I would introduce my comments on technique with the general statement that in working with early adolescents I apply the analytic method at the point of the first meeting and maintain it throughout the analysis. As with children, I endeavor, however, to adapt my technique to the degree of ego maturation which has been attained and to the particular phase-specific areas of anxiety and narcissistic sensitivity; and I also try to consider the content of my interpretations in the light of the phase-specific tasks to be accomplished. This last applies not only to interpretations which are made but also to interpretations which deliberately are not made lest they hinder rather than augment the developmental processes.

The analytic method obviously presupposes that the analyst present himself, at the outset, in his appropriate role, one which encompasses interest and empathy but which does not deviate from neutrality and which respects that aspect of the adolescent which is trying to achieve autonomy. By definition, then, it precludes any nonanalytic interventions or manipulations with respect to the patient himself or his environment. I have thought the establishment of this attitude to be essential for the noncontamination of future transference manifestations, and also for the development of the therapeutic alliance, since it sets the stage for the early adolescent's perception of the reality of the analyst as separate from the infantile objects.

It is within the context of the analyst's neutrality that I shall discuss my first thought concerning technical problems in the initial contact.

As we know, the adolescent rarely, if ever, comes for his first appointment with an accurate conception of the analyst's role. In general, we are most aware that we may be viewed as an extension of the parents, as a personification of the old rather than the new, and thus as reflecting old superego standards and a perpetuation of dependence. What we may tend sometimes to overlook is that the early adolescent's picture of the analyst may also be one that carries the attraction of support for instinctual gratification. And this can only mean that this attraction ultimately will be a threat to that part of the adolescent which is seeking instinctual control.

I have thought it is just because we know so well how the resistances to analysis are often especially marked in early adolescence that we may be overzealous in our efforts to establish rapport. This zeal, then, may trigger countertransference intrusions so that we may unwittingly present ourselves as apart from the primary objects by means other than our adherence to neutrality. For example, we may unconsciously imply, in a manner not always easy to pinpoint, that we are on the side of the adolescent's negativistic and hostile aggressive strivings against the parents, that is, on the side of those strivings which (as I have earlier implied) I believe are rarely if ever totally devoid of some anxiety and guilt. This may result in engendering in the adolescent a spurious sense of power, with the analyst an accomplice, if not the instigator, in his acting out. Or, by trying to convey to the adolescent our understanding and nonjudgmental attitude toward those activities usually condemned, in some measure, by adults, in an equally subtle way we may appear to him as participants in superego corruption.

None of us would dispute the fact that there is no other time in life when the two opposites—regression and progression—draw each other out and set each other in motion to the extent that they do in adolescence. The early adolescent may use his peers as a mainstay for regression in any one or all three of his psychic systems and to bolster him in his battles against his parents. But we know it is a quite different matter if he sees an adult, in this case the analyst, as being in an analogous role. In the latter instance, there is an almost invariable concomitant which either immediately, or as a delayed reaction, will increase rather than lessen his suspiciousness and fears. He may feel he is slipping under the influence of someone who, more powerful than himself, may promote instinctual license and simultaneously seduce him into revealing his sexual fantasies and activities; or, and particularly in those instances where there is a history of an actual childhood seduction, there may even eventuate the unconscious fantasy of this being repeated with the analyst.

I would add it is primarily in those adolescents who are most rebellious and antagonistic, and who may come to the analyst with a manifest and explicit request for support against their parents' restrictions, that the underlying wish to achieve ego control is often especially strong; and that the basic fear of superego and id seduction is often especially marked. Of paramount importance in such cases, then, is that the analyst focus on this wish for control as one of the motivations, or the motivation, for analysis, and that he scrupulously avoid any involvement in the adolescent's externalization maneuvers.

For example, a 13½-year-old girl obviously had come to my office under coercion. She rested a pad on her knees and wrote for the entire hour. I tried hard, but only once did she speak, when she angrily snapped her answer that she was writing an essay on the evils of the establishment. She made it quite clear that I was in this category. At the end of the hour, I verbalized my agreement that she wished no help at this time and left the way open for her to telephone me should she change her mind.

Over a year later, she requested an appointment on the basis that her parents were "driving her nuts." She was obviously upset and I had the sense that her externalization might be a friable one and more in the nature of a face-saving device.

In the course of two interviews, it became apparent, through her derivative communications, that one of her central problems was a fear of loss of control linked to her masturbation conflict. The scenes she provoked with her parents and her older brother were clearly aimed at drawing them into her arena of sexual excitement. Her frequent refusals to go to school were not solely an expression of defiance, as she would have her parents believe, but were associated with the anxiety she experienced at having to sit still in a classroom when her intense sexual excitations threatened to overwhelm her. In a paradoxical way, her emphatic complaints that her parents were exerting too much control and grounding her repeatedly were, unknown to herself, also her way of saying that they were, in fact, depriving her of control; that is, "driving her nuts." For, in her scheme of things, her only means of handling her instinctual pressures was to discharge them through almost unceasing activity with her peers. Yet, by providing her with derivative but anxiety-arousing masturbation outlets, these activities served to perpetuate rather than alleviate her tensions.

This girl opened the first session with a long series of complaints against her parents and an explicit, insistent demand that I advise them to treat her differently: that I recommend she be allowed to go into Central Park and to ride the subways whenever she chose, and that she have no curfew imposed upon her. I listened to her story impassively and when she had finally finished, I said she had told me of her external problems, but I wondered about her internal ones, since it was to these that my kind of work pertained. I maintained this attitude consistently in the face of her alternations between revealing her inner conflicts and then reverting to her demands, which at times were tantamount to threats, for an alleviation of the external. She was enormously relieved when, at the close of our second appointment, we had established between us her need to understand what was going on "inside" so that she could control her feelings instead of allowing her feelings to control her.

Now, in the first hour, when this girl seemed on the verge of speaking of her "hangups," and then hesitated, I suggested it was difficult for her not to regard me as a member of the establishment. She spied a package of cigarettes in an outside flap of my pocketbook and helped herself to one, underscoring that her parents did not know she smoked; and she proceeded to tell me how she had smoked pot, how she *might* decide to "go straight," and indirectly revealed her concern lest she be tempted to try hard drugs. In the course of her second appointment, she told me I should not have made my remark about the establishment. She explained this implied that I was not an adult; it would have been more appropriate had I implied that I was not her mother. The ostentatiously innocent and earnest manner with which she thus chided me was, in one sense, all part of her provocation; but she also had made a valid point. I had felt challenged by this girl, who did not present so easy a picture as I may have depicted. At the moment of my allusion to the establishment, I had been overeager to gain her confidence, and there very likely had been a subtle element of seduction in my manner or voice. Later, in speaking of her decision to accept treatment, she again warned me to maintain my appropriate role by paying me a dubious compliment. She compared me favorably with another analyst with whom she had begun analysis two years previously and with whom she had broken off contact after only a few months of treatment. This other analyst was "not a very good one," she said. She had allowed her to break appointments and leave her hours whenever she wished; and, she added, she also had let her "bum her cigarettes!"

My second thought regarding the initial contact pertains to the adolescent's anxiety, as well as his shame and guilt, with respect to revealing his inner life. It has seemed to me that we are so attuned to the threat that this carries for him, so attuned to his narcissistic vulnerability, and so apprehensive lest we frighten him away that our reluctance to set foot in troubled waters may sometimes deprive him of a valid relief.

The early adolescent who is willing to consult with an analyst often has conceded that there is a discernible reason for taking this step. He may well fear, however, that there is another reason. To take an oversimplified example: In the case of an underachiever, the discernible reason may deal with his learning problems. The inner, feared reason may derive from his unconscious castration complex and express itself in a generalized feeling that there may be something "terribly wrong" with him which makes him different, and which the analyst will perceive and thus verify, so that he will be doomed.

If, in the initial contact, we detect this inner reason, and if we are able to bring it out into the open, we may have taken a first step which is no mean one. The underachiever will probably be more relieved than not if we find a suitable opportunity to obtain his acknowledgment that he sometimes feels unsure of himself in ways that transcend the academic area; that these feelings are not easy to define but are confusing and disturbing and amount to his feeling all wrong about himself. His relief will come from our attitude and tone of voice which imply that, in our experience, this sort of feeling is neither unique nor irreversible, but is a problem to be analyzed.

I trust that what I have said will not be construed as my advocating that we abandon caution in our approach to the early adolescent patient; or that I am overlooking the fact that we must be guided by our own experience, sensitivity, and intuition. But I do mean that if we are too ready to augment or even instigate avoidance maneuvers, we may lose rather than gain.

I shall now turn to my two thoughts which relate to problems that I have encountered in the handling of the transference in early adolescents.[2] My first remark regarding transference manifestations concerns the consequences of a technical error which I made when I failed to perceive that the main theme of the analysis, at a given time, was the expression of the patient's transference. In this connection, it is relevant to inject that there have been times when the cathexis of the early adolescent has appeared to be so much vested in his school activities and his peer relationships, or in his initial and experimental attempts at assuming a heterosexual role, that I have not alerted myself sufficiently to the transference manifestations that have nonetheless been active and pertinent.

A boy, not quite 15, had been in analysis for a year and

[2]I should here inject for the sake of clarity that in this paper I am using the term transference in its strict meaning to denote a repetition of past events and experiences, and am not extending it to include all of the patient's attitudes toward the analyst.

a half. An only child, he had entered into a relationship with me in which he strove in manifold ways to elicit those responses which he saw as a means for correction of the emotional deprivations and destructive responses that he felt had been inflicted upon him by his parents; and it should be said that his grievances had some reality basis. His mother had frankly wanted a girl, had lamented repeatedly her inability to conceive again after his birth, and had never welcomed his active, masculine strivings. In his preschool years, he had spent most of his waking hours with a maid who had paid little attention to him. Throughout his childhood, and up to the present, his father had been away much of the time on long trips and, when he was at home, he had been depressed and withdrawn.

I commenced this boy's analysis with the resolution to resist both his overt attempts to force me into gratifying those needs which he felt had never been fulfilled and his, at other times, artfully disguised methods to lure me into this role. By the end of the first year of analysis, it seemed that these tendencies had been much lessened. I should add that he was somewhat obsessional, with a proneness toward isolation when his ideational contents became anxiety arousing.

At this time, the boy's main preoccupations had to do with his first serious attempt to have a steady girlfriend (whose name was Jane). I cannot elaborate on the content of the analytic hours with which I am here concerned save to say that they had to do primarily with his uneasiness in this relationship, an uneasiness which was traceable to his castration complex and his related doubts about the adequacy of his genital. These factors we had already openly touched upon in the context of his masturbation. In any event, for a number of hours, he now offered his own interpretations, mainly through his dreams, of what he saw as the causes for his uneasiness with Jane, linking these to his castration anxiety.

He also relied heavily on symbolic meanings (and I feel impelled to say that he did not learn these from me) on which to base his often complex and even fanciful interpretations. His way of thus engaging in what was largely a pseudo self-analysis was highly intellectualized, and I saw this as part of his isolation tendencies when faced with anxiety. For this reason, I interpreted what I thought to be the relevant defense. No sooner had I made this interpretation than I knew I had inflicted a painful narcissistic hurt; and so I indicated I knew he had taken my interpretation as a criticism. But by this he also felt criticized because I had, as it were, criticized him for feeling criticized.

I next endeavored to speak to his extreme narcissistic vulnerability of the moment in terms of the painful inadequacy we both knew he was experiencing with Jane; and of the inevitable intensification of these feelings at this time, when his anxieties about his genital were in the foreground. However, in my efforts to help maintain this boy's narcissistic equilibrium, I was too unrestrained in the almost soothing understanding I showed as I paved the way for the interpretations I made in subsequent hours. It was not long before he began behaving like a contented child, interspersing his associations with expressions of how "great" analysis was, he was "so much better already," and of how much he liked my office and also me because I understood him so well. It was then that I realized the extent to which I had been gratifying him.

When I had rearranged my perspective, I could see it had not been his defense of intellectualization that had been the important factor of the moment. He had been, in fact, manifesting a transference resistance in that by enacting his intellectual gymnastics before my eyes, he had been repeating his futile attempts to gain his mother's admiration of his phallic exhibitionism in his oedipal phase. Further, in my ill-

chosen ways of trying to undo the narcissistic injury which
I had inflicted by repudiating his phallic advances, I had
fallen into the trap of encouraging his regression and of
providing, on a preoedipal level, that very emotional corrective experience I had cautioned myself to avoid.

We would all agree that certain elements of corrective
emotional experiences are probably the *byproducts* of all analyses. It also might be interesting to speculate on how much
the search for a corrective emotional experience may be
phase-specific in adolescence and the various ways in which
this may, in general, be implemented. Nonetheless, I believe
many of us would agree that the main purpose of analysis
is to make the necessary corrections by genetic constructions
and the working through of the infantile conflicts. And I
have offered this brief sketch to show not only how I allowed
an early adolescent's manifest preoccupation with outside
activities to obscure my awareness of the transference, and
thus to lead me to make a misinterpretation, but also how,
in my efforts to undo my apparent yet incompletely understood error, I momentarily ceased to function in my proper
role of analyst.

My second thought is concerned with a problem contingent
on insufficient understanding of all the ingredients of a given
transference resistance. It has relation to an area which has
continued to interest me and on which I elaborated some
years ago (Harley, 1961a). Specifically, I have in mind the
individual who reaches early adolescence already burdened
with an ego which throughout childhood has never overcome
a sense of uncontrollability and helplessness in response to
instinctual excitations and whose ego-instinctual balance has
always been an uncertain one. These are children who, because of one or several combined genetic factors, usually
rooted in the early preoedipal period, but then continuing
in new forms or new combinations in the oedipal and even

postoedipal periods, were never able to attain the relative respite from instinctual pressures more commonly associated with the latency years. I am referring to those children who were subjected to excessive and repeated premature genital arousal and who, as will be recalled, were the focus of some of Greenacre's (1952a) earlier studies.

The point I should like to make here has to do with the sometimes enormous threat to the early adolescent of this type, which arises from his anxiety lest he be unable to contain his instinctual excitations and associated body sensations and feelings. To say this in other words, it is as though the instinctual changes of puberty, with the attendant assault on the already precarious ego-instinctual balance, threaten to activate the memory traces of the early states of extreme organismic distress arising from the fact that the massive stimulation had exceeded the immature organism's capacity for discharge. It is further relevant that in these cases there tends to be a perpetuation of the excess of aggression linked with the early and premature genital arousal, which not only results in an increased sadomasochism, but which also contributes to the preservation of the ego's primary, as it were, sense of helplessness in the face of genital arousal.

I learned that in certain situations it was my failure to perceive and comprehend this factor in the early adolescent's fear of his libidinal strivings in the transference that led to an impasse in the analysis. I shall attempt to illustrate this by recalling the patient who first helped me to understand it.

This was a 14½-year-old girl who, in early prepuberty, had erected constricting defenses against her instinctual strivings, and who was approaching the end of her second year of analysis. Up to this point, I had been unable to loosen her defenses against her affects. Suffice it to say that I knew, both from the history and genetic constructions which we had already arrived at, that this girl belonged to that group of overstimulated children of which I have been speaking. She could remember her compulsive masturbation in early latency and recalled how one day the insides of her thighs were so inflamed that she could not wait until her mother had vacated the bathroom; she had barged in to ease her burning sensations with cold water, even though in so doing she risked revealing the fact of her masturbation to the mother. She had no awareness that she had thus been seeking her mother's aid in controlling her excitement rather than in augmenting it. This I then interpreted. She had hinted at her latency masturbation fantasies when she spoke of the picture games she had played with herself in these childhood years, but insisted that she could remember only the fact that she had imagined a variety of things—that the content of her imaginings she could not possibly recall; I believed her. Nor did she deny my suggestion that she wanted to keep these fantasies buried away as a means of avoiding the excited feelings they might evoke; but this suggestion yielded nothing further. She was equally insistent that her latency masturbation seemed long ago, like part of the Dark Ages, and that she now experienced no genital sensations and no desire to masturbate. This, too, I believed.

With this reserve fund of material, I listened to the following dream:

> I was playing football and Harry—a boy in my class—made a pass at me; and I seemed to have forgotten how to play the game and thought it was dodge ball, so instead of catching the pass I dodged it.

She immediately saw the dream pun but seemed not to see the coincidence between the dream boy's name, Harry, and her father's name. Hesitatingly, she said that she thought the dream had to do with the Friday evening, two weeks hence, when Ernie, a 16-year-old boy, was to take her to her first dance; and she now volunteered her anxiety lest she not know what to do should he try to kiss her goodnight. I approached this anxiety at first in its simplest terms, that is, her uncertainty regarding the expected behavior for her age on her first date with a boy. This yielded no result; nor did my attempts in subsequent hours to approach her underlying sexual fantasies by reference to the forgotten game in the dream, and to her wish to dodge all the picture games of her imagination. She only said I did not understand and that she herself did not understand enough to tell me. But, if Ernie kissed her, she was afraid she *would not know what to do.*

There now ensued a shift in the analysis, the cause of which she easily understood. She turned her attention away from Ernie to me, which obviously meant that she sought safety from the heterosexual (Oedipal) dangers in a preoedipal mother relationship. At this juncture, we came up against a period of powerful resistance after she had confessed she was beginning to have "liking feelings" for me, which she feared would increase. In the course of many weeks, I attempted every possible means that I could devise to understand the specific contents of this resistance. For example, I tried to deal with the implied regressive threat in her turning to me for comfort and security; with the fantasy that, as her mother had done, I would increase her excitement rather than help her control it; and I gave interpretations in derivative form of the homosexual implication in her "liking feelings" for me and of her possible fears of merging into me. Finally, she verbalized her concern that she might even have the urge to hug me. But when I remarked that perhaps she feared she would not be able to control this urge, or even that I would permit her to act upon it, she was convincing in her assurance that she knew full well this urge would not lead to action. She then repeated that I did not understand; she could not explain, but if she "let her feelings come," she would not know what to do. At that moment, I recalled that she had used this same phrase, that is, *that she would not know what to do*, in the context of the goodnight kiss from Ernie. It was then that I suddenly understood; and I told her I thought she feared most of all that her feelings would become so strong she would not be able to stand them. Her relief was unmistakable.

After we had repeatedly linked this fear to those early states of intense excitement which she had sustained when she was so little, and when it was understandable that she must have felt almost as though her little body would burst with such strong excitement, she ultimately dared to experience that immediacy of feeling provided by the positive and negative aspects of the transference; she could then allow her sadomasochistic primal scene fantasies to emerge in conjunction with her genital sensations. It was also now that she could understand that it was what for her amounted to an almost overwhelming strength of her feelings that lent such reality force to these frightening fantasies. In short, it was her comprehension that her basic fear lest she be unable to contain her feelings was, in one sense, an anachronism that seemed to provide her with the courage to proceed to analyze the pregenital and preoedipal components which had led to her unresolved oedipal problems.

My final remarks have to do with the technical handling of perverse masturbation practices and the problem of passive homosexuality in the early adolescent boy. In this connection, I have in mind those boys whose future psychosexual development appears to be endangered by rather constant perverse inclinations that often have predated the onset of adolescence and that in themselves are indicators of strong pregenital fixations rather than of temporary drive regressions.

There is fairly general agreement that, in the more usual

course of affairs, it is not too difficult to enable the early adolescent boy to speak of the act of masturbation, especially when we approach this in the context of the phase-specific body feelings that a boy of his age is experiencing. More often than not, he will at first deny any concerns, but once the fact of his masturbation is an open one between us, we can slowly proceed to the various anxieties involved. The early adolescent, however, whose masturbation activities are consistently, or for the most part, of a perverse order will usually strenuously resist any direct mention of masturbation. He may repeatedly make sly references to it, but usually will hastily retreat when we try to pursue these. Yet, in the three such cases I have worked with, I have thought it has been largely this very problem that has kept the adolescent coming.

I would here inject that my findings in respect to the adolescent's attitude toward his perverse masturbation practices are very much in accord with those of Laufer (1968). Laufer states the problem most aptly, I believe, when he suggests that in his cases masturbation could not serve "the function of helping the ego reorganize itself around the supremacy of genitality" (p. 115). He further sees the adolescent's anxiety as arising not only from his belief that this behavior is a confirmation of his abnormality, but also from his awareness of his inability to use masturbation as "trial action" for adult sexual behavior.

In order to provide a setting for my comments on the question of the technique involved in dealing with these and related problems, I shall draw on one more case description as my starting point.

A 13-year-old boy eagerly accepted analysis. From the vantage of both his biological development and his general demeanor, he had the appearance of a 15- or 16-year-old. He was depressed; although an A student, he was still concerned about his schoolwork, and although president of his class and a surface participant in most peer activities, he inwardly felt isolated and uncertain of his position in the group. He also had been intensely afraid, since early prepuberty, that older boys and men would attack him on the street or in his room at night. In contrast to his urgent request that he commence his analysis as soon as possible, he opened his first hour with what became an oft-repeated refrain for months: "Do I have to come?" No matter how I attempted to deal with this refrain analytically, he retorted that he had to come; he was trapped. He also reiterated that his youth was slipping away too rapidly, that he was not preparing adequately for the future. He emphasized how he wanted to be on his own and counted the years until he could drive a car. Yet he also told, rather wistfully, of his desire to have life remain unchanged; and how, before leaving for weekend or vacation trips, he hid a bottle top in the kitchen so that when he returned it would still be there as a confirmation that "things" were the same. Initially, I saw his mild depression, and his conflicting desires to retain his status quo and yet to move forward, largely as part of the developmental processes of mourning (Root, 1957; A. Freud, 1958) and of the interplay between regression and progression.

The first material in the analysis dealt with his disparaging, well-nigh annihilating hostility toward his father, which soon showed itself as his attempt to obliterate his strong negative oedipal ties. In this context, he portrayed his deep affection for his mother, appearing more childlike when he spoke of her and seeming to regard her more in the light of an all-giving, protecting preoedipal mother than as a positive oedipal love object. Toward me he was formal and polite, an attitude which was in marked contrast to his fury that betrayed itself as he shut the door behind him at the end of each hour. He vehemently heaved it with one hand and then caught it with the other just before it could slam. So violent was his action that one day, unknown to himself, he actually dislocated one of the door hinges. It is noteworthy that behind his defensive exterior his extreme castration anxiety was almost invariably detectable.

It was some time before I realized that his expressed fear and underlying wish to be "trapped," although doubtless related to at least two genetic happenings,[3] at this stage reflected his fear and wish to reveal the perverse nature of his masturbation. His aversion to change reflected his fear of losing his perverse activity, while his concern that he was not preparing for the future was his awareness that this perversion

[3]Some of the characteristics and the genetic material of this patient coincide with Greenacre's (1953) findings regarding fetishists. Until he was five years old, he shared a room with his sister, 11 months younger than himself, and this would seem to have been one of the determinants in his proclivity for primitive identification, with a "bisexual splitting of the body image even antecedent to the phallic phase" (p. 92). In the pregenital as well as in the phallic-oedipal phases he sustained traumas of a "castrative type" (p. 89). At two years of age, he was alone with his mother in her bedroom and witnessed her spontaneous abortion. This occurrence, described to the patient by his mother at the outset of the analysis, facilitated his use of it to screen a later traumatic experience in the phallic-oedipal period. When he was four years old, he visited his maternal aunt and six-year-old cousin at a country farm. The cousin fell over a barbed wire fence which pierced his crotch. He was carried bleeding into the house by his mother (that is, the patient's aunt) who placed him on the bed, leaning over him to dress his wound. Not wishing the frightened younger child to wander around unsupervised, the aunt insisted that he remain in the room while she tended the cousin. In looking back on this experience with his cousin, my patient described how he felt "trapped in a chamber of horrors"; and the event became linked with his mother's admonishment of him for masturbating. It was interesting to observe how, in his analysis, he was frequently prone to confuse the image of his aunt bending over his cousin with that of his (castrating) mother; and how, as we worked with this material, a further distortion eventuated in that he began to insist it was his cousin, and not himself, who had been rebuked for masturbating. Throughout the analysis, he manifested a marked body-phallus equation; his body suffered "*in toto* or in its various parts all of the distresses of castration anxiety" (Greenacre, 1955, p. 192).

was preventing him from keeping abreast of the forward march of events. His fury against me, which broke through only at the end of almost every hour, was aimed at the negative aspects of the preoedipal mother, now transferred to me: I was the vengeful, castrating, phallic mother who, in this instance, would rob him of his perversion.

For the time being, I shall leave this patient to outline the principles of technique which I found helpful in working with him with respect both to the perverse nature of his masturbation and the passive homosexual fantasies and behavior he also revealed. These principles are essentially the same as those I have used fairly consistently in dealing with passive homosexual problems in early adolescents, albeit in this patient the problem was more a bisexual one in that his masculine strivings and attendant heterosexual stirrings could, on occasion, assert themselves more genuinely and forcibly than they could in other such boys.

The first principle I have derived from Anna Freud's (1952) findings through which she demonstrated that the unconscious fantasy of the passive homosexual was an active one since through his active partner he sought to retrieve his lost masculinity.[4] From this she arrived at her formulation that the promise of a cure was a castration threat. In dealing with problems of perverse tendencies, then, I am first of all mindful of the fantasied castration threat implicit in the ad-

[4]These findings were nicely demonstrated by a 13-year-old boy whom I saw many years ago and who taught me a great deal, especially so since I drove him away from analysis by pursuing too avidly his passive aims. He came back finally when I told him, over the telephone, that I had made a mistake in not conveying to him that I also knew how much he wanted to be big and strong. Soon after his return, he presented me with a series of daydreams, the gist of which were that he was cared for and even "mothered" by famous baseball players. The ending to these daydreams, however, was that through this close contact with these athletes he himself eventually became a great ballplayer.

olescent's abandonment of his perverse strivings. At this point, I shall return to my patient with the perverse masturbation practices.

When this boy was not far from his fifteenth birthday, and after repeated indirect approaches, I dared to confront him with the possibility that his extreme anxiety in speaking of masturbation stemmed from his feeling that his ways were different from many other boys'; and that this might mean to him that he was strange or abnormal. His spontaneous response was: "I knew I was trapped, I can't tell you." To this I countered not only by underlining both sides of his conflict over whether to tell me or not, but also by saying he might fear that analysis would take away this problem before he was certain he wanted to give it up; and I added it might be hard for him to realize that ultimately it was he and not myself whose power it was to decide whether to change something in himself or not. To this, he blurted out: "I'm a transvestite. Goddamn it, if I give up my paraphernalia, I'll lose my potency." He now told how he put on his mother's underpants and blouse, lay on his back, and fondled his penis through the underpants, at that moment consciously identifying himself with a girl; whereupon he removed his paraphernalia, as he called it, lay on his stomach and, now identified with the male role, masturbated to the point of ejaculation, which he could not achieve without these preliminaries. He also now told how he had initiated this practice in prepuberty soon after discovering his mother's blood-stained underpants in the clothes hamper. Weeks later, he confessed his frequent urge to hug and kiss his parents' men friends and his associated fantasies of anal penetration.

The second principle I have derived from Freud (1931) who, in speaking of activity and passivity, cautioned that we have "no right to assume that only one of them is primary and that the other owes its strength merely to the force of defence." He goes on to ask: "And if the defence against femininity is so energetic, from what other source can it draw its strength than from the masculine trend . . . ?" (p. 243).

I endeavor, then, to apply infinite care in the analysis of passive homosexual problems to respect openly the boy's attempts at active, masculine behavior, usually refraining from any mention of its defensive purpose save at those times when this is also apparent to him. Even then I remind him that, defensive or not, this is nonetheless also a mark of the way a significant aspect of himself wants to be. I agree very much with Fraiberg's (1961) observation that it is far easier, with early adolescents, to interpret their passive behavior as a defense against their active aggression than it is to uncover and analyze the passive *aims*. But in my experience I have, nevertheless, found it possible sometimes to bring these passive aims into the analysis and, in some measure at least, to assuage the concomitant narcissistic hurts by utilizing the opportunities afforded to acknowledge the boy's simultaneous wish to move forward and to claim his active strivings. If he gives danger signals of regressing to the point of a surrender to his passivity, I try to counterbalance this by emphasizing the other side.

In referring to the analysis of passive aims, I do not mean that it is not equally important to analyze the destructive, aggressive fantasies which so often are directed first and foremost against the mother, thus enhancing her phallic, castrating image and furthering the identification with her. For example, my "transvestite" patient, who was now 15½ years old, recounted his "baby fantasies." He would experience rage when thinking of infants because they "just screamed for their bottles and their mothers"; and he would imagine himself sticking pins into them to torture them. What aroused his most violent rage was that they had not learned control, so that he could never make them obey him. The fantasy was, of course, overdetermined: The infants reflected his younger sister with whom he had vied on a preoedipal and negative oedipal level, as well as that passive, infantile aspect of himself which he both cherished and loathed; the pins were the shots he had inordinately feared since early childhood and his turning of passive into active; yet, at the same time, he satisfied his almost boundless masochism by identification with his tortured victims. Yet the uncontrollable infants also stood for his own enormously aggressive impulses which he feared might become uncontrollable. When I interpreted this last element, his association was that he masturbated each day before coming to his hour because somehow he felt that by so doing he would protect me. He took pains also to masturbate before taking a girl out for the same reason, that is, as a protection to her. While masturbating, he felt "aggressive and bad"; when he had ejaculated he felt "passive and good," and quenched his thirst with cold milk. He experienced no aggressive masturbation fantasies, he said, but confirmed my suggestion that he had to keep them away by recalling that while masturbating, he kept popular tunes running through his head over and over again.

In a later hour, he closed his eyes, was silent for only a few moments, startled as he opened his eyes, and explained in surprise that he thought he had fallen asleep and had dreamed his fantasies were not his own but made in a factory. I agreed this might be a comforting dream. At that moment, however, I felt his need for ego support and so I remarked that it was, nonetheless, often easier to understand and therefore easier to modify or design anew what one had wrought with one's own hands than to do the same with what others had put together by machine. His ultimate response was to disclose his "little people fantasy," in which he held tiny women in his hands and humiliated them by ripping off their clothes; thus he felt that he had complete control over them, almost as though he had power over a world of women. The transference allusions in this derivative masturbation fantasy he volunteered without my help; and he also volunteered that it had entered consciousness only twice, but each time as he approached my office.

While we all know by now how rarely, if ever, we can predict whether an adolescent, and especially an early adolescent, will manifest an overt perversion in adulthood, I believe it is of prime importance to begin to analyze these perverse strivings, if possible, in early rather than in later adolescence. We hope that this will help to loosen those pregenital fixations which are the cornerstones of the perverse fantasies and their invariable concomitant of unusually strong sadomasochistic tendencies; and we also hope it will help to reinforce the ego's alienation from the underlying omnipotence fantasies and thereby lessen the danger of their more lasting integration. These narcissistic problems obviously cannot be viewed as those temporary ego regressions of adolescence which ultimately support the forces of progression. It may also be, as I have mentioned elsewhere (Harley, 1961b), that when previous development has predisposed the adolescent toward a weak genital organization, the maturational forces, which now push toward a shift in drive organization, may, in one sense, augment the analytic work.

Further, since it is the constituents of these perverse pregenital fixations which have not only contributed to the unsuccessful oedipal experiences of these patients, but which also tend to bind him to his primary objects, they may prove to be of tremendous hindrance when he is faced with the task in later adolescence of finding new heterosexual love objects. I have more than once been fascinated to note how, as we begin to work through the pregenital conflicts, the analytic hours are sometimes sprinkled with undistorted positive oedipal strivings which seem not to serve defensive aims but which seem rather to force their way spontaneously and fleetingly into the mainstream of the hour. And I have wondered if somehow, somewhere, the adolescent may not know that the attainment of an undistorted positive oedipal position is essential to his forward movement.[5] This idea may be related, though perhaps very distantly, to Anna Freud's (1958) observations on those war orphans whose adolescence was preceded by a further search for a mother figure, and for whom the "internal possession and cathexis of such an image" seemed "essential for the . . . normal process of detaching libido from it for transfer to new objects, i.e., to sexual partners" (p. 266).

I shall not attempt to summarize my thoughts on a few technical problems which I have encountered in the treatment of early adolescents. I would rather emphasize that the kinds of patients to whom I have largely referred, and the samples of analytic material which I have included, may imply that my analyses of early adolescents proceed into depth more easily than is the case. My most outstanding omission has been the often seemingly endless hours in which the analysis appears to be well-nigh stalemated by the adolescent's preoccupation with his peers and his current crises; and when his apparent uninvolvement with us and the aims of analysis is sometimes more than discouraging. I have also failed to mention his sometimes crafty and ingenious methods for concealing his private life, and his not infrequent adeptness at "playing dumb," so that it may not be until two or three years later, when he is more settled and a little more at home with his changing self, that we learn of the things we failed

[5] I have been repeatedly reminded over the years of K. Eissler's (Chapter 2) comment that adolescence affords a "second chance" for the solution of the oedipal problem.

to perceive at the time, or of the fact that our subtle interpretations, which we thought had gone far afield, had actually hit their mark. And more than once, I have thought
that an early adolescent had quit his analysis because I had
been undercautious in approaching his fantasy life, only to
discover, when he returned in later adolescence, that his leaving was related to his conviction that I suspected him of a
specific bit of acting out in which he was engaged, when in
reality, this possibility had never even crossed my mind.

In closing I would emphasize that I find myself taking
increasing care in determining whether or not the early adolescent's seeming inability to engage in analysis warrants a
decision to interrupt the treatment until he is older. Such an
interruption may at times be quite necessary. But there are
also instances, I think, when he may be assimilating more
than we realize, when our work with those defenses which
might prove to be permanently crippling may be more effective than we know, and when we may be laying a more
substantial basis for future analytic work than either he or
the analyst is always able to recognize.

5

INTRODUCTION

Preventive Intervention in Adolescence, by Moses Laufer

The task of providing psychiatric assistance to adolescents is complicated by a number of factors—some resident in the patient, some in the professional would-be helper. Among the former are the reluctance to acknowledge distress, the penchant for externalization, and the frequently shifting character of mental organization. Among the latter are a lack of clarity about developmental norms and expectations, vague criteria for assessment of pathology, and the absence of valid data about the relative efficacy of specific therapeutic interventions.

In his essay Laufer describes the efforts he and his staff have been making to study and deal with these areas of uncertainty and to offer help to troubled adolescents. Paramount in the design of the program he has developed is the role of *assessment*, which, he makes clear, may itself have a significant therapeutic function. With a shy, confused, or fearful adolescent the very act of talking about himself may provide significant relief of tension and feelings of shame. In any case, such careful evaluation is a necessary prelude to the provision of what Laufer calls "nonintensive treatment," by which he appears to mean supportive or focal psychotherapy of a short-term nature.

117

Laufer is concerned with the prevention of "breakdown" in adolescents, or at least with the amelioration of its consequences for further developmental progress. The range of conditions covered by the term seems rather broad, but would appear to include acute psychotic reactions which do not portend a chronic schizophrenic disorder, as described by Miller and Feinstein (1980). The kind of walk-in center Laufer delineates here would seem to represent a valuable instrument for early intervention in the crises of adolescent life.

5

Preventive Intervention in Adolescence

Moses Laufer, Ph.D.

Preventive intervention in adolescence is an area of work about which we still know very little, and about which there exist various and contradictory views. Some people believe that the most that should be done during adolescence is to support and counsel. Others believe that intervention should, when necessary, include intensive treatment. Some people state categorically that the process of adolescence and the tasks facing every adolescent are such that it might actually be harmful to intervene before the person has reached adulthood. Others seem less sure about this; they believe that a short period of intervention revolving around specific problems may be useful.

My own views are that, even though the process of adolescence is not well understood, psychoanalytic theory and practice has made available to us important guides which can be used to help many adolescents whose problems may range from transitory disturbances to acute mental breakdowns. However, my own experience, as well as that of colleagues

Reprinted by permission from *The Psychoanalytic Study of the Child*,30:511-528, 1975. New Haven: Yale University Press.

This paper was originally presented at the Hampstead Child-Therapy Clinic, October 1974.

who work with adolescents, indicates that it is not only our limited knowledge which hinders us in this work, but that the somewhat haphazard application of what we do know about mental functioning and about adolescence *to the problem of assessment* adds to our difficulties. Many of the new and the so-called more modern ways of helping adolescents are based on the belief that technical changes have hidden in them the cure, and that we only need to go on developing ways of getting to people—a belief based on the implied assumption that everything else will follow from there. I do not, with these remarks, wish to dismiss the outstanding work being done by a whole range of professional people who, through a variety of services in the community, work with and help many very disturbed and vulnerable adolescents. I do think, however, that it falls upon those of us who are psychoanalytically trained or psychodynamically oriented to provide the leadership in understanding and in the application of this understanding to work with the disturbed, the vulnerable, or the ill adolescent.

When we set up the Brent Consultation Centre and the Centre for the Study of Adolescence, we were aware that the service and the research we were planning would be expensive and would very likely, for a variety of reasons ranging from lack of staff to lack of money, be difficult to duplicate. Nevertheless, we felt that there was an important place for an organization such as ours. The interrelationship between service and research would enable us to apply what we do know to helping many different adolescents who were experiencing a crisis in their lives, and at the same time would make it possible for us to study, in depth, a number of adolescents who present a type of psychopathology that is often associated with this period of development.

The experiences in preventive intervention which are described in this paper come from the work at the Brent Consultation Centre and the Centre for the Study of Adolescence which has been going on for just over six years. The Brent Consultation Centre is a walk-in service which is supported by the Education Department of the London Borough of Brent. This means that the London Borough of Brent votes us an annual budget—a budget which is used almost totally for the employment of a part-time staff of psychoanalysts and child therapists who carry out interviewing for assessment and who undertake the psychological treatment of adolescents. In effect, the way our service is set up means that any person (but we hope mainly adolescents) can walk in and be assured of being seen by a member of our professional staff. During the period that we have been open, we have seen somewhat over a thousand adolescents and young adults.

Related to, but actually separate from, the Brent Consultation Centre is the Centre for the Study of Adolescence, a research organization which was set up by us at the same time as the Brent Consultation Centre. The main function of the Centre for the Study of Adolescence is the study of mental breakdown in adolescence. The data for this study are obtained from the analysis or intensive psychotherapy of a limited number of adolescent patients.[1] Until now, our funds for this research have come from foundations and private contributors, but recently we received an award from the Department of Health and Social Security to undertake a broader, statistical study of those adolescents who come to us for help. The Centre for the Study of Adolescence is staffed by the same people who work at the Brent Consultation Centre, which means that each member of the staff has some responsibility for the service and for the research.

[1]The ideas underlying this research have been described more fully elsewhere (Laufer, 1973).

When we set up the Brent Consultation Centre as a walk-in service for adolescents, we began with the assumption that there must be a large number of young people who are in immediate need of help, but who, for a variety of reasons, do not make use of the existing services. We also assumed that if we could get them to seek help, we could intervene at a time in their lives when the interferences in development may not yet have seriously disrupted their lives. We assumed that people's fears of mental illness, their guilt about their own thoughts or actions, or their beliefs that they may be irreversibly damaged would keep many of them away from the more formal agencies, and that very likely they would seek help only following, *rather than before*, a severe and obvious crisis. Our day-to-day work takes such factors and anxieties into account: For example, we have no formal procedure of intake; all information is obtained in the course of the interview (the information about an adolescent's life will vary enormously, depending completely on what the interviewer considers appropriate to discuss, to ask about, or to investigate). We have no waiting list; an adolescent is seen within a matter of days, or immediately if he requests this or if he or we feel that it is urgent. Our assessment procedure varies; we may see an adolescent for assessment once or twice or 15 times, if necessary; the interviewer himself decides at what point he has enough information about the adolescent's present and past functioning to make an assessment and to suggest the most appropriate help. Adolescents are discussed at regular weekly staff meetings, which are attended by all the interviewing and assessment staff, who make a final decision about intervention.

Before describing further what we actually do at the walk-in Centre, I shall give more details of how we function from a staff point of view, because there is an important relationship between the people we see, the kind of work we do, and the expectations which the staff members have of themselves. With the numbers of adolescents who come for help, clearly one of the facts is that we see many very disturbed young people who are either experiencing an acute crisis which may include their families, their friends, their future plans, and so on—crises in which we may be able to help, even though we may feel that our intervention is very limited and perhaps only of temporary benefit. At the same time, we see quite a large number of young people who are obviously at risk and for whom something may have to be done carefully and quickly. I do not want to give the impression that we are a "crisis service"—we are not—it is simply a fact that by being a walk-in service which is available to anybody, we inevitably will see people who are at risk. This means that a member of the interviewing staff may, in one week, see adolescents who are doing quite well but want some help for an acute problem, without there being too much demand on that staff person; during another week, he may be faced with a need to try to do something about a number of adolescents who are seriously at risk.

In such circumstances it may easily happen that we begin to feel that everything we do carries with it an air of urgency or, worse still, that what we are going to do will save the adolescent or change his life. While some of this may be true in some cases, such a tendency carries with it the potential danger of creating an air of omnipotence and the accompanying belief that we can do something for everybody. Some work with disturbed adolescents lends itself to such a belief, especially if there are no built-in safeguards. We have guarded against such a development by (1) our weekly staff meeting in which members are expected to present their work; (2) the arrangement whereby all staff is part-time, with the implied expectation that everybody will continue to do work away from the Centre, *including intensive treatment*; (3)

the requirement that all staff will, in addition to their work with adolescents, work with or treat children or adults. Contained in these requirements or these limitations which we place on ourselves is the awareness that work with adolescents, and especially continuous or too much work with adolescents, carries very serious dangers which can be detrimental both to one's work and person—I have already mentioned the air of omnipotence which can be created and perpetuated; other dangers are the unconscious demand to be idealized by the adolescent; the living out, via the adolescent's sexual life, of one's own neurotic difficulties; the need to be the perfect parent, or the savior; and the implied denigration of the adolescent's parents. Such dangers also exist in work with children and adults, but I believe that the specific dangers I have mentioned are greater in work with adolescents, mainly because of the adolescent's own developmental needs and conflicts.

The range of problems for which adolescents seek help is very wide. However, I shall concentrate on a few of the things we have learned and on some of the areas where important questions still need to be answered. I shall discuss some of the problems in assessment with which we are faced repeatedly; our experience with adolescents who present "hidden/urgent" problems; special practical problems in the assessment of adolescents whose lives are at risk; and our experiences with the nonintensive treatment of a number of adolescents.

PROBLEMS AND FUNCTIONS OF ASSESSMENT

Some of the difficulties we encounter in assessment reflect our uncertainty about the meaning of certain forms of behavior in adolescence; some are more related to the kinds of young people who come to us. Some adolescents who come in appear to be quite sophisticated about themselves and their problems, and are capable of describing their lives in ways which enable us to know what is going on. Others who also may be worried about themselves have little or no ability to tell us what is wrong. They know that they are worried or different, or that they are isolated and unable to stay on a job, but their relation to their own internal life is such that they are surprised and threatened when we say we want to know about this. These adolescents often feel helpless and bewildered by what is going on; we, too, may feel this way because there may be little likelihood of creating an awareness that something is wrong and that it comes from within themselves. Of course, in every assessment, we take into account a whole variety of external factors which may be important, but finally we must try to understand what is or is not going on internally. For some adolescents, such an approach is either foreign or too threatening, and we get nowhere. But there certainly are also adolescents who can tell us about themselves.

From a technical point of view, I believe that the whole procedure of coming to the Centre, of being interviewed and being encouraged to talk about himself, can be a very important experience in the life of that adolescent. For this reason, I will not only want to find out what I must know for assessment, but I will, when appropriate, encourage the adolescent to participate in the assessment procedure. For example, if I ask a question, I will explain why I have asked the question and what I will do with the answer. I will try to show the adolescent how I go about deciding what I think is wrong and what I think can be done to help. This may seem to be a seductive procedure, but it need not be so if the interviewer conveys his awareness of the adolescent's anxiety. It helps to remove the bewilderment and some of the frightening magic of "assessing"; it also enables the adolescent to begin to feel less terrified of being labeled and of being told that nothing can be done. Many of those who seek help have never before talked to anybody else about their problems, nor have they acknowledged consciously the extent to which they have been and are burdened by what they believe is wrong with them. By the interviewer and the adolescent jointly formulating what is wrong, the frightening unknown becomes a little less powerful and at the same time the adolescent can begin to feel hope that somebody understands what is wrong and may be able to help.

If the adolescent allows me, I will scan his whole present life—his social relationships, his schooling or work, the relationship with his parents. But inevitably I want to be able to establish the severity of the structured pathology which may be present and the extent of interference in the developmental process (A. Freud, 1958, 1962; Laufer, 1965). In other words, I will try to establish whether the disturbance is transitory or neurotic, whether I can spot an established psychotic process or the beginnings of what is a break with reality. How do we do this? And what weight do we give to what we find out?

The way in which the adolescent is responding to the developmental tasks (the change in the relationship to his parents, the change in the relationship to his contemporaries, his reactions to his physically mature body) are of primary importance in assessment. My own bias in assessment is to place the greatest importance on learning about and trying to understand what is going on in the adolescent's relationship to his own body, and in knowing about the central sexual identifications which exist. I will, therefore, want to know how the adolescent is responding to the fact that his body is now physically mature (that he can produce semen and impregnate a female; or that she ovulates and menstruates, i.e., that she can become pregnant and grow a child in her own body). In optimal circumstances, I will be able to get such information from the adolescent's description of his relationships to people of the same or the opposite sex, from a description of his masturbation activity (including his masturbation fantasies), and generally from the way in which he takes care of his body. The intricate details of the adolescent's relationship to his own body not only can be one of the main means of establishing the extent of the interference in the developmental process, but it can be one of *the* means of establishing the severity of the pathology, and especially whether there are the ingredients either for a "breakdown" (which I shall define later) or for psychosis.

As I mentioned earlier, getting the information which we must have for assessment is often difficult. Sometimes we do not get it, and we may then be stuck, not quite knowing how to proceed. But as has already been implied, my method of obtaining information is an active one, in which I will carefully ask the adolescent questions related to all aspects of his life. I am aware of the dangers inherent in such a way of working, but I believe that this way of getting information need be neither traumatic nor anxiety-provoking, especially if we keep in mind that there may be times when it is *not* appropriate to ask too much. I will then not only note the content of the person's reaction, but I will also pay attention to the way in which the answer is given.

AWARENESS THAT PROBLEM IS INTERNAL

For example, a young man said that he had been worried about himself for a long time, but he could not make himself seek help because he thought it might be embarrassing and unpleasant, and in any case he was not sure whether it would be of much use. He became very worried, however, when he realized a short time ago that he had walked to a nearby railway station and had thought of killing himself. But he suddenly thought that he should not do it because he had told his parents that he would never do such a thing. He was dressed shabbily, he kept on glancing away from me, he giggled and blushed when he talked of this. My first impression was of a very disturbed young man—when I went to fetch him from the waiting room, I thought he looked like some of the schizophrenic adolescents I had seen in the acute admissions ward of a hospital. I started the interview by saying that he looked quite worried when I came to the waiting room, and I wondered whether he had been worried about what he might want to discuss with me.

His first answer assured me that his pathology might be less severe than I had assumed. He said that he had felt troubled for years; he had nearly given up; but he had been hoping that I might do something. He talked of his loneliness, of his difficulty in having a girlfriend, of his sudden failure at school after having had a long record of being one of the best in the school, and now of working as a clerk (after he and his family and his head teacher had all assumed that he would go on to a leading university). I acknowledged the feeling of failure, the shame and anger with himself, and the hopelessness.

It was when he could tell me about his masturbation activity that I was able to understand why he presented such a disorganized and shabby picture of himself, and then it was also possible for me to decide that the pathological process was not a psychotic one, even though it reflected the presence of severe interference in functioning. He talked of his long-standing inability to touch his penis, of his humiliation when he could masturbate only by using a vibrator, and of his belief that he was irreversibly abnormal. He was able to describe how he worried about himself, but there was no concern about ominous body changes or weird feelings from his body over which he had no control. In telling me all this, he stared at me to see how I responded, and he could say, with some encouragement from me, that he thought I might be disgusted and that I would confirm that he was a pervert.

From the point of view of assessment I felt that my primary function was to establish the extent of disturbance (and to assure myself that the process was not psychotic in nature), and also to prepare him for the need for long-term intervention (which we could not offer at that time, but which we would try to arrange for him). With this young man the question of treatment was not a difficult one to discuss, because he was very much in touch with his anxiety and with the extent of his isolation. That the problem was an internal one was easy for him to perceive, as a result of which the idea of a period of treatment was quite acceptable to him. Discussing treatment with him also gave him the hope that he could change.

THE HIDDEN/URGENT PROBLEMS

At the Centre we see a group of adolescents who present special problems in assessment and who may, from a practical point of view, be in urgent need of help of some kind. These adolescents also say that they are worried, but they do not quite know why. In describing their day-to-day lives as well as their immediate past, they create a picture of suffering or despair that contains a pervasive feeling that everything is worthless or hopeless. I am describing not only the severely depressed adolescents, but those who feel that nothing has changed for years and that nothing will ever change. The depression which they present may not be the neurotic or psychotic type of depression; rather, it is characterized by a feeling that the possibilities of something altering in their lives are nonexistent. Nevertheless, they have not given up completely, and often they come to the Centre thinking that this is a last try. The hidden/urgent problems which these adolescents come with are hidden from themselves, and the urgency is something of which they are not at all aware when they first come to us. With these adolescents one can easily miss the severity of the existing pathology or of the impending danger to their lives, and it is an important function of ours to know when to be concerned and why.

Breakdown

The feeling of worthlessness or hopelessness is, I believe, a reaction to something they experienced earlier in adolescence—an experience that bewildered and terrified them. Some of these people, I believe, felt that they either were mad or might go mad; they felt disorganized by their uncontrollable regressive thoughts or actions—thoughts or actions which were directly linked to the feelings coming from their sexually mature bodies. In assessment, some of these adolescents then describe themselves as dead, not caring, feeling hopeless, hating themselves, and not knowing what to do with themselves.

In such instances the assessment serves a function that goes beyond eliciting the information we need to understand the severity of the pathology. The assessment can be used—very effectively, I believe—to enable the adolescent to try again to come into touch with the anxiety which at one time overwhelmed him. More specifically, the mere act of putting into words his despair, his shame, and his wish simply to give up can be a highly significant step forward. In assessment interviews it is very often not possible for us to determine what these thoughts *really* are about, to what extent the interference is of a secondary nature, or whether the existing pathology is reversible or not. Nevertheless, it is of the utmost importance to establish whether earlier in adolescence there took place what I can best describe as a "breakdown"—an overwhelming of the personality, that is, the experience of being overwhelmed by feelings and the accompanying belief of having lost control of the ability to do anything about it. These adolescents recall the "breakdown" as a time when they had temporarily lost the link with reality—*and it is this which terrified them*—but at the same time they had some awareness that what was happening to them was not really true. The behavior, thoughts, or feelings which these adolescents describe often create the diagnostic impression of a psychosis, but I believe it is more appropriate to categorize them under the headings of "breakdown" because such a description contains the idea of the reversibility of the pathological process (despite the many unknowns inherent in it).

It is my conviction that this kind of "breakdown" regularly occurred in adolescents who attempted suicide (assuming they are not psychotic). They present a special problem of assessment and management, to which I shall come back. The other adolescents for whom "breakdown" is an appropriate description are those who suddenly fail badly at their exams, who suddenly seem to be paralyzed by the experience of going to university, who suddenly isolate themselves and refuse to go out with friends. Less obvious and less clear signs of a "breakdown" are seen in the adolescents who slowly withdraw from the outside world, who drift into drug use and then become dependent on drugs and unable to risk giving them up (as one boy said, "Why should I be mad and empty when I can feel that I have friends?"), or who adopt beliefs or behavior which make them into total aesthetes. These adolescents may be viewed as making use of normal adolescent defensive maneuvers; they are often described as neurotic or, more colloquially, as eccentric. But such descriptions help deny the severity of the disturbance which may be present and the extent to which nothing has changed in these people's lives from early adolescence on.

Jane, aged 19, explained to me that she could not concentrate. She had been thinking of seeking help for some time, but she decided to do something about her difficulties when she found that she was refusing time after time to accept invitations from boys to go to parties. Instead, on Saturday evenings, she would read, listen to records, and then just go off to sleep. Once, when she did go out with a boy and he tried to kiss her, she felt disgusted and had to spend a long time when she came home washing her face and looking in the mirror to see that there was nothing unusual about her looks. *She was aware that this behavior was ridiculous*, but she *had to* do it. At present she did not have many friends—she preferred to spend her time alone.

In response to my questions, she described how she hated herself when she first began to menstruate, how she cried and felt that her father would never love her again as he used to. Instead of saying anything which might help her to see what the conflict was about, I said that this must have been an awful time for her, and I wondered whether she continued to have trouble about menstruation. With much embarrassment, she told me that her periods had been irregular for four or five years, but now they were alright.

After I explained why I wanted to know about these things, she went on to tell me about her isolation, her thoughts of suicide which had haunted her for some years, and her feeling that something had happened to her which left her with the feeling that part of her mind was detached from the rest of her. She had given me a number of signals in the interview that something had indeed gone wrong earlier in her adolescence, and when I asked her to describe further her feeling of disgust when the boy tried to kiss her, she casually talked about her eating difficulties in the past. These turned out to be anorexia nervosa—at 17 her weight had dropped from 115 to 70 pounds; it was a time when she felt fine because her body was dead and she felt weak and ugly. She had almost no feelings, so there was nothing to be worried about.

I responded by saying, "You were very right to have come to the Centre. You've been very unhappy for a long time, but you couldn't do anything about it because you were too ashamed. But now that you've come for help, you *must* do something about your life." This experience at the Centre was very important for Jane. Not only could we recognize that her past difficulties were, in fact, an illness, but it was possible to convey to her that she could be helped and that some change could take place. It was as if she now had an ally in her fight against something which until then had simply been terrifying.

Adolescents Whose Lives Are at Risk

The other group of adolescents who come to us with hidden/urgent problems are those who have attempted suicide. Very often, the actual suicide attempt may have taken place some time prior to their seeking help, and often we learn about it only in response to our questioning rather than because the adolescent tells us about it. It is also remarkable how frequently such information is not given to us either by the parents or by professional people (if these are the persons who are first in touch with us). We may be told that the adolescent is feeling depressed, or does not want to work, or is behaving in an odd way, but very often there is no reference to a previous suicide attempt.

My own view about adolescents who have made a suicide attempt is that they have, *at the least*, had a "breakdown" (sometimes the attempt may have been part of a psychosis). Even though the adolescent may tell me that now everything is fine, and that what he is really worried about is his job, or not having a girlfriend, or feeling sexually abnormal, and so on, I react to the information of a past suicide attempt as if it were an urgent crisis, *no matter when it was that the actual attempt was made*. I make it quite clear to the adolescent what view I take of the attempt and why, and I always let him know that I think he is still at risk of repeating it.

From a management or practical point of view, I always involve the parents of the adolescent who attempted suicide, conveying to them as well my view of the seriousness of the situation. Of course, some of the adolescents and parents think I am making a fuss about nothing, and they may try to dismiss what I say. But on the basis of my own experience with the psychoanalytic treatment of adolescents who have attempted suicide, as well as that of colleagues who have analyzed such adolescents at the Centre (as part of our research into mental breakdown in adolescence), I am convinced that from an assessment and practical point of view it is correct to consider such an event an urgent crisis and to make it into a family crisis. To do less than this is to deny the power of the omnipotent fantasy which may temporarily be kept under control but which can, under certain precipitating circumstances, again seriously interfere with the adolescent's reality-testing function, and result in another suicide attempt (Friedman, Glasser, Laufer, Laufer, and Wohl, 1972; Laufer, 1974).

THE NONINTENSIVE TREATMENT OF ADOLESCENTS

I mentioned at the beginning of this paper that our funds for the walk-in service come from the London Borough of Brent. When we first started this service, we insisted that adolescents from anywhere should be able to be seen for assessment. This was agreed, but it was decided that treatment would be reserved only for adolescents from the Borough of Brent. This means that the adolescents coming from outside the Borough of Brent who are in need of treatment have to be referred to other services in the community.

Initially, it was our policy to limit nonintensive treatment to once-weekly sessions for up to one year. This was, at the time, determined primarily by the fact that our budget was very limited. Recently, however, we decided to alter this policy, partly because our budget for the service has been increased substantially, but also because our once-weekly treatment for a limited period was not working out well. Our present policy is to offer up to twice-weekly treatment, without any time limit. While I cannot yet say how this will work out, I shall describe how we go about deciding to offer nonintensive treatment, and in which circumstances I think it to be of use.

A decision about treatment is made at our weekly staff meeting. The reports of all the interviews with the adolescent are circulated in advance of the meeting. It is then up to the staff members attending the meeting to formulate the nature and degree of psychopathology and to recommend the most suitable form of treatment. Whenever the question of nonintensive treatment arises, we encounter much uncertainty about its applicability to adolescents as well as real differences of opinion about its aims and its effectiveness. I find it difficult to decide which factors would account for this—whether it is that we do not understand what intervention does during a developmental process, whether it is our assessment which is at fault, whether the uncertainties reflect our ignorance about the period of adolescence itself, or whether the aims of nonintensive treatment are such that we must expect a good deal of failure. These are some of the questions which we are studying at the moment.

Although we still have a long way to go before we can clarify these problems, I would single out as one of the factors that clouds some of our work the description of our intervention as "treatment." As psychoanalytically trained people, we have certain expectations when we undertake "treatment"; the expectation may be that we can bring about structural change or that we may be able to undo the pathological process which is present. The description of nonintensive intervention as "treatment" superimposes expectations which are different from what I believe such intervention should set out to do. I do not wish to give the impression that I believe that nonintensive intervention in adolescence is not worth doing—far from it. Although such intervention cannot undo the pathological process, it can contribute something of much value to the present and future life of the adolescent. What it can contribute—and I do not think that we should expect anything beyond this—is to help prevent the existing pathology from interfering with the ongoing developmental process; that is to say, it can make it easier for the adolescent to confront the specific developmental tasks, thereby enabling the developmental process to proceed. If we can do this, then we have done something important.

The main developmental tasks of adolescence involve the change in the relationship to the parents, the change in the relationship to contemporaries, and the change in the attitude to the body. More specifically, we assume that the period of adolescence (that is, the time from 13 to 21) will normally enable the adolescent to use experiences in the outside world as well as those related to his internal world (I include those which are specifically related to his own body) in ways which help him with these developmental tasks. If, due to internalized conflict, the adolescent is isolated, or is unable to obtain sexual pleasure from his body, or is unable to risk disapproval from his parents, or is convinced that he or she is socially and sexually inadequate, then the danger is that the failures during the adolescent period will strengthen the already-existing interference in development. When this person reaches the end of adolescence, he will have missed his *once-only chance* to change his relationships to his internal objects, a change which normally would result in his acceptance of the fact that he alone is responsible for his sexually mature body (Laufer, 1968). I use the description *once-only chance* because I believe that the period of adolescence has a specific developmental function which, if interfered with through internalized conflict, cannot simply be undone or caught up with in adulthood. On the contrary, the results of developmental interference or damage in adolescence inevitably have repercussions throughout one's adult life.

If my assumptions about the function of nonintensive intervention are correct, then it follows that the roles of assessment of psychopathology and selection for nonintensive intervention are especially important. The dilemma with which we are constantly faced is that a number of those who come to the Centre for help are very disturbed people, and we know that we may be able to do little for them via nonintensive intervention. Nevertheless, the other side of this is that many of these adolescents are only just beginning to be in touch with the reality of their existing disturbance and to sense the impact of their internalized conflicts on their present and future lives. We know, or believe, that if their psychopathology hinders them in involving themselves in age-appropriate experiences, their infantile fantasies will continue to exert a dynamic power because these fantasies will persist unaltered if they are not tested and checked by reality experiences.

A period of nonintensive intervention can sometimes be of great help to some of these people, but at the same time we cannot lose sight of the fact that we work with many limitations. One of the built-in dangers of offering nonintensive intervention is that we may easily lose sight of the presence of these very important limitations; it is as if the urgency of adolescence as a developmental period makes us want to blur the differences between what takes place in nonintensive intervention as compared to intensive treatment. I have in mind the differences between insight on the

one hand and the internal reality of the transference neurosis
and working through on the other (Stewart, 1963). But these
issues require much more intricate study, and I hope that
our work at the Centre will help to clarify further some of
these differences.

Implied in my remarks about nonintensive intervention is
that we are still quite unsure about what we are doing, whom
we can and whom we cannot help. In our staff meetings we
are very careful to define the aims of our intervention, and
do not offer such help to adolescents who are clearly either
too ill for this or who have no relation to their internal lives.
Yet, in selecting patients for nonintensive help we have until
now relied on such general criteria as severity of the disturbance (which presupposes our ability to rule out the
likelihood of an ongoing psychotic process), the adolescent's
awareness (even if this is only slight) that his problems exist
within himself, the extent of the adolescent's suffering, and
the adolescent's conscious wish to do something about his
present life. This means, in fact, that the adolescents whom
we have so far selected for nonintensive help vary enormously from the not-too-disturbed to those who are obviously
very disturbed and at risk. I can best summarize this aspect
of our work by saying that we think that such intervention
is an important part of our service and can be of great help
to some adolescents, but we do not yet know which criteria
in assessment can help us to be more selective, nor do we
know which technical procedures work and which do not.

Summary

In this paper I have described mainly the work of our walk-
in service for adolescents. I have not described our research
into mental breakdown in adolescence which is being carried
out through the Centre for the Study of Adolescence. I am
aware that I have avoided discussing a number of important

issues related to adolescent development and psychopathology, including the many gaps in our knowledge about adolescence—unknowns which hamper our work severely; the pros and cons of various forms of intervention; the suitability of the various psychopathological categories which are often used to describe what is wrong. Nor have I mentioned our work with parents. Instead, I have chosen to describe a few specific areas of our work which are related to assessment and to intervention. By focusing on what I consider to be the main work of the walk-in Centre, I have also tried to describe what we have learned from this kind of work.

6

INTRODUCTION

The Function of Acting Out, Play Action and Play Acting in the Psychotherapeutic Process, by Rudolf Ekstein and Seymour W. Friedman

Perhaps the most taxing problem in the treatment of the severely disturbed adolescent is that of finding a channel for the establishment of a therapeutic relationship. Too old for the play techniques of early childhood, the adolescent has not yet evolved the cognitive and self-observing capacities that will permit him to use the free association approach of adult analytic therapy, and is, in any case, a frequently unwilling patient, oriented more to action than to reflection as a means of reducing tension and warding off anxiety.

Ekstein, another product of the Vienna school, has long been concerned with the application of psychoanalytic approaches to the care of borderline and psychotic children. Building on the foundation of Aichhorn's work, he has conceived a method based on what he has called "interpreting within the metaphor" (Caruth and Ekstein, 1966), i.e., accepting the patient's defensive displacements and avoiding translation of the assumed primary conflict until the child indicates his ability to tolerate it. The paper "Observations on the Psychology of Borderline and Psychotic Children"

(Ekstein and Wallerstein, 1956) provides the rationale for this way of working with the psychotic child.

In the present paper Ekstein and Friedman describe in extensive detail the use of a similar approach with an adolescent who many would now consider "borderline." The therapist follows the patient in his shifts from "acting out" through more tempered levels of "play action" and "play acting" as he gains increasing mastery of his profound conflicts and ego deficits. The therapist's flexibility is reminiscent of Eissler's idealized model (Chapter 2); the technique carries with it, however, risks that few would be prepared to assume outside the structure of a highly sophisticated residential setting, such as the one that served as a laboratory for this experiment.

6

The Function of Acting Out, Play Action and Play Acting in the Psychotherapeutic Process

Rudolf Ekstein, Ph.D., and Seymour W. Friedman, M.D.

THE THEORETICAL AND TECHNICAL ISSUES

In the psychoanalysis of adult neurotics, acting out is considered a substitute for recollection (Fenichel, 1945), while thinking is regarded as experimental action (Freud, 1911). Our clinical material, derived from the treatment of a neurotic delinquent adolescent boy, suggests that *acting out is a form of experimental recollection*. Play action and play acting, both facets of play to be differentiated later, may be thought of as containing both the elements of acting out and those of thinking. Freud's reference to the dream as the royal road to the unconscious has been often quoted whenever the classical technique applicable to adult neurotics is discussed. The royal road to the unconscious of the child patient is his play (Erikson, 1940), his best means for the communication of the unconscious conflict. Nevertheless, as one knows from the

Reprinted by permission from the *Journal of the American Psychoanalytic Association*, 5:581-629, 1957. New York: International Universities Press.

treatment of more severely disturbed children, it is not always possible to create a situation which permits the use of play (Ekstein and Friedman, 1956), just as many borderline adult patients are not capable of the use of free association.

Play requires a certain maturation of the ego organization and is therefore possible only in those situations where these achievements of maturation are fairly stable and are not excessively invaded by more regressive precursors of thinking such as acting out, a more primitive mode of attempted problem solving. In order more clearly to understand the differing functions of acting out, play action, and play acting within the structure of the therapeutic process, we must review certain facets of ego development.

In the genesis of the psychic apparatus one observes that the main mode of functioning consists of instant need gratification. The first, most primitive "problem solving" of the human mind consists primarily of instant impulse discharge, and even the attempts at hallucinatory gratification by means of vivid fantasies are but substitute means of instant need gratification. The preverbal period of personality development, in which motility and motor development are dominant, takes place usually in a symbiotic relationship. The mother is used as the auxiliary ego which not only gratifies and prohibits, but also thinks for the infant who, in a certain sense, is capable of a kind of "thought" only as is expressed through impulsive action whenever need arises. As the psychic apparatus develops, modes of problem solution grow richer and impulsive action is supplemented by, among others, play action.

Accompanying this change, more advanced thought is developed in spoken language. While action is an attempt to master reality immediately, to make it subservient to the needs of the individual, play action actually is delayed action as far as reality is concerned, and combines the quasi-gratification of the play with an attempt at resolution of conflict. Although the child's play has been considered his first great cultural achievement (Freud, 1920), through which he is capable of giving up immediate gratification, it still is near the primary process mode of thinking.

The model example illustrating the original function of play and demonstrating it as an attempt to master the separation from the mother can be found in Freud's *Beyond the Pleasure Principle* (1920). This first achievement by the child of impulse delay is an unstable one and frequently cannot be maintained. If too much inner or outer stress burdens the child, he cannot use play action in order to counteract increasing anxiety and he must return to earlier modes of mastery or pseudomastery such as emergency measures extending to panic reactions. Panic could be considered as a form of action since one of its meanings is to summon up the rescuer. Parenthetically, we may say that the replacement of play by action does not always necessarily mean ego regression. If play is considered a form of trial thinking, action may well represent the final carrying out of a task which has been successfully thought out. We might well then differentiate between acting out—the unconscious repetition of a conflict—and action—the conscious solution of a conflict situation.

As the mental development of the growing child continues, he will slowly replace more and more elements of play action with expressed fantasy and higher forms of thought. Pure nonhallucinatory fantasy could be considered as standing between play action and secondary process thinking in the hierarchy of prevalent modes of thinking. The stages of mental development—action without delay, play action, pure fantasy, play acting, reality-oriented secondary process thinking—should not be seen as distinctly separated from each other but as arrangements in which any of these modes of thought might be dominant while the other, coexisting modes are more or less submerged. Psychosexual development (Greenacre, 1954; Hartmann, 1954) is similar in that it contains not distinctly different phases but different dominant expressions of instinctual life. Hartmann's concept of phase dominance (1954) is applicable to ego development as well as to instinctual development.

For example, although action may be the outstanding mode of expression for the one-year-old child, we assume that other forms of problem solving or pseudo problem solving such as vivid imagery, the first beginning of language, and simple reality testing are present. Action, though, may be his dominant means of problem solving and of communication. Play action is already a very complex mental phenomenon which includes the act, the fantasy, advanced elements of language, and frequently strong aspects of reality testing. The child knows that he plays rather than acts and may criticize the adult who assumes that the child takes his play fantasy seriously in the sense that he cannot test outer reality. But even if the secondary thought process is in command, we know that it is accompanied by more primitive forms of mental functioning.

In this communication, we shall attempt to develop the concept of acting out as experimental recollection, of play action as the slow replacement of impulsive and inappropriate action by a more advanced form of thinking, of play acting as an initial identification with a fantasied object in order to master the future experimentally, and of fantasy as a higher form of play action in which the need for action is given up. Whatever the patient produces, acts out, plays out, or talks out, is to be understood within the framework of psychotherapy as the communication of the unconscious conflict that has driven the patient to seek the help of the psychotherapist. Since acting out is an attempt to resolve an unconscious conflict of the past, it is neither appropriate in terms of current reality testing nor adequate in the forming and maintaining of present object relationships. In structural terms, one may say that it expresses the dominance of id over ego, while secondary thought process constitutes the dominance of ego over id. In terms of the capacity for object cathexis, acting out is a manifestation of a more narcissistic personality organization, while secondary process thinking usually implies the capacity for more normal object relationships.[1]

The precursors of acting out in the genesis of the psychic apparatus are found in the preverbal period of the child's development (Greenacre, 1952b; Carroll, 1954). Greenacre (1952) suggests that a child who learns language from parents whom he basically cannot trust will not rely on speech as a means of orienting himself to reality and is apt to regress in later life to preverbal forms of communication, that is, to acting out, in order to find a better means of reality adaptation. Acting out, it can be said, originates in the impulsive act of the infant, his only means to obtain gratification, to "call" the helper. Later acting out contains a variety of elements. In common with the impulsive act, the first way of the baby to meet his needs, it contains the quality of impul-

[1]These comments on the hierarchy of different forms of thinking, of different aspects of the psychic apparatus, have their usefulness if understood within the framework of psychotherapy. The concept of acting out is used in a different framework if it is applied simply in order to describe asocial behavior. Even from a social point of view, however, acting out may consist of socially laudable action. We use the concept here in order to describe and explain certain behavior which is to be understood as repetition of an unconscious conflict, as the patient's only available way to communicate this conflict. The repetition of the conflict is possible only under the condition of the distance device of acting out. The function of distance as a psychological concept and its role in the psychotherapeutic communication has been discussed in preliminary form in earlier papers by Ekstein and Wright (1952) and Ekstein (1956).

sivity and the lack of sufficient capacity for reality testing. In this latter sense it can be considered as inappropriate action. Together with play, it contains certain elements of thought and action which attempt to bring about recollection. And since it is usually fairly well rationalized, it also contains elements of advanced thought, an attempt at integration with those elements in the personality which are capable of reality testing. The impulse and the frustrating environment thus may be thought of as the "parents" of acting out.

In classical adult analysis, acting out has always been considered a major form of resistance (Fenichel, 1945), as a substitute for remembering and for the free-associative process. Attempts are usually made to stop it through interpretation and occasionally through taboos if the acting out seems to make the psychotherapeutic process impossible. For certain adults whose character structure included excessive acting out before the beginning of analysis, it has been suggested that analysis might not be the preferred method of treatment (Spiegel, 1954) but that such patients may require serious modifications of the classical technique.

The free-associative process has been replaced, particularly in younger children, largely by communication via the play (A. Freud, 1946). Thus recognition has been given that the less mature ego organization of the child is not capable of using the free-associative process as expressed in the requirement of the basic rule and must make use of other forms of communication. The play of the child has been likened to the dream of the adult, and the opportunity for play action bears many similarities to and differences from the opportunity for free association in relation to different dream elements.

Just as the adult neurotic is unable to associate freely for considerable stretches during the analytic process, we soon find that the child is unable to play freely and that play interruptions (Erikson, 1940) take place which are indicative of increased resistance, increased defense against overwhelming anxiety and inner instinctual demands.

In order to go beyond the mere descriptive aspects of acting out, we conceive of different states of acting out, seen here as a complex phenomenon which may partake of elements of different components in the hierarchy of the thought organization. We owe to Dr. Helen Sargent (personal communication) an attempt to schematize the concept of acting out in relation to developmental stages of impulse expression, mastery, and utilization in problem solving (see Table 1).

The vertical axis of the schema represents the theoretical normal evolution of impulse control from immediate action through stages of delay, internalization, substitution, modulation, and eventual balanced adaptive direction and mastery.

The horizontal axis defines states of impulse expression within the context of mastery mode, thought development and reality testing, and characteristic level of ego organization.

This schema may have generic value in determining the specific stage of acting out in the dynamic interplay during psychotherapy and certainly proves a valuable aid in following our patient during the recovery process.

Our clinical observations are concerned with a type of play interruption in which the play, rather then being replaced by silence or by the change of topics, tends to erupt into acting out. Play action may become so stimulating, so powerful, that it threatens to lead to genuine acting out and impulsive action. The unconscious conflict, then, is not reenacted via the play but tends to be reenacted in actuality. One may liken such a child to an actor who plays a dramatic part on the stage only to find himself being driven to living out

TABLE I

CONCERNING THE CONCEPT OF "ACTING OUT" IN RELATION TO STAGES OF IMPULSE MASTERY AND EGO DEVELOPMENT

Levels of Communication	Impulse Expression	Mode of Mastery	Thought Development	Reality Testing	Ego Organization
	ACTION	Immediate gratification	Hallucinated object	None	Symbiotic
Regressive "call for help or control"	PLAY ACTION	Rudimentary replacement of impulse by thought	Trial thought; primary-process dominated	Play solution as reality test	Struggle against symbiosis
Experimental recollection: past directed; inappropriate to reality	FANTASY	Gratifying object internalized	Thought substituted for action: primary and secondary	Temporary decathexis of real object	Autism and/or temporary internal gratification
Elements of thought and reality testing; future directed	ACTION FANTASY (PLAY ACTING)	Preconscious trial solution	Rudimentary secondary-process domination	First attempt to master *future* by role taking	Beginning of autonomy; identification by imitation
	DELAY AND ADAPTIVE DIRECTION	Resolution in thought and adaptive action	Secondary process established	Object relationship and reality testing established	Ego identity; mature ego

COMPONENTS OF ACTING OUT

this part in actuality. Such a turn of events indeed creates special technical problems for the psychotherapist since communication via action more than any other form of communication tends to destroy the psychotherapeutic situation. In the clinical case from which we derived our material, however, we encountered the problem of treating an adolescent boy with strong tendencies to act out his conflict and for whom the capacity for verbal communication and free association in a psychotherapeutic setting was so limited as to be almost unavailable to him as a means of therapeutic communication. Since acting out and play action dominated his language development, it seemed necessary to permit his use of this language in the therapeutic situation until his development enabled him to turn to verbal language and made possible his use of the more conventional form of psychotherapy of an adolescent.

THE PATIENT'S BACKGROUND

Frank was brought to Southard School by his parents when he was 13 years old, as an alternative to detention in the Juvenile Hall of a large Eastern city after he had been caught by the police following an act of petty thievery. On their way home after committing the crime, he and two other boys of his gang had been discovered carrying dangerous weapons. One boy had concealed a switchblade knife on his person, while Frank had a piece of lead pipe. For Frank, admission to the residential treatment center was a welcome event that climaxed a succession of delinquent acts of petty thievery, truancy, and running away from home, and was, he hoped, a final refuge from an unbearable home situation and the last resort to save him from what seemed to him his inevitable fate of ending his life by "frying in the hot seat."

Unwanted by both parents from the time of his conception, Frank started life as he fantasied it would end—in an atmosphere of violence, treachery, hatred, faithlessness, and futility. His father, an irresponsible playboy barely out of his adolescence, had impregnated his mistress while Frank's mother was pregnant with Frank. Frank's father acknowledged the affair but refused to accept responsibility for both the illicit pregnancy and its outcome. The same irresponsibility, aloofness, and rejection characterized the father's attitude toward his son and his marriage, which from its very inception had also been unstable and turbulent. The father's infidelity was but another incident that poured fuel on an already seething marital discord and added to the mother's fury and desire for revenge. A bewildered, confused girl of 17 when she had married, Frank's mother found her abrupt plunge into motherhood an impossible task to carry alone. Already burdened with one child, a daughter born one year before Frank, she had immediately become pregnant again only to seek refuge in a threatened miscarriage and in a variety of illnesses throughout her pregnancy. Immature and deeply troubled, she had married mainly to assert her independence and to express her defiance of her own father, who characterized her marriage as an act of a "screwball" motivated "only by a biological urge."

Into this marital setting of increasing strife and neglect Frank was born five weeks premature, a cyanotic baby unable to breathe spontaneously, sucking and feeding only with the greatest difficulty. An object of pity to his mother and the target of his father's scorn, contempt, and hatred as a weakling, Frank was described by the mother as a baby who refused cuddling and developed slowly. Anxiety, experienced as being caused by his poor state of nutrition, led his mother to force-feed Frank until by the end of his first year he had become overweight and fat.

By the second year he demonstrated his greater need for eating than for cuddling by developing an almost insatiable appetite and an immense craving for sweets. On the advice of a pediatrician, his mother began to deprive him of food, with the result that Frank began to raid the refrigerator and cupboards at night devouring everything edible that he could find. Food, having once been the only supply that his mother had given him freely, now had to be taken forcibly and by stealth.

Goaded by his mother's withholding of and his intractable hunger for food, he turned to garbage cans for nourishment, and at the age of two poisoned himself by ingesting rat poison in a neighbor's chicken house, necessitating emergency treatment in a hospital. By the age of four his scavenger activities led him to his mother's purse in search of money, an action which, interpreted by his parents as stealing, resulted in brutal spankings and more deprivation of food by his father. Frank, in retaliation, turned to the neighborhood groceries for food so that by four and thereafter his practice of stealing food, candy, and soft drinks had become a well-established repetitive pattern.

The combination of his apparent general retardation, clumsy motor development, stealing, ravenous greed for sweets, and his indifference to reward or punishment further strained his relationship with his parents to such a point that Frank was regarded by his mother as emotionally inaccessible and unreachable. Attempts at imposing discipline and toilet training were futile and Frank remained enuretic until he was eight, even continuing to wet and soil occasionally when he was 13. Thumb sucking, which enraged his parents and could not be stopped by restraints, beatings, scoldings, or food withdrawal, also persisted on occasion until the age of 13, when it was replaced by biting and gnawing of his nails and knuckles.

Throughout his first eight years, the continuity of his physical contact with his mother was broken by repeated moves, living with grandparents, and the abortive efforts of a succession of maids to care for him and his sister while his mother sought to achieve a professional career. Regarding his desperate loneliness and the bleak and dreary emptiness of his early childhood that he could not emotionally communicate, Frank remembered an incident in which he saw himself sitting alone, waiting for what seemed like hours for his parents, until in a panic he went in search of them at the home of a friend. Relieved to discover them, he ran to them only to be scolded and rebuffed and ordered to go home. Another memory of his loneliness, as he described his mother's habitual absence from home, involved a Sunday outing in the park with a neighbor's family that left him with a deep yearning for his mother but with only a sense of hopeless futility and resigned indifference about his capacity ever to win her love.

Frank's early emotional reactions of silent withdrawal, inaccessibility, or sulking changed to overt temper tantrums, rages, and aggressive outbursts against his mother and favored sister following the parents' divorce when Frank was five. Relieved to find that his father would no longer be able to terrorize him, Frank was at the same time confused, puzzled, and disappointed by the meaning of his father's desertion, which he remembered only as a casual announcement by his father that he would be leaving for another city and would probably never see the children again. But what he failed to express verbally and affectively of his deeper feelings regarding his father's abandonment of him, he enacted in his intensified stealing activities and further estrangement from his mother and hated rivalrous sister.

His mother's remarriage when he was nine rekindled the dwindling hope for a loving father. A brief attempt to court the stepfather soon ended in disappointment, pseudo indifference, and resignation, as well as intensified stealing and running away as Frank found his stepfather wanting in the qualities and characteristics that he fantasied of the ideal father; nor could he tolerate the stepfather's flourishing relationship with his sister. In quiet desperation, Frank expanded the area of his thievery from food to clothes and finally to any object that was not attached or assiduously guarded and accounted for. He became a problem child in school and was repeatedly threatened with expulsion. Falling below his superior intellectual capacity in his failing school performance, he also provoked and taunted the teachers and principal with his boisterous swearing, obscene tricks and jokes, and unruly and defiant behavior. When finally he began to rifle the purses belonging to his female classmates in reaction to his sister's entrance into the same school, the school authorities demanded that his parents take some drastic action about him.

Attempts by the parents to foster his interest in YMCA and church activities, and to supervise and encourage his association with children of their professional friends led only to his furthering his contacts with other delinquent boys, one of whom was soon detained in the Juvenile Hall for robbery with a gun. Unable to cope with the rising tide of his delinquent behavior, his parents finally acceded to the community pressure by requesting psychiatric help, first in a child guidance clinic, which was soon relinquished as allegedly ineffective, and finally with a psychotherapist who was both a social friend and professional colleague of the parents. Although he was helpful in a limited capacity for a year and a half, the therapist's relationship with Frank was soon interrupted when Frank's detention in the Juvenile Hall placed the final disrupting touch upon his treatment and in effect made it impossible for Frank to remain at home.

Frank's view of the Juvenile Hall, as a haven of safety for him until he could reach 21 and forever escape from the hated and intolerable life at home, was conveyed both to the examining psychiatrist during his evaluation at Southard School and to the psychotherapist in his first therapy sessions. He described the state of affairs at home in the following way:

> I am angered by my mother and sister. They fuss at me all the time. Both stick up for each other and nobody sticks up for me. I feel alone against them. I have a temperamental temper and almost always I have mean thoughts about my mother. My folks say I shouldn't swear but I'll be damned if I care. Maybe I steal to be a big shot or just to oppose them. I do almost anything I can think of just to oppose them. I steal, get on the loose after curfew, stay out all night. I used to steal things right and left. I just went ahead and did it without thinking. I got so I wasn't careful. I got caught. I wanted to get to Juvenile Hall. I thought they would keep me out of trouble and that would also give me a chance to get away from home.

Despite his glib manner, the gravity and desperation of his situation did not escape him as he acknowledged that things had gotten to such an "extreme urge and necessity that a very radical step had to be made" so that he was finally brought to Southard School. But on reflection he thought he was "going to like the place" and that he was "going to latch onto it." Frank lived up to this prediction and stayed at Southard School for five and a half years, undergoing psychotherapy three times a week over a period of five years.

Frank could not have had a more perfect alibi for the police who caught him stealing and the judge who ordered his detention than his lifelong traumatic background with its history of alleged chronic parental neglect, deprivation, cruelty, and desertion. For the staff of the residential center as well, his dismal, miserable life at home, devoid of parental love and care, could readily be accepted as the whole explanation of his difficulty. Overidentification with this miserable and appealing boy by those responsible for his care and treatment, as well as the tendency to overlook his loss of capacity to use a home and intimate, stable contacts, could well justify a program which would visualize his treatment only as providing a new and more loving home environment geared to meet his emotional needs. The importance of understanding and treating his intrapsychic conflicts by intensive psychotherapy could, under these circumstances, be quite readily considered unnecessary.

The living power of Frank's plight to depict his victimization by his parents and family circumstances as an "alibi" for his delinquent behavior immediately became evident from the character of his initial relationships with the staff personnel. Failure to receive letters from home or the arrival of a brief cold note from his mother evoked the deepest sympathy from the staff and tended to arouse their furious indignation over the injustice of his neglect and desertion by his family.

In interviews with his social worker, he would freely discuss his disturbed behavior at the school, his stealing from local stores and in the residence, his abortive runaways from the school, and his exhibitionistic pranks and swearing in the classroom. Then he would break into tears or sink into depressive apathy as he would silently make a plea for understanding and acceptance. After destroying his own possessions and clothing as horrible reminders of his past, or impulsively squandering his allowance on one spending spree, he would recall to the staff his "inadequate background" and excite their sympathy with his unfortunate fate and desperate situation.

Increasing awareness by the staff personnel that almost his

sole source of contact with his family lay in the maternal
grandfather's financial support of his treatment at Southard
School stimulated them to try to reach him and make themselves more available to him for closer relationships. In his
hunger for such relationships, Frank repeatedly reached out
to every available adult, and the initial impression he made
was that of a child who, "given a chance" and given love and
adequate fulfillment of his basic needs, could blossom into
emotional health.

It soon became evident, however, that despite his hunger
for close relationships and despite the immediate availability
of the setting to him, Frank could not avail himself of people.
His relationships would immediately break down shortly
after his initial contact with adult parental figures. He was
unable to relate himself to other children as well, but would
form a close, parasitic type of relationship usually with a
younger boy whom he could exploit and who readily lent
himself to Frank's exploitation (possibly a reversal of his expectation as to what would happen were he to turn to an
older person). His emotional withdrawal became increasingly
evident as he would sit in what seemed like a depressive
stupor at times, his head on his chest, or his slumped body
crying out the despair, hatred, and loneliness within him,
refusing to participate in any activity or respond to any ministrations from the staff. At these times his impoverished
relationships and apparent vacuous emotional life gave the
first overt glimpses of the depth of his illness and of the
difficulty in reaching and helping him which had been revealed in the psychological tests and psychiatric examination
during his evaluation.

The examining psychiatrist was impressed with Frank's
rapid shift of moods from initial apparent apathy and depression to lively animation as the examination proceeded. He
seemed like a boy who, having left a "prison," was now dis-

covering that he could breathe more freely in a hoped-for, newfound freedom. Southard School was seen by Frank as at least an improved version of the Juvenile Hall, of the "Big House." But there were many signs that this freedom, too, would soon become threatening and disappointing to Frank.

Sometimes under pressure of speech, he glibly rationalized his stealing, his defecation in his pants, and a host of antisocial acts, seriously expounding with pseudo insight upon his many problems. He freely acknowledged that his delinquent behavior, so troublesome to his parents, was intended as revenge against them. With quasi insight he discussed his detention in the Juvenile Hall as a means of demonstrating what a "big shot" he was.

His self-concept was unusually self-deprecatory and he described every aspect of himself in derogatory terms:

> I'm too fat; I've got big feet. The only brains I have are those I eat. Oh yes, if you'd crack my head open and you'd fry what you got out of it you'd have scrambled eggs. My ears are always dirty and my teeth are no good. They're crooked, chipped, and yellow. Not scared, they're not scared, just yellow. My hands are no good either. I bite my fingernails too. My chest isn't any good either. It mixes in with my stomach and my stomach's too fat.

He perceived his mother's contribution to his self-concept as follows: "She would like to get rid of me but doesn't want me out of her sight. She says I cause her to fuss. She says I shirk my work. I don't like her and she likes me even less. It all started when my father went away." His view of his previous treatment was blandly stated with finality: "It was a waste of money. The therapist was a family friend. I was awfully sorry to put my stepfather to so much expense. It did give me a chance to be away from home though."

Regarding his hopes for help at Southard School and for the immediate future, Frank expressed a rather dim view: "I don't know if it will do any good or be a waste of time. I hope it will do good. It won't stop me from doing things." But what he alone felt would help was: "One person, me, myself, and I. I'd like to stop. Heck, who wouldn't. I don't want to end up in jail. Most you could do though is to find out why I act the way I do."

On the psychological tests Frank showed almost superior intelligence, but with only a limited capacity for affective response. Strong aggressive impulses could be expressed only in fantasy or in acts which had the purpose of reassuring himself about his own ability and of inflicting punishment upon and exacting revenge from the parent figures. Severe anxiety stemming from deeper conflicts and the fear of retaliation appeared to impair his intellectual efficiency. The Rorschach reflected his critical evaluation of situations, his lack of trust in others, and his preoccupation with missing parts of bodies, crawling creatures, and crouching animals. Prominently seen in the Thematic Apperception Test was his callous disregard for the feelings of others and his secret pleasure over his success in defying parental figures. The diagnostic impression of the evaluating team was that of a behavior disorder with neurotic features.

THE BEGINNING OF PSYCHOTHERAPY: THE GANGSTER GAME

Frank's efforts to communicate with the therapist mainly by verbal means in the initial interviews failed to establish a productive psychotherapeutic atmosphere. Silences associated with strong inhibition, blocking, and distant withdrawal frequently interrupted Frank's tenuous contacts with the therapist, and his verbal productions appeared against the background of an emotional vacuum. To create an optimal therapeutic atmosphere, Frank was given the opportunity to communicate via play action those inner struggles that he otherwise could not relate.

The therapeutic setting then became a scene of play action, a conspiratorial meeting between the patient who became "Jocko the Monk, the Big Boss" and the therapist, the "Doc" who, having served 10 years in prison for practicing medicine illicitly, had joined the Big Boss as a gangster lieutenant or as a doctor and who could provide either a gangster or medical type of service depending on the wishes of the Big Boss. The gang met regularly to discuss the plans to pull the "Big Heist" which, starting out with Frank's fantasy of holding up an armored car and then a bank, extended into a gigantic criminal operation which aimed to overthrow the rule of the current administration and to seize power and land, with final control of large cities and states. The following is a sample interview as the patient was taking hold of the play technique and was in the process of discussing the gang's plan to move into a new area and to seize control of it to further the plans for the Big Heist:

Frank came to the interview with the news that there had been a slight hitch in the plan. He excitedly reported that even though we got most of the bulls, some of them had gotten away. He explained that some stoolies must have been at work and that the plan had been sabotaged. On second thought, maybe the real reason that our plan had not worked completely was that we had not thought of something very important rather than because of a stoolie. We had forgotten that there was a day shift of bulls and that these bulls were not in the formation at the police academy when we had bombed it. There must have been at least a hundred bulls out. He had already thought of a plan to get rid of them, but believed that it would be better to wait because the remaining bulls would be on the watch for another attack and we wouldn't be able to pull this plan so easily.

I mused that since we had delivered a knockout punch they would be dazed and in shock.* Maybe we could follow up with another attack before they could reorganize and get reinforcements. He agreed it would be a good idea and immediately had a plan to get rid of the other bulls. We would have to get more planes, bomb each precinct police station, and strafe the whole area around it with machine guns. Satisfied with his plan, he gave me the order to call the airport and to have 16 planes ready within two hours. I went through the play motion of following his orders and complimented him on his ingenuity. I told him that when he pulled this heist we would from then on have no more bulls to oppose us. We would own the city and run it.

Frank picked up the fantasy with a rather satisfied grin and began to talk about owning the city of New York and how he could exploit it and capitalize on it. Once we had taken over the city the bulls would have to kowtow to us. We would be the police force. Nobody could leave the city except by paying $1,000 ransom. I wondered why the boss was acting like a piker, making them pay only $1,000 when we could bleed them dry as long as they were at our mercy. Frank instantly agreed and said that their fine would be $50,000. They would have to pay in order to get out.

As the discussion about the plan to complete the Big Heist continued, Frank began to show signs of anxiety and wondered about the possible opposition to the plan. He was afraid that the U.S. Government might oppose our plan, that they might send in detectives who would be even harder to spot than the bulls who wore uniforms. I assured him that no matter what opposition he had from anyone else, he had my full support.

Anxiously, Frank wondered if the plan could succeed, and

*Editor's note: The therapist in these interviews is not identified.

then after considerable thought suddenly broke out with a beaming expression on his face as if inspired by a wonderful idea: "You remember the deal where the Indians sold the deed of Manhattan Island for $24? That deed is still kept on exhibit in a museum." He had thought that if we could steal the deed to the city we would have legal and lawful possession of the city. On the other hand we wouldn't even have to steal it but could leave $24 for the deed and this would give us possession of the city legally without any fuss or trouble. I complimented him on the ingenuity of his plan but wondered whether the bulls would see eye to eye with us and whether they might not oppose this. He said, in a grand manner, that we could leave them a Century note and this would be more than enough to pay for the deed which was worth only $24 in the first place. I protested that we needn't give the bulls any more than we had to. If the deed were worth $24 originally, then maybe that was all it was worth now. It didn't seem to have gotten any more valuable since it was originally signed.

As we continued to discuss our plans to pull this Big Heist, Frank thought of the final step of rounding up the remaining bulls and putting them in jail. I wondered again whether this was not dangerous, that maybe it would be better to rub them out since there was always the possibility of their breaking out. He said that wiping them out quickly would be too good for them. This was too peaceful a means to get rid of them. I thought that maybe the Boss had a good point and that his revenge was important. He suggested that he could keep them in jail and guard them heavily, but starve them slowly and weaken them so that they could never break out. He again became anxious and thought it would be better to knock them off quickly. He didn't have such cruel feelings toward them that he wanted to torture them. I said that the Boss took pity on the bulls and was pretty nice to them even after they had let him go hungry for so long, but whatever he wanted to do with them, it was alright with me. We ended the hour as Frank took out a package of Life Savers and we toasted the new heist with them.

In the following hour, Frank's enthusiasm for the Big Heist continued to be tempered by his marked anxiety that led him to question the wisdom of every step that we were about to take and led him to introduce a variety of obstacles that he expected would result in the failure of the heist. He ordered the therapist to call the weather bureau and then announced that weather conditions would make flying impossible. The heist would have to wait. As the therapist confronted him with his fear of his wish to eliminate all the bulls, he coped with his mounting anxiety only by a pseudo bravado and a feigned enthusiasm for the heist, and then actually missed the following hour.

With his anxiety reduced because of the missed hour Frank could announce in the subsequent hour that the heist had gone off well. We were in possession of the big city and everything seemed to be going as arranged. He thought, however, it would now be necessary for the gang to wall itself in and just stay put until the heat was off. He fantasied that the F.B.I. might bring in its entire force and the gang would be in the desperate position of having to defend its new gains. Maybe it would be better to avoid an outright battle with them by collecting huge taxes from the businessmen so that after accumulating $1,000,000 the Boss could pay for the city by selling the deed back to the government and thus make everything legal and straight. If necessary, he would re-nounce his citizenship and secede from the United States. The F.B.I. would then not have any right to make war on the Boss since he was no longer part of the union.

The therapist questioned whether the F.B.I. would accept these terms and the Boss insisted they would have to or face

another more terrible atomic war. When the therapist wondered aloud whether the F.B.I. would accept this deal, Frank
turned to another solution. This solution entailed the cessation of all gang activities and the return of the city as well
as of the deed to the United States if the government would
only return the original $24. This $24 he would not even
keep but would give to charity. In the meantime all members
of the gang would have to become respectable and honest
citizens. When the therapist asked if this were not a plan to
buy the F.B.I. off, the Boss protested that he didn't like to
think of it as a bribe but just as a smart deal. The alternative
to the deal was to risk an atomic war with destruction for
everyone. The therapist assured him that his loyalty was first
to the Boss, but he had to think of the gang too. He was
beginning to wonder whether the gang would go along with
this plan of becoming respectable citizens. It might sound
crazy to them and make them wonder whether the Boss had
not gotten sick. As far as the therapist was concerned, if the
Boss decided to change his plans he might need more help
and the therapist was ready to stay by him either as a Doc
or as his henchman.

Relieved of the pressure aroused by the fantasy of destruction and of dreaded retaliation, Frank turned to a verbal
account of his trip to his grandfather and told of a pleasant
visit with his uncle. He confessed that while on this visit he
was tempted to heist something from him, but decided
against it because his uncle was such a nice guy.

These samples from the initial phase of psychotherapy may
be considered a prelude of things to come, and permit us to
observe *in statu nascendi* the major defense operations used
to cope with the unconscious conflict and the ensuing anxiety.
In the patient's struggle to reveal the unconscious conflict to
the therapist and to himself, as well as to keep the unconscious
conflict repressed, he utilizes a variety of means which offer

a model of operations that permits predictions of the process to follow.

As he starts to talk about himself, anxiety increases and stops ordinary means of communication through thought. Thought may lead to recollection and threatening imagery which have to be warded off under all circumstances in order to cope successfully with anxiety. Increasing anxiety leads then either to silence or, as we have seen in these samples, to the imminence of acting out. Talking out is replaced by playing out, which threatens to erupt into acting out. Playing out and acting out keep the unconscious conflict repressed, but at the same time permit the patient to reveal the unconscious conflict on a more regressed level of mental functioning.

The psychotherapist recognized the conflict by noticing the pattern of the play fantasy, the play act, and the emerging acting out in the psychotherapeutic situation. As the therapist understands the patient, and confronts him with his inability to destroy the policemen even in fantasy, at the same time letting him know that he accepts his material, the patient feels understood although he cannot understand himself in terms of thought. His displaced negative transference, directed against the "bulls," is unconsciously compared by the boy with the actual therapeutic situation in which he finds himself working on his problems accompanied by a friendly, understanding, and accepting psychotherapist. He leaves the playing out and returns to talking out, discovering now that he does not want to steal from a kind and friendly uncle. The interpretations by the therapist have to be understood against the background of the patient's inability to give up displacement at this point. Therefore, the therapist must avoid interpreting the displacement, but may freely interpret as long as this safeguard against anxiety on the part of the patient is respected.

These initial moves permit anticipation of future trends in the therapeutic process. One may assume that the beginning months of psychotherapy will show an overwhelming use of action and play, a lesser use of pure fantasy, and a very moderate use of secondary process thought. The interpretive work will help the patient to resolve his conflict in the manner that has been discussed in the model. As the months go on, however, one may be certain that the amount of play action will decrease and will be taken over more and more by verbal communication typical for the chronological age of the patient. Concomitantly, we may also expect to observe a regressive process manifested by actual or imminent acting out.

While play action in the therapy proceeded as has been described in the first interview sample, we learned about an experience Frank had not reported to his psychotherapist that reflected an aspect of the transference situation and culminated in genuine acting out. He had visited his grandfather during a holiday and found him unusually loving and giving. Under the influence of alcohol his grandfather made numerous erotic advances toward Frank, heaped kisses on him, and made frequent promises of gifts and eternal support and affection. Shortly following this incident, Frank stole a knife from the dime store. Characteristically, he arranged that the theft be discovered as he freely exhibited the knife to the personnel in the residence and hinted that he had stolen it. How this acting out became a direct part of the psychotherapeutic process is illustrated in the following interview:

Frank followed me into the office with a slight sneer in his voice as he began to complain contemptuously about the way things were run at Southard School. He thought that the kids ought to get together to write a constitution to guarantee that "No R.T. could enter a person's room without a search warrant." He went on to complain that the police could break in any time and there was no privacy or protection against them. Then quite abruptly he remarked that being the Boss of a gang was getting a little bit wearing on him.

He had decided to plan no organized heists any more but to let the members of the gang go on their own free heist. The therapist retorted, "Well, Boss, if the job is getting too big for you then maybe we ought to turn it over to someone else. It looks like the Boss hasn't been doing such a good job of being a Boss lately anyway." Frank's face expressed a faint trace of relief as he asked how I had come to that notion. I reached into my pocket, pulled out the knife that he had stolen from the dime store, and said, "This shiv, for instance, Boss, this stinking, worthless little shiv. When you pulled that heist didn't you know you were putting the gang's neck in a noose? The bulls could have come down on our tail and then what would have happened to the big heist that we've been working on for so long?" Frank immediately took the knife, opened the blade, and kissed it, appearing surprised that I had it. He placed the knife in his belt and said he was certainly glad to see it back. Then he grinned broadly and said that no man should be without his weapon. This was really a wonderful weapon. I retorted, "A wonderful weapon! That little tin shiv? A worthless piece of junk! What protection can the shiv give you compared to the kind you can get from the really big weapon, Boss, the secret weapon we're working on here?" Frank became anxious, removed the knife from his belt, and began to reflect. He fingered the blade and said nothing. I continued, "The Big Heist is too important to both of us, Boss. We've got to protect it even if we've got to make sacrifices for little things. Compared to the Big Heist everything else is just small potatoes and we're not going to let anything like a tin shiv stop us from pulling it right."

Showing annoyance, I asked him what had been the price of the knife and Frank meekly answered that it was worth 89 cents. I said, "Okay," and pulling a dollar out of my pocket added, "we've got to undo that little heist and keep the bulls off our tail and from interfering with our big plans. You want the shiv, you can keep it, but here's the dough, and you're going to take it back to the man." Frank said he was beginning to see what I meant. Maybe the thing to do was take back the knife. He didn't want the money and he didn't need the knife. It was just a lousy little weapon that was no protection compared to the protection that the big secret weapon could give him. He would put the knife back and that would square the account.

He leaned back and with a trace of emotion in his voice as well as with some conviction said that he realized what I meant and could see what I was driving at. I had hit the nail on the head. The shiv was worthless, but the Big Heist was the most important thing. We had to protect it at all cost. He sat back and seemed tense as he held the knife in his hand. He looked at it fondly and said that it was a nice shiv though. For the next 20 minutes Frank debated about what to do with the knife. At one time he was sure it was a good weapon and a good shiv and at another time it was just a worthless piece of junk that ought to go back to the store. Finally, with determination, he agreed that this was the only thing to do and wondered how it should be done. He thought he could do it alone, and I told him that this was something between us and maybe we ought to pull it together. He suggested that maybe we could take it back tomorrow. I said, "Today, Boss, two o'clock." He agreed this would be okay.

A few moments later Frank expressed his concern about the future of the gang. Even if he should be caught by the cops, we would have to keep the gang together and the plans for the Big Heist alive. I told him that no matter what happened, the gang would always be behind the Boss but that he should remember that if we pulled our Big Heist together in our own stronghold then no cops in the world could ever get to us. Frank nodded his head in agreement and reflected that after the Big Heist was pulled we would have complete and real freedom. I said that he had come upon a very wise thought. It sounded like the Big Boss talking now. Frank said, "Who wants to be dodging bullets coming down your ass?" I retorted, "Yeah, Boss, it's a strange kind of freedom that makes you have to run all the time to dodge bullets. It's a kind of freedom that makes a guy sometimes even prefer to go to jail to escape those bullets. Maybe the Heist can bring real freedom for the Boss, so that he never has to be afraid that he'll always have to dodge bullets or wind up in the hot seat."

At two o'clock as we had arranged, I accompanied Frank downtown and we went into the dime store where he surreptitiously replaced the knife on the counter and I stood guard. As we walked out together he remarked that our mission was accomplished. We had walked through heavy snow and Frank complained of having wet feet and feeling cold. We stopped at a soda fountain in the store and had hot chocolate together. When I left him at the school Frank thanked me for having come along with him on the mission.

The friendly image of the good uncle, which had permitted him to curb the impulse to steal from the uncle, is here fused with the overwhelming, noxious image of the threatening grandfather. Both images are the expression of the strong ambivalence in a transference situation. As he runs away from the threatening transference situation and as anxiety mounts, Frank cannot maintain play action but saves himself by delinquent acting out. As he is attracted by the friendliness, acceptance, and understanding of the therapist, implicit in the therapist's way of dealing with the gangster game,

Frank wishes to give up stealing and to undo the acting out. Diminished anxiety in the psychotherapeutic situation permits him to move from playing out a problem to talking it out and to resolving it in a reality-oriented manner. Increased anxiety, however, reduces the effectiveness of the ego organization, forces regression to a lower level of communication, and leads to acting out. The increase of instinctual pressure that may be caused by inner or outer stimulation in seduction is the decisive factor that leads to increase in anxiety and to a use of less mature ego organizations which thus may be considered as an SOS signal, a flight reaction during the therapeutic process.

THE FUSION OF PLAY AND ACTING OUT

The clinical material also demonstrates how increased anxiety is intimately and with predictable sequence related to regression and to the tendency to act out. In Frank, however, we observed a peculiar modification of this familiar sequential relationship, in contrast to what can be expected in the ordinary situation. In normal or neurotic individuals, increased anxiety often leads to more rational, though more restricted, seemingly more highly adaptive behavior, while in Frank, the reverse was true. One possible explanation for this phenomenon is that in the hierarchical organization of the ego, recent, more appropriate, and more highly adaptive functions can operate simultaneously with more primitive, outmoded functions because they are cathected by energy, which itself is differentiated into hierarchical systems. These systems are differentiated by virtue of the quantity of neutralized or deneutralized energy available for their cathexis, or upon any combination of these energies lying at any point intermediate to the opposite polarities. A more mature ego organization under the dominance of neutralized energy cathexis is less prone to resort to acting out as a method of problem solving than is the more primitive organization which is cathected mainly by deneutralized energy, i.e., by sexualized and aggressivized energy.

Apparently, it is the extent of the deneutralized and neutralized energy cathexes which determine what portions and levels of the ego organization will come into play. Under pathological conditions of personality development, certain aspects of the ego organization fail to become consolidated at an optimal specific time. Under similar conditions, there is a failure of development of the neutralized cathexis. But as soon as the energy cathexis is neutralized, then the lower levels of functioning fall under the aegis of the adaptive functions rather than remaining a part of the expression of the neurosis.

As Frank's anxiety about continuing the Big Heist diminished, and as he could permit himself to take hold of the therapeutic situation, now seen as less threatening despite his perception of it as an apparent encouragement to him to act upon his murderous fantasies, he began to plan the Big Heist with the aim of acquiring the proper weapons and tools for its execution. It soon became apparent to the Big Boss that in order for the gang to carry out the Big Heist it would be necessary to have guns and blackjacks. How the fulfillment of this aim was carried into the therapeutic situation by the medium of play action and acting out to the point where these two means of expression became fused in the therapeutic process is demonstrated in the following excerpts from sample interviews:

On the way to the office Frank told me where he could get a real rod, one that shot real bullets. I asked him where. He said that the head man in his outfit had swiped it from him and had kept it in his hideout. He thought he could heist it from the head man by getting the moll (Frank's social worker) into the operation. He thought she could be trusted by this time. I didn't think it was a very good idea to let anybody else in on our heist because it could get around too far and the bulls would be down on us. He insisted that we see the moll anyway and proceeded to get an appointment with his social worker through the receptionist. As the hour ended he assured me that the moll was alright. She had been in the racket a long time and he was sure she was on our side and could be trusted. I told him I would leave it up to his judgment and go along with him since he was still the Boss. (The therapist's questioning of the soundness of his being the Boss seemed to be clearly understood by Frank as a question regarding his capacity for reality testing and was not construed by him as adverse or belittling criticism.)

On the afternoon of the preceding interview, Frank met me as I was about to leave the school and told me he had arranged with the moll to case the head man's hideout. He had discovered where the blackjack had been stashed away. I fell in with his plan to pull the heist there and then, and we entered the Director's office. Frank immediately went to the closet where his BB pistol had been put for safekeeping, and we also discovered a homemade blackjack that Frank had once carried around with him. Together we stealthily reached my office across the street where I suggested that we keep the weapons in our own arsenal.

This phase of psychotherapy shows a significant change as a consequence of the therapeutic technique employed. In the earlier phase the child could handle the increasing pressure when stimulated by play action only by play interruption on the one hand, or by delinquent acting out on the other. He could see the psychotherapist only in terms of the good and friendly uncle or of the drunk and seductive grandfather. As the psychotherapist permitted the child to express himself through play action and fantasy by entering the child's world and becoming part of it, by creating a bearable situation in allowing a transference situation to develop in which initial projection of narcissistic problems was possible, the child could combine play action with a modified form of acting out within the psychotherapeutic process. The stealing of the gun from the Director's office, taking place as it were within the psychotherapeutic process, within the limits set by the psychotherapist, is remindful of the stealing of the knife but at the same time shows some of the significant aspects of play action inasmuch as it included a form of reality testing. True enough, the reality testing employed depended actually on the auxiliary ego of the psychotherapist who set and provided the limits and who let the boy know the difference between those actions that create danger and those that still can be used in order to work on a problem through trial action. He who steals from someone with intention of being discovered does not actually steal but communicates his concern about the consequences of delinquent behavior.

The child's activities are also attempts to test the psychotherapist and to test the limits newly gained. As the play action continued, Frank wished to know if the psychotherapist would be willing to go beyond the boundaries of the school, beyond the four walls of the therapy office, and whether he was really ready to follow the boy in his quest for an answer to his problem. In the samples just cited we see a fusion of play action and acting out but with a preponderance of play action.

Increasing anxiety in the therapy process suggests that new aspects of repressed material are pressing toward consciousness, and one very often has the feeling that acting out threatens to overwhelm play action. It is during these phases of psychotherapy that the skill and patience of a psychotherapist are taxed the most, and that the danger exists that the psychotherapist's interpretive language within play action and play fantasy may carry him away to a form of counter-acting out with the patient either through a form of delinquent participation or a form of oppressive forbidding, both technical mistakes mentioned by Fenichel (1945).

Clinical case material not infrequently fails to be convincing enough to clarify per se its technical framework and basic strategy. Too often it may give the impression that the choice of a technical method used is the result of an arbitrary decision by the therapist, who seemingly imposes upon the patient the atmosphere of the therapeutic process and the mode of communication to be used within it. In Frank's therapy, the inference might be made that the therapist imposed the techniques of play action and acting out upon the patient, that he preferred to plan robberies and play act the role of a gangster. The inference could be carried to the point of Moreno's (1964) conviction that since his stage is the equivalent of the therapist's analytic couch, he is within his prerogative as the therapist to choose the technique of play acting as the means of communication between himself and the patient. It is our conviction that ideally the choice of communication belongs to the patient whenever this is possible and that it is the patient who decides upon the language that he can best use to convey his thoughts and to make contact with the therapist. From the many cues that he gave the therapist and from the therapy process as it developed, Frank clearly conveyed that this was his choice of communication, a message that the therapist understood and accepted.[2]

Play action within the limited setting of a therapy office in a residential setting changed to a combination of play action and acting out in the therapeutic process as the therapeutic

[2]In some instances, however, even the therapist of this conviction must decide upon the language form of communication, as when he cannot use the mother tongue of the patient and forces him to use a second language in which the patient necessarily says and conveys much less about himself and his deepest basic problems (Greenson, 1950).

situation or the Big Heist moved into the community. In the search for weapons and suitable game for the operations of the Big Boss, Frank and the therapist began to play out the gangster activity of "casing" the pawn shops and jewelry stores in the downtown section of the city. The following material is from another therapy session:

As we reconnoitered the downtown district for suitable victims for the gang operation, our drive took us through the north side of town which aroused Frank's anxiety. Discovering that this wasn't familiar territory to the Doc because it was the territory of the North Side Gang, a rival gang of the Big Boss, Frank became fidgety and suggested that we ought to move through it quickly. Along the way to the airport, Frank practiced shooting it out with the bulls while I was instructed to practice making a quick getaway so that we could time the whole operation in case the gang would get hot and would have to take it on the lam by plane or train.

In a subsequent session, the casing operation evoked in Frank paranoid suspiciousness about women who might actually be bulls in disguise.

On the way to the heist, Frank opened the door of the car and pretended to be shooting it out with the bulls. He was sure that the bulls were cruising around in their prowl cars and although he knew it was smarter to keep the rod concealed, he thought it was smart to be on guard to be able to get the drop on the bulls. I veered to the side as a woman driver moved out of a parked position and Frank cursed at her and called her a dumb moll. He thought she might be a bull trying to head us off. There followed a determined plan to shake the moll by turning into a side street and then getting behind her so that she wouldn't be in the position of trailing us.

As we entered the jewelry store on the pretext of getting the Doc's watch repaired, Frank pointed out the wall safe.

Casually we looked it over and overheard a woman talking to the clerk about this very old safe. Frank eavesdropped on their conversation without appearing to pay attention to them and then, as we left, announced that he really wasn't interested in the joint at all. He knew of another good joint that we could case. I remarked that that dame was innocent looking enough but maybe she was working her racket too. Frank said he didn't know about that.

As we returned to the therapy office to deposit our weapons in the arsenal, I offered him some brownies that I had brought from home. He said he was hungry after the heist. He reached into the bag and took one and I ate one with him. He reached in again and I told him to help himself. He took all of them.

In a subsequent hour, we moved in on a Federal job, a postal truck carrying unregistered mail containing money. Armed with a BB pistol and a blackjack, we had played out casing a postal truck in front of the capitol building and we had agreed to pull the heist that morning. First the pawn shop would have to be heisted for the rod and this was in readiness because the Boss had planted Slippery the Ox in the pawn shop. Frank immediately began to suspect Slippery. Maybe he had squealed and had given the heist away or had been fired because the owner might have become suspicious of him. We would have to call the heist off and lay low.

As an anxious expression crossed his face, Frank attempted to assume a pseudo-bravado air but could not conceal his anxiety. The therapist said, "Boss, you've got plenty of guts, real guts. You wouldn't have gotten so far without guts. But I have the funny feeling that when we go on these casing jobs you become troubled. Maybe you're not satisfied with this heist and want to pull another one." Frank grumbled sadly, "Sometimes too much guts gets you into trouble." I said, "The kind of guts you've got sure carried you a long way.

But I hate to see the Boss so unhappy and I'm beginning to wonder if casing these joints and pulling these heists hasn't been making you dissatisfied and unhappy. I still know a little bit about this doctoring business that I used to do before they caught up with me and put me in stir. Maybe you'd rather I worked for you as a Doc than as a gangster." Frank insisted that it wasn't the casing jobs that made him dissatisfied. He wanted to pull a real heist.

Deciding on a sporting goods store that carried rods and ammunition, we found a parking place in front of the state capitol building. Sighting the capitol building, Frank blurted out that he had an idea. We could go up to the dome of the capitol and case the city from up there. We took the trip up to the capitol dome and on our way down stopped to visit the chambers of the Supreme Court and the state legislature, which was in session. We ended up discussing the difference between the legislative and judicial branches of government and partaking of refreshments in a drug store. Frank sniffed the air and remarked that the place smelled like a sewer. Finishing our refreshments, we drove back to the school as Frank again played at shooting it out with the bulls.

As the operation of the Big Heist broadened into the scope of a syndicate that extended its plans to murder, robbery of armored cars, and the plunder of federal agencies, the need for weapons to carry out the heist continued to carry the therapy process into the community jewelry stores and pawn shops in order to enrich the gang arsenal with guns, holsters, and knives. The fine line between play action, acting out, and carrying into action his primitive impulses became so thin that Frank had begun to experience mounting anxiety bordering on panic. With increasing paranoid projection of his internal threatening images onto even the most innocent external figures, he suspected strangers on the street and even the maids in the residential setting of being bulls. The tension in the transference situation could be dealt with only by externalizing and by removing the threatening figures of the stoolies and the bulls from the immediate therapy situation, since the therapy office, the hideout of the Big Boss, had now become suspect and dangerous as well. Nevertheless, the office continued to serve as the base for the therapy situation, the Big Heist, as each hour started and ended in the office.

The Discovery of the Core Conflict

To safeguard the operation of the Big Heist, i.e., to maintain the transference situation, Frank conceived the notion of establishing a hideout and an arsenal which he called a stash-out somewhere in the country on the outskirts of the city. The further extension of the gang's operations into blackmail when Frank announced his plan to take pictures of the school staff walking into a whorehouse, and the recognition by the therapist of this plan as a "shakedown," enhanced the need to remove the base of the gang operations to an old abandoned house somewhere on the outskirts of the city.

As he confessed his intention to make a big business out of his camera, a business which evidently was to be a mixture of delinquent and legitimate activities, he related his anxiety about the sex play that was going on among the children at the school who would strip before each other and exhibit themselves. He belittled this behavior as kid's play and felt that when a guy got older he wanted to go a lot farther than that. He didn't think it was right for boys his age to have intercourse. That was for married people. But when older people got married they didn't seem to get much fun out of sex either. They got more fun out of having children. Since he had come from a family of five kids he could speak with some authority.

He felt especially sorry for his stepfather who was really a good guy and who had married into the family when there were two kids but wanted more children of his own. He had tried very hard to make the family happy but he seemed to be up against it. Besides working hard, he took many special courses at the university in order to get ahead so that he could do more for his family. But look what happened. Hard times had befallen him and his family. There was a lot of sickness in the family and his stepson was in jail. Frank felt sorry for him because he was such a real good guy, and more than anything else wanted his children to like him and to be happy. He had worked like a slave for them and they had let him down. And the hardest thing for him was having his son in jail.

Frank became genuinely remorseful as he continued his rueful lament about his stepfather's unhappy plight. The therapist empathized with Frank's plight too, and remarked that his stepfather probably didn't know how much Frank also wanted to like him and how much this whole business had been so tough on him too.

We reached the abandoned house and cased it before we entered. Stealthily making our way through an open window, we played out the act of breaking into the house in order to burglarize it. The sight that greeted us recalled the bleakness and dreariness of Frank's past. Amid dilapidation and dirt was an array of broken-down furniture, packed trunks, and household belongings in sordid disarray. It was as if a family had suddenly taken flight and had abandoned and deserted their home. Rats' nests and droppings, cobwebs and beehives stuck out from the walls while a pile of intimate family correspondence dating back to the early years of the century attested to the historic past of this abandoned house. Frank walked about exploring the house in a desultory and bewildered manner, picking up and discarding a number of items.

For many minutes he appeared as if in a trance and could not be contacted.

In our second excursion to the abandoned house we conversed about many things. Frank said that his new photography racket would be a front for our heists just as my doctoring business was my front also. With both of us having a respectable front we could go on the heist without too much trouble. We might even end up in hell. I said, "At least we go down there together, Boss." Frank grinned and appeared anxious.

Frank proposed that we pose as respectable people looking over the house so as not to arouse the suspicions of people in the vicinity. We could pretend that we were artists who were making sketches of the house. I complimented him on his clever idea and suggested as an alternative that we could pose as architects interested in old Topeka homes that had their heyday back in the golden days. He responded with another alternative, namely, that we could pose as realtors looking over the property.

As we drove past the college campus we talked about college education. Frank said that he had heard that college education was quite expensive, but he thought it was a good thing for people. Quite by coincidence I noticed the Rabbi crossing the street and pointed him out to Frank. He thought it was a nice thing that people who went to college could get some religious education also. He used to attend the Episcopal church but reflected that he didn't like the hypocrisy of people who went to church on Sunday and then disobeyed the Sabbath law by working that day. There was something hypocritical even about the minister preaching on Sunday since this was work and was opposed to the Commandment to observe the Sabbath. When he found out that the Rabbi headed the Congregation Beth Sholom, and when translated for him that it meant the House of Peace, he reflected that it was a good name and that there should be more of it. There wasn't enough peace in the world and not enough people had it. He confessed that at one time he had thought of becoming a minister. He had been very much interested in religion but gave it up. He thought it was a noble profession since many ministers worked and died for the sake of others. But what was the use of sacrificing oneself for others?

Once he thought he might be a bull too. Bulls often gave up their lives for the sake of others. But that was some stupid idea that he had long since given up. When the therapist reflected that Frank had been doing a lot of thinking about what he wanted to be, Frank agreed that he had, but right now he would like to be a traveling salesman. He would like to go out and see the world.

Quite abruptly he said he wasn't going to be president. The therapist said that maybe he had been thinking that he would like to be president. Frank was quite emphatic in his denial. If he were president, the country would be involved in six different wars with Russia and families would be involved in 15 different wars among themselves and there would be a hell of a lot of trouble in the country. If he were president he would really make a mess of things. He had made a mess of things already. Frank moodily reflected on his thoughts as we arrived at the abandoned house, slipped under the dense thicket of dead brush, and climbed through an open window.

TOWARD A NEW IDENTITY

The shift in the process of identification from more primitive, narcissistic to more advanced object relationships coincided with Frank's search for his identity, with the quest for the person that he wanted to be. As reflected in the preceding interview, this process continued for some time and was associated with increased capacity for communication by means of verbal language and the use of secondary process thought. The following interview illustrates Frank's preoccupation with the nature of his identity and its complex unintegrated structure, composed, as it were, of a variety of conflicting individuals:

Frank greeted me with a reserved "Howdy" and went to his usual seat. I wondered whom I was addressing today. Was I talking to the Boss or to Frank? A little surprised by this, he grinned and in a swaggering, bragging manner said he would let me in on a secret. The Boss and Frank were the same person. I said that in a way I knew this too but thought in some ways that they were also different persons, just as a person had different feelings about himself and would have different ambitions at different times. Puffing out his chest in a swaggering manner, Frank said that he was really the Boss, and Frank was one of his aliases. I told him that I had heard that he went under many aliases. He said it was true. He also went under the alias of F. C. Smith. I told him I had also heard that he went under the aliases of Frank Charles Smith and Frankie Smith, as well as Frank. With a broad grin he said, "They're all me."

I said that sometimes I wasn't sure to which Frank I was talking. And I thought that he must be unsure to whom he was talking when he was with me, the doctor who was once a reputable physician or the doctor who had been released from stir. I usually had a hunch as to which Frank I was talking, though. When he planned his heists I knew he was Jocko the Monk, the Big Boss. And when he was a reserved, growing-up 14-year-old boy, I thought he was Frank Charles Smith. When he was a boy talking about his ambitions for the future who wanted to make something of himself and could talk about justice and current events and could make a public speech, then I thought of him as Frank C. Smith. And there was the Frank Smith who didn't quite know what he wanted to be and wasn't himself certain who he was, so he would put up a show like a grown-up person and feel that he couldn't quite fill those shoes yet. And there was little Frankie who longed to be even younger than his years and wanted very much to be like a young child but also found this kind of person out of place. Frank listened attentively and nodded his head slowly and somberly in agreement. He said that he knew he was in an awful dilemma but didn't quite know what to do about it. He fell silent and seemed to be groping for something else to talk about. When he began to talk again, it soon became evident that while the original topic seemingly had been dropped, actually Frank had returned to it in the metaphor of a play production that followed.

In the discussion that ensued we made plans to produce a great play. Between ourselves we would combine the roles of producer, writer, director, actors, propmen, and audience. Frank's enthusiasm became fired as we discussed the plans for this great production. He suddenly announced that he had an idea and immediately briefed me on the plot. He would be the proprietor of a liquor store who was to be held up by a stickup man at the close of a busy day. I was to play the part of Liquor Louie, a small-time mug who had been robbing liquor stores for weeks, unmolested by the cops. Frank set the stage and we proceeded to act out our roles. The play ended as Frank, the proprietor, was shot to death. His dying words were for the criminal, Liquor Louie, with whom he pleaded to make his getaway before the cops could descend upon him.

In the following hour Frank was full of venomous criticism of the food that was served in the residence. His thoughts turned to the then recent atomic spy trials and he supported the President's demand for the death sentence. Nothing was worse than a spy or a traitor. They deserved to die. With increasing animation he became vituperative against deserters. The guy who ran away in combat and deserted his buddies deserved to die. The therapist took the view that deserters might be intensely troubled and frightened and perhaps needed help rather than the punishment of death. Frank expressed some doubt that men could be helped after they had deserted and then categorically passed the judgment that he had no use for draft dodgers either.

His thoughts turned to the recent event of the firing of a famous general by the President. Frank supported the view of the general that the then current war should have been pushed on to the mainland of the enemy's country. It was the only possible way of winning the war. But instead of being rewarded for his intentions he was fired as disobedient and insubordinate. Frank emphatically insisted that if the war were going to be won it would have to be pushed.

But Frank's dilemma, like that of the general, seemed insoluble. Not to push the war meant to lose the war but to pursue it vigorously was to incur humiliation and disgrace. To find a solution for this dilemma Frank again turned to the big production as he expressed his dissatisfaction with the scene that had been enacted the previous hour. He announced the name of the big production: "The Bulls March On," Scene I: "The Beginning of the Last Holdup." In a crucial moment, as we reenacted the scene, Frank announced that he was F. C. Smith, the dick. He revealed that he was a detective who had been trailing and had now caught up with me, that lousy mug, Liquor Louie. He fired point blank into my body and ignoring my plea for the croaker as I lay dying, he contemptuously and venomously retorted that I didn't need a doctor any more and that my criminal career was over. What I needed was the police, and if I lived at all it would be in jail. He had no pity for me as this was the fate and deserved punishment of all crooks. Shortly after this

therapy session the staff found circulated around the residence the following circulars: "Wanted for Murder, Dead or
Alive, Jocko the Monk, Alias Frank Smith."

At this point, when the patient begins to modify his identification with the criminal gangster, the negative, threatening paternal introject, to one in which he wishes to play
the part of the detective, and thus to ally himself with the
positive forces of culture, a further comment should be made
on the psychological nature of play action. Our material suggests that we can differentiate between two different forms
of the play, one of which will be called play action, the other,
play acting.[3]

In his play action, Frank unconsciously repeats the original
conflict, identifies himself with the aggressor, the negative
paternal introject, and "resolves" the conflict through pseudomastery and identification which is experienced as complete and which permits no compromise. (As expressed in
Frank's fantasy, "Traitors deserve to die.")

Play acting, however, refers to an activity in which there
is no complete identification with the role the person acts but
in which he rather tries to master the problem by cue-taking
and by imitation. He now wishes to take the part of the
detective, the honest citizen, the defender of our societal
structure against subversion. However, he takes these roles
with tongue in cheek, as it were, and tells the therapist that
they are merely to pretend, that they are merely acting, as
if they were to put up a front in order to hide the true selves.

In our case, play action is oriented toward the past and
represents the repetition of the unconscious conflict. It thus
constitutes an attempt at recollection. Play acting, however,
attempts to modify a past identification and constitutes

[3]The concept "play acting" is used in the text because of its descriptive
usefulness. In the genetic schema we speak of fantasy action in order to
stress the genetic and functional difference between play and role playing.

Frank's first attempt to master the future, to trial act, as it were, the future role with which he wishes to identify himself. He thus unconsciously repeats ahead of time the future rather than the past. He adopts the world of the psychotherapist on a trial basis without permanently committing himself as yet. Play action serves the past while play acting is in the service of adaptation, of future growth. Behavior which is primarily based on imitation, on acting a role, could be considered regressive in comparison to behavior which is dominated by more complete identificatory processes. Inasmuch as this behavior stands in the service of trying out the future, however, of testing a new role, it can also be considered a progressive move within the psychotherapeutic process.

One month later, as Frank was in the throes of anxious suspense lest his grandparents withdraw him from the school and from treatment, he heralded the end of the Big Heist as a gangster game in the following interview:

Frank seemed very uneasy and did not look at me. I slowly walked to the window and then very casually said, "I guess you're convinced that what I say to your grandmother on Tuesday will make all the difference about your staying or leaving here, and you don't feel that you can really depend upon me." Frank silently nodded his head in agreement.

I went on, "I can understand that you feel you can't really trust me yet." With considerable irritation Frank retorted, "I wouldn't say that exactly. If I didn't trust you I wouldn't tell you anything. I wouldn't talk to you at all." I said, "That's true, Frank, you do have more trust in me than you did, but I think you feel you can't trust me to come through for you all the way and to stick by you in a real pinch." With deep conviction and with unbiased candor Frank said, "That hits the nail on the head, that's exactly the way I do feel." I said, "I certainly appreciate the way you feel about your grandmother's visit on Tuesday. The outcome means a great deal to you." Frank found it hard to continue and fell silent. I said, "It's just as hard for you to say that you like being here and that you depend on Southard School and me as it is impossible for you to trust me completely. But I expect that, and I wouldn't believe anything else. Something that has been a problem to you for so many years can't be overcome that quickly." Frank grinned and slowly nodded his head in affirmation. I casually remarked that maybe he thought I would have to prove myself to be the kind of person he really could trust. Maybe he would have to find out what kind of person I really was.

Frank slowly went back to his seat, restlessly searched through the drawer of the desk, and drew out the BB pistol. He cocked it, took a shot at the wall, and then began to shoot at a distant target. I remarked that he was hitting the target much better now. Slowly and deliberately he looked the gun over and then with heated disgust exploded, "This goddam gun isn't worth anything. I don't know why I bought it. I spent three dollars for it and I don't know why. It's caused me nothing but trouble since I bought it." With considerable remorse and self-condemnation he went on, "For six months I've done nothing here. I thought that it made me a big shot." And then with explosive condemnation he said, "But I'm only a big shit." I said, "I remember not so long ago when that gun was the most important thing to you, Frank, so important that you could think of nothing else and you had to have it." Frank said, "I'm going to take this thing apart and get rid of it. Do you have a screwdriver?" Finding a paper clip as a substitute for a screwdriver, he went to work on the gunsight and with a vicious gesture removed it and laid it on the desk. He remarked that this was as far as he could go now. He would need more tools to take the gun apart completely.

I wondered if it were the gun itself that he had needed so much. I remembered that once he had told me that the gun had as much value as the U.S. Treasury because it had buried within it an extremely important secret, George Washington's secret. With considerable anger in his voice he said, "I made one mistake." Cocking the gun and looking down into the barrel, he added, "Living. That was my mistake. Being born was my mistake." Again he viciously attacked the gun and with intention of ripping it apart. I said, "Maybe we'll get to the secret in that gun, sometime after all." As he laid the pieces of the gun on the desk, he sat back silently, and as if in a distant trance, nodded his head in confirmation. He sat in silent dejection and contemplation until the hour was up.

The vicissitudes of the patient's acting out during the psychotherapeutic process have brought us to a stage during the recovery in which a new facet of the problem of acting out becomes visible and requires clarification. While he still acts out and travels along with the therapist in order to accomplish the Big Heist, to plunder the abandoned house, we find that he himself attempts to cover up his delinquent activities and ambitions, his destructive fantasies and wishes, by trying to create an impression that he is really like everybody else. He challenges the psychotherapist and wants him to help him so that they both may appear as decent law-abiding citizens, that they may act as if they belong to the community while underneath a solid front they would continue with their undercover activity.

This turning point in the psychotherapy in which he toys with the choice of a variety of noncriminal professions gives one the feeling that the reversal of the process is taking place. At first it seemed that the psychotherapeutic process could be maintained only if the psychotherapist was willing to play act with him, to put up a front as if he himself were a criminal, the Doc who helps the Boss. This situation in which the psychotherapist imitated the child seemed to be the only way in which Frank could express himself and could move toward the nuclear conflict.

As he moves toward the basic conflict, and as anxiety increases, he wishes more and more at least to act like the psychotherapist actually is, like his teachers, and like those who take care of him. But underneath he wishes to maintain a life of his own. He wishes to impose on his rich and destructive fantasy life an imitative façade, a crust, which could be considered a precursor of identification with the love object. One may see in this development an increase in the strength of genuine object relationships, whereas previous object relationships were overburdened with the projection of narcissistic affects.

Two facets of the material deserve special comment. On the one hand, via the new object identification, via the effort to assume at least an imitative front, he suddenly discovers a new image of the stepfather, now described as a disappointed man who did his best and wanted nothing more than the love of his children, but instead had the bitter experience of having his stepson in jail. The delinquent pattern is exchanged for neurotic symptomatology, the capacity for and the necessity of increased guilt. One may predict that the acting out process may soon come to an end, or rather, that its occurrence will be less frequent.

The second facet which deserves our consideration concerns the disappointment which he experiences when he finally enters and conquers the forbidden abandoned house, the symbol of the unconsciously hoped-for childhood home. He finds nothing there but a few old letters, like expected letters from home that he never received, and thus discovers that the Big Heist ends in his unearthing of a heap of abandoned dust. One is reminded of one of Freud's beautiful similes in which he describes the power of the unconscious, and suggests that if the unconscious conflict is brought to the surface, it loses its effectiveness, in very much the same way that a mummy, excavated from the ancient tombs, falls to dust as soon as it is exposed to the light of day.

As soon as he can give up past longing as well as longing for the past, the acting out—the delinquent but neurotic reconquest of that which is now abandoned—becomes meaningless. Recollection of the past, achieved via the acting out and expressed as an unconscious memory through the conquest of the abandoned house, thus can be understood to be in the service of the reconstructive process. Some theoretical implications of this concept have been discussed elsewhere (Ekstein, 1954).

Frank is now ready to take another step. The potential love objects of the present, who have been no more than objects of imitation for him, now receive new meaning. The original capacity for identification, documented in the different image that he now has of his stepfather and well illustrated in earlier wishes for positive, helpful professions, is restored, and can be set in motion.

From time to time as disappointments occur one may expect that he cannot help but fall back on old defensive and adaptive devices which are predominantly primitive acting out mechanisms. These acting out devices, however, are now in the service of a more mature personality organization and in part, at least, have an adaptive function which primarily will help him to some extent to master reality, and will only secondarily serve the purpose of the repetition of past unconscious conflict.

As the psychotherapy proceeded, Frank developed the capacity to maintain contact and to communicate with the therapist almost exclusively on a verbal level. Play action and acting out within the therapy process were replaced by talking out and thinking out, even those fantasies dealing with a variety of inner conflicts that were mainly concerned with Frank's efforts to cement the identification with the therapist as a nonthreatening masculine object. The symptom of stealing and the wish to steal were relegated to the background of his psychic life and had started to subside completely. What acting out occurred was experienced on the fringe of gang activities within the residential setting with his adolescent peers who bullied the younger children and engaged in defiant, boisterous, and sexually aggressive gestures against the residential personnel.

After a number of months of this phase of his therapy, Frank again began to feel the inner pressure which he ascribed to repeated disappointments about his family. He very rarely received mail from home and was under constant tension lest his grandfather carry out the threat of removing him from the school because of financial reverses. These circumstances, associated with the approaching date of his birthday and the anticipated visit with his parents during the holiday season, again stimulated strong wishes in Frank to possess a real gun. For many months Frank struggled with his conflict about the wish to possess such a gun and the fear of the consequences of this responsibility, and many therapeutic sessions were concerned with the means of obtaining such a gun.

During one point of this phase of his therapy, Frank hit upon the plan to borrow money from the bank with the therapist underwriting and guaranteeing the loan. Frank and the therapist went through this procedure and obtained a loan of $250. Its effect, rather than elating and gratifying Frank, was to intensify his anxiety, as if he had been discovered in a forbidden act with the therapist, and as if he had revealed a secret mission to the loan officer who appeared to him as a terrifying and threatening figure. The fear also that he would not be able to repay the loan and would damage the credit and reputation of the therapist led to his immediate repayment of the loan with the loss of two and a half dollars of unused interest. Action and acting out had been replaced by a new symptom which we might consider to be the precursor of a phobia.

Frank's desperate and compelling wish to possess a real gun was finally fulfilled in a legal manner after he had managed to save a sufficient amount of money from his allowance, a no small feat for Frank. Together with the therapist he purchased a gun which was registered with the police by the proprietor of the gun store, and was kept under lock and key in the therapist's office. The gun became the symbol of a trusting, loving, and accepting relationship between Frank and the therapist, and on one level served as a source of play gratification as a number of therapy hours were spent shooting at targets along the river.

Frank glowed with pride at his achievement of overcoming his fear of guns; he fantasied himself the master of that which he once dreaded. His self-esteem rose, soon to be dampened by the renewal of his conflict about the possession and shooting of the gun with the therapist, until he began to express doubt as to whether this was what he really wanted and whether it was a source of enjoyment to him after all. At this point in his treatment he declared himself ready to enter a boarding home and to enter public high school.

The positive relationship in the transference situation was paralleled in Frank's immediate and gratifying state of acceptance and positive feelings in the boarding home. Although he made many complaints of a feeble nature about the boarding home mother, he basked in the newfound relationship with the boarding home father. For the first time in his life, Frank declared that he had met a man who made him feel that he was a person, worthy of respect and dignity. With guarded astonishment he confessed that it was the first time that something like this had ever happened to him. The feeling of being trusted and respected was experienced as the arrival of his day of glory.

But the brittleness and fragility of this newfound identification with the male love object, and of the trusting relationship for which he had searched so long, soon became evident when Frank experienced a homosexual panic that drove him back to Southard School and forced him to relinquish the boarding home. The panic was provoked by keen disappointment in the boarding home father when he expressed distrust of Frank's possession of the gun. Frank had been certain that he would be trusted with his own pistol since the boarding home father had trusted him with his own hunting rifle and they had enjoyed using it together. When the boarding home father, with some justification, expressed his fear of pistols, and did not permit Frank to keep his in the boarding home, Frank experienced this rebuff as an expression of deep distrust. If the father with whom he had identified himself could not trust him, he could not trust himself. Fear of his own aggression and erotic impulses coupled with his perception of the boarding home father as one who could not trust him in the active masculine role brought on the panic. For Frank, denial of the right to possess a gun symbolized the fear that the father could not trust his control over his aggression, but could accept him only as a passive child, as one who would therefore have to surrender, to submit, and to be castrated in order to be accepted.

Paralleling this same experience in the transference situation, Frank, in a panic, broke into the therapist's office one night, stole the gun, and ran away. He had left the following note which was readily discovered by another boy in the residence: "Dear Doc. I am very sorry that I went back on your trust about the gun but it was the only thing left to do. I feel shitty all over anyhow. Frank Smith." Although he was found in his room the following morning, depressed and almost inaccessible, he later revealed that he had walked the streets all night, gun in hand, full of rage and bitterness, desperately hoping that he would not encounter the therapist who he had expected would look for him and who actually had carried out a futile search during the night for runaway Frank. Frank's reaction again was to destroy the gun as being a source of nothing but trouble. He vowed that never again would he have a gun and gratefully accepted the therapist's help in selling it, again with a loss of money but with great relief to Frank. The public school situation also collapsed as Frank found it impossible to continue attendance when he experienced a most profound panic and paralysis which made it impossible for him to enter the high school building. The abrogation of acting out symptoms had led to the appearance of a genuine phobic symptom, a form of "inverted acting out."

Frank's runaway note confirmed our speculation that the panic situation in the boarding home had been a displacement of the transference situation. The therapist, like the boarding home father, was suspected by Frank of accepting him only in the pseudomasculine role, expressed in the act of carrying a gun, which the therapist, however, controlled and kept from Frank's possession by keeping it locked in his office.

In the ensuing months, Frank on two separate occasions again experienced the all-compelling and irresistible wish and impulse to possess a gun, a wish that he could gratify only in forbidden secrecy with another boy in the residence. On one occasion the illicit possession of the gun culminated in remorse and self-condemnation with the violent dismantling and destruction of the gun, the flinging of its parts into the river, and the loss of his highly cherished monetary investment. In the second incident Frank concealed the gun for a number of months in his room and then brought about its discovery and confiscation, but with the additional feature that this time Frank participated in its legal disposition, again with a loss of money, but with the conscious choice on his part that he would have to sacrifice the gun in order to enter a second boarding home.

These incidents paralleled and climaxed his agonizing inner struggle over his holding onto or finally rejecting the bonds that attached him to his family. Frank compared his dilemma regarding his relationship to his phantom mother to the futility of a dead-end street. Desperately he pinned his hopes on the fork in the road that would lead him in another direction, but just as desperately he felt the incapacity to trust that this fork could lead to anything but a dead end as well. The abandoned house that yielded nothing but rubble, dirt, and memories of a token love in the past now entered his conscious thinking in the form of the dismal awareness that his hopes for a loving and reawakened relationship with his mother, the hope to return to his family, had also crumbled into a heap of dust. He saw his dying hopes in the fantasy of himself as a ship's captain, dutifully remaining with his ship as it went down to the bottom of the ocean; and as one who once had pathetically held on to a spark with the futile hope that he could kindle it into a flame.

The relinquishing of his narcissistic relationships and the cutting of his ties with the past, facilitated by the increased capacity for new object relationships and more genuine identifications with his love objects, culminated in the second and now successful attempt to live in a boarding home, an event in which Frank actively participated from the planning stage. In the psychotherapy, play action and acting out ceased and gave way to the conventional form of treatment of a neurotic personality. Secondary process thinking largely replaced primitive play fantasy and acting out.

Frank reentered public high school and was able to maintain an excellent academic performance, despite the residual
of his phobic symptom which made it extremely difficult for
him, particularly, to give reports in front of the class. He
became interested in religious training and seriously considered entering the ministry. After graduating from high
school, he maintained the bond with the boarding home, at
the same time loosening it to some extent, terminated psychotherapy, chose a university he wished to attend, and took
a part-time job in the interim before entering the university.

With a positive and more realistic view of his helpful and
supporting grandparents, he had now created for himself
new introjects upon which to rely, introjects which gave him
new purpose in life and had the power to help him overcome
the early difficulties in which adults were seen to be unde-
pendable, treacherous, deserting, and criminally negligent.
Limited originally to aggressively taking from society that
which he felt was always withheld from him by troubled and
immature parents, he had come to a new self-concept as a
young adult now in the position to help others.

How the core of the acting out personality remains active
despite advancement in the hierarchy of personality organization is illustrated in an experience of genuine neurotic
acting out toward the end of his treatment.

Frank had become a member of a church and was an active
and enthusiastic participant in a young people's group. During one particular discussion led by a woman group worker,
the subject of the rightness and wrongness of stealing under
various circumstances came up. The group leader felt that,
in the case of a Czech boy who during the Nazi occupation
of his country was forced to steal in order to maintain himself
and his family lest they starve, it was not considered wrong
to steal. Frank took violent exception to what he considered
a lax and hypocritical judgment on the part of the group

leader. He strongly felt that under no circumstances was it considered morally right to steal and quoted as his authority the Commandment "Thou Shalt Not Steal." He insisted that only this rule in the Bible could determine the rightness and wrongness of the act. The judgment of the group leader had troubled him greatly.

The therapist interpreted his need to maintain absolute and infallible rules of rightness and wrongness that could not be compromised by human beings, and his need to place trust only in such rules when he felt that the word of a human being could not be relied upon as a guide to reality testing in extreme circumstances. Frank's response was to confirm the interpretations by acting out in the following experience. That same evening he took the boarding home parent's car with his permission and drove it along an icy street. Looking in the rearview mirror, he found that his rear window was steamed up and he could not see outside. The impulse to have fun by "gunning" the car led him to drive for two blocks with the car swaying from side to side until he was suddenly halted by a police car. Frank was chagrined, but was able with the boarding father's help to go through the court experience with dignity and with increased understanding of his failure fully to accept his responsibility as a driver.

In the therapy session, it became clear that he was acting out his perception of the unreliable internal image that hid itself when he was tempted to obey a primitive, dangerous impulse, but which made its presence known only after he had exposed himself to danger so that he was made to pay the penalty for his primitive and illicit gratification. The acting out confirmed the therapist's interpretation, carried him back to the past conflict with the parents, and served to further his insight into his conflict in a way that contributed to a more effective resolution in the future. In this view, the acting out could be seen as a positive attempt at a new resolution.

SUMMARY

A case has been described in which the prevalent mode of communication during psychotherapy for large segments of the process consisted of acting out behavior, play action, and eventually play acting. In adult neurotics, acting out is considered a form of resistance to be removed by interpretation or by suggestion and injunction. In this case, the assumption was made that the acting out, play action, and play acting, rather than being merely a substitute for recollection, represented *experimental recollection*, a primitive mode of the ego to bring about reconstruction, which is in the service of adaptation. The unavailability of sufficient neutralized energy cathexis for higher forms of ego organization was considered a contraindication to the use of technical tools applicable to adult neurotics.

The acceptance by the therapist of whatever means of communication the patient could use made it possible for the boy to imitate the therapist and finally to identify himself with him, thus complementing the predominantly negative introjects of the past with positive introjects. Acting out was given up, substituted for at first by phobic attitudes, and replaced finally with a genuine and stable adolescent personality whose obsessive-compulsive adaptive devices were now in the service of reality testing rather than merely the repetition of unconscious conflict. An attempt was made to relate technical considerations to a psychic structure that was dominated by acting out, the function of which has been described in terms of newer concepts of ego psychology.

PART II

Residential Treatment

7

INTRODUCTION

Notes on the Theory of Residential Treatment, by Joseph D. Noshpitz

Although a number of the earlier chapters dealt with treatment of adolescents in residential settings, the emphasis was placed on the techniques of individual psychotherapy. In the sections that follow, we shall be dealing with a wider range of factors that embrace the total experience of the young patient in such situations. Thus such matters as institutional design, staffing, and interdisciplinary collaboration begin to move into central focus. Perhaps the *locus classicus* for the formulation of these issues is Alt's (1960) book *Residential Treatment of the Disturbed Child*.

In the paper that follows, Noshpitz distills the essential elements in the process of residential treatment, placing them within a psychoanalytically grounded historical context. His major emphasis is on the modes of intervention that have evolved in the wake of psychoanalytic ego psychology— particularly, what he refers to as "ego support," derived from the nature and structure of the milieu itself; "ego interpretation," provided by way of informed confrontation by all staff members in contact with the patient; and "psychotherapy" in the traditional sense, directed primarily to the patient's intrapsychic conflicts. Noshpitz also considers alternative ways of dealing with the omnipresent problem of the rela-

203

tionship between "therapist" and "administrator," for which there appear to be as many different models as there are institutions that concern themselves with it (see Stanton and Schwartz, 1954).

7

Notes on the Theory of Residential Treatment

Joseph D. Noshpitz, M.D.

We are now developing a variety of methods and, inevitably, a group of parallel theories to account for how and why we do things in residential treatment. These theories will very likely differ from each other more and more as time goes on. This is not in itself a bad thing. What might be unfortunate would be a tendency to form sects which will sail along indifferent to or at odds with each other's contributions. It therefore seems useful to consider some of the current theoretical aspects of such treatment side by side and see what each has to offer; for we may well hope that as the many new practices have begotten new ideas, these new ideas will in turn beget still better practices, and that the intermingling of our theories will result in mutual fructification rather than collective inhibition.

Historically, some of the theory of residential treatment came into existence as an outgrowth of child analysis. The early child analysts found that the child's environment (in the sense of parental attitudes, school experiences, interac-

Reprinted by permission from the *Journal of the American Academy of Child Psychiatry*, 1:281-296, 1962. New York: International Universities Press.

tions with certain groups of associates, etc.) influenced the movement of treatment to such a degree that some type of extratherapeutic handling had to be undertaken, either by the analyst or by someone associated with the analyst. As a result analysis began to come to grips with the problem of children whose disturbances were such that they could not live at home. A separate environment had to be created for such children and it was here that the seeds of one type of residential treatment were sown.

As they began to accept institutional children or to consult on such cases, analysts laid down certain requirements. These in turn led to the emergence of a theory of residential management that considered residential work effective to the extent that it made a child available for therapy. Aside from the treatment hour, whatever happened to the child during his daily living was to be handled in a more or less common-sense supportive way in keeping with sound mental hygiene principles. Some attempt could be made to imitate the qualities of a pleasant home, but there was no anticipation that factors within that environment (unless by their capacity to impede progress) would determine the course of the treatment in any major way.

This method had its complications. For example, if the child did not want to go to his hour, there went the entire *raison d'être* of the establishment. Or if he decided he liked someone in the milieu better than his therapist and insisted on telling his secrets to that person, a very real issue had to be faced.

The relation of the analyst to the staff of the residence was never simple. The analyst might be completely unconnected with the residence proper. He might have occasional contacts with the director in order to acquaint that individual with the general direction of treatment, or, possibly, to complain about some of the things which were happening to his patient.

At times, he might ask for certain supports from the environment. In general, however, the secrecy of the therapy material would be considered very important in such a setting, and the therapy had to be seen as something special, different, and apart. Aside from the active avoidance of doing things wrong, such as seducing or brutally handling the child, the use of the milieu directly was seen chiefly by its funneling—that is to say, the practice of actively directing many bits of information and many of the child's relationship bids toward the therapist. In essence, one might say that this was a style of therapy that attempted to imitate the traditional situation in a healthy home, the child being taken to see the analyst.

We might call this arrangement the "purely" analytically oriented residence. To look at a polar opposite for a moment, we might next consider a type of residential setting that arose quite apart from the influence of psychoanalysis, one in which the question of therapy was never primary, and in which sometimes, indeed, no form of therapy was ever contemplated. Here the child would be placed because his difficulties were sufficiently severe that his parents or the community felt that he could not remain at home. The philosophy of such a residence would generally be that benign, kindly understanding and common-sense handling were the cure for most childhood emotional ills. In such an environment a gentle but consistent punishment pattern was likely to be regarded as the best technique for coping with aggression, and a lot of good, warm, common-sense mothering the counter to regression. Scarcely an institution of this sort exists that cannot name a long list of troubled children who have left its precincts, only to write letters for years thereafter to this housemother or that athletic director saying how much help they had received and how their whole lives were changed by the opportunity to know so and so. We might guess that the thing that helps children here is the opportunity to form better identifications. This is no mean lever for change in childhood. It is probably true that more children are helped in this country each year by being supplied with more adequate identification figures than by any other single means.

From the scientific point of view, the great problem with this approach is that we do not at this point know what in fact are the precise conditions under which the most wholesome and appropriate identifications can take place and what are the preconditions for changes in identification. We know something about these ideas, but not enough to study a child and say that if the following conditions are set up, the following identifications will follow, and then list them. We often say that if a certain predelinquent youngster is sent to a reform school, his delinquency potential will probably come to its fullest flower in short order. So much we are able to predict, and probably with fair accuracy. But in terms of sharp and delicate decisions, our knowledge is still pretty crude. Those whose task it is to choose particular boarding homes or foster homes for problem children, and those who must assign children to cottages in the course of admission to large treatment centers know something of how difficult such decisions can be. They have to face the vital issue of other children as identification objects as well as foster or cottage parents. Thus, when a child is sent to a kindly and humanely organized residence, the best one hopes for is that exposure to benign people will "somehow or other" cause the right identifications to follow. From our point of view the weakness of this approach lies along two axes. First of all, the "somehow or other" creates an essential area of uncertainty which must always be present. The very nonscientific character of the approach makes it difficult to predict which child will be helped and which child not, and how much.

The second, and perhaps more important, area of difficulty is the whole question of exactly what is the nature of improvement and growth in such disturbed children. Is identification really enough of an answer for them? That is to say, how necessary is it that other processes of repair take place (and even have priority over identification with one or the other of the treatment people) as the road to health, growth, and improvement? Here we have a major area for further research and study with an enormous body of data already available. There are literally hundreds of graduates of these benign types of residential centers, many more who emerge from such centers almost every month, and there is the likelihood of a host of such individuals continuing to be treated in such centers for some time to come. The techniques of measuring the nature and process of improvement, while perhaps not too well advanced, are still not so primitive that we could not obtain a great deal of very useful data by a close study of the impact of this type of environment on such youngsters.

We can assume, then, that among the things a residence does to help children toward recovery are: in the first setting described, hold onto youngsters while they are in treatment in such a way as to promote the course of the therapy, and in the second, provide objects and conditions favorable to the formation of new identifications. Next, however, we must ask ourselves: What other techniques do we know about that can be made part of residential therapy? This is in a sense the major question confronting the field now. To the extent that we seek answers to this, we are looking for new methods, new approaches, and, in short, "breakthroughs."

Fortunately, during the past half century, we have seen the development of two lines of approach in residential treatment. Each of these approaches should have a profound bearing on the techniques that are employed during the period immediately ahead of us. Both will need a considerable degree of further refinement and explication before they realize their potentialities to the full, but both are ready to offer much to the sick child. We can classify the two areas as (1) ego support and (2) ego interpretation. Their theoretical underpinnings are the more recent developments in ego psychology: They take into account the concept of various distinct ego functions, the notion of damage to individual ego functions, the possibility of the repair of such damage with appropriate techniques, the role of the character defenses as essential elements among these functions, and the basic concept of character interpretation alternating with content interpretation as the avenue along which treatment must flow. In a way, both of these techniques might seem to be diametrically opposed; one is an ego-rebuilding technique, the other an ego-analyzing technique. In fact, however, they can and must be used side by side, for each of them copes with a different aspect of the child's functioning. Let us consider each of these techniques in detail.

Ego support implies a group of treatment tactics aimed at strengthening, consolidating, and giving sharper outline to an ego which lacks the type of integrity that should have come with normal maturation. Thus the readiness to confuse fantasy with reality, the inability to delay gratification, the readiness to be overwhelmed by emotion, distortions of object relations, all the attributes associated with an early phase of normal development are found at much later stages. Obviously, such ego weakness is central in the psychopathology of schizophrenic children, or in some severely neurotic youngsters in the latency period. In a more punctate and local sense, it is discernible in severely aggressive, hyperactive, impulse-ridden youngsters. Techniques aimed at ego support for this type of problem have recently received considerable documentation and one need only point to a few items in the literature to illustrate this. We think here, for example, of a very moving passage in *Love Is Not Enough* (Bettelheim, 1950) which describes the awakening of a child in the morning. Scarcely anyone, either in this work or, I imagine, out of it can read that passage without having an enormous empathic reaction to the sense of pain and stress experienced by the children, as well as a considerable respect for the sensitivity and the appropriateness, the clinical rightness, of the techniques employed in response to the child's need. Here we have a situation where a weak ego is confronted by a stress with which it cannot adequately cope; the environment moves in to offer the child the techniques and support that will enable him to come to grips with this stress, master it, and pass beyond it with a reasonable degree of success. It is clear in the course of this work that no interpretation is employed and that all the techniques invoked are aimed at increasing the child's sense of contact with the human environment, freeing the child from a certain feeling of fear and anticipation of danger, assuring the child that giving up the more comfortable and gratifying state of being in bed under the covers does not mean merely a chilling plunge into a hostile world but into the gratifications the world offers as well. The child is lent channels, provided with compensations, and proffered handholds, as it were, along which he can begin to make the laborious climb from the one state of being to the other. In sum, we can say the staff is giving him support. It is to be hoped that, with the passage of time, the various ego functions involved both in the youngster's state of paralysis and in his capacities to free himself from this shut-in situation will become more and more exactly enumerated and evaluated. One way to go at this is by examining the techniques which originally become established through the intuitive and sensitive clinical responses of director and counselors, and then breaking these methods down into their various elements, each of which meets the failure or the inadequacy of particular ego functions in the child's makeup. At present, this work is often almost necessarily of a trial-and-error character; one knows in general what one wants to do, but the specific details have not been worked out with sufficient accuracy to permit exact methodological approaches to each and every situation. The element of innovation is still strong within us and the burden rests upon us to study our innovations and the situations that evoke them and begin to specify which does what to which part of the ego. Redl's work (Redl and Wineman, 1951, 1952) abounds with the details of various techniques for the support of the ego that cannot control impulse, that cannot handle stimulation, that cannot cope with emotion, and that is constantly and repeatedly overwhelmed. The experience of observing a huge bout of some affect washing over a child's ego and disorganizing it is one that any practitioner of residential treatment encounters repeatedly and one to which he becomes very sensitized. Much of residential work, in fact, is bound to be:

1. an anticipation of the type of situation which might threaten to overwhelm patients (e.g., unexpected visits, sudden shifts in personnel, inadequate protection from bullying or blackmail, etc.);
2. the structuring of an environment which tends to head off and prevent, or at least minimize, the occurrence of such stimuli and their resultant reactions;
3. an alertness for the early signs, the premonitory warning indications that such a phenomenon is about to occur;
4. the rapid moving-in as a response to such signs (and how much staff training that requires!) with some

emphasis on the techniques necessary for that mov-ing-in, e.g., the quiet word or silent gesture that acts as an external signal to the internal defense patterns, the quick offer to talk with or to play with the youngs-ter, action to divert the other child on the scene who is the provoker, etc.;

5. the techniques of management that become necessary for cutting one child out of the herd, what to tell the other children, the availability of preplanned alter-native program devices, etc. The state of our knowl-edge being what it is, it is inevitable that there will be a sufficiency of instances when the child does become overwhelmed, when, in spite of our most skillful ef-forts and our most alert responsiveness, situations will arise which will provide too much stimulation, too much frustration, or too much of whatever it is that triggers this reaction;

6. the techniques appropriate to responding to the overwhelmed child, the appropriate degree of iso-lation, comfort, containment, and control, or what-ever it is that this type of youngster when overcome requires;

7. finally, the method of working toward a gradual re-building and restructuring of the youngster's com-posure and control until he is once again ready and able to work at his optimum.

It is clear from the above instances that the task of pro-viding ego support is an extremely complex one and requires an enormous amount of information about the individual child, a solid body of theory about the nature of ego oper-ation, a highly trained and capable staff familiar both with theory and with the individual child's vagaries and needs, and an incessant imaginative attention to the search for ever-surer ways both to prevent and to treat the various types of emotional flooding that the child may experience. The keynote of this type of work is specificity.

This approach, indeed, gives us one of our strongest arguments against untrained staff no matter how talented. Having someone manage the child in a "common-sense" way may act as a considerable hindrance to the careful observation of exactly what elements go into such a relationship and the really thorough comprehension of what is taking place. A certain obscurity and lack of clarity seem inevitably to follow on the heels of turning well-intentioned but untrained staff loose with a very sick child; sooner or later they establish some method of living together, but it then takes an enormous amount of work to get a full picture of what is being exchanged between staff and child in the name of support, where the successes are and where the failures. In addition, having established a *modus vivendi*, it is hard for the unsophisticated staff person to shift as the child improves and to alter techniques to meet new needs and new capacities.

Ego interpretation is quite a different issue. Here we are dealing with a concept reasonably familiar from the technique of psychoanalysis, the concept originally referred to as character analysis or character interpretation. There is a great deal of "misbehavior" or "symptomatic behavior" that is part and parcel of the image of many disturbed children in a residential setting. Some of this behavior, the inquisitiveness, playfulness, and acting up that are symptomatic simply of the patient's age rather than an expression of pathology, is a function of the normal *esprit* of childhood. Some of it results from becoming overwhelmed as noted above and requires techniques appropriate to that. Much of it, however, has quite a different flavor. It represents a characterological pattern, a style of operation geared in antisocial or parasocial directions, and carries with it a strong tinge of pleasure,

usually of directly erotic character. Much manipulative behavior falls into this category, as does bullying and sexual
aggression toward other children, some stealing, some running away, and a host of other vandalistic and exploitive acts
generally included in the area of behavior problems. Many
of these acts are fairly simple pleasure-seeking activities; but
they are often intermixed with other strivings which are
either directly or in part designed to protect the child from
the awareness of certain infantile impulses, regressive wishes,
anxiety-producing thoughts, oedipal struggles, and the like.
The counterphobic defense is the perfect example. When
this defense is utilized, if the unconscious wish is to be coddled
and babied, the behavior includes spiteful aggressivity and
running away; if the unthinkable fear is castration and bodily
injury, the conscious act is that of provocative challenging
and bullying. Such behavior comes into being and persists
in large measure both because of its defensive function and
because it is a source of gratification. The problem of the
staff then becomes that of calling attention to the nature of
this defense as a defense, and the labeling of the child's search
for pleasure as problem behavior. If a 10-year-old with a
normal I.Q. insists on clinging, sitting on laps, and soiling,
then, like water dripping on rock, the staff can direct a steady
delicate stream of interpretative remarks toward the child
aimed at making the infantile behavior a forbidden pleasure,
something that defends and helps the child hide from some
feeling. Sometimes less play would be given to the overt act
in itself than to the quality of the affect with which the act
is done or to the nature of the ego envelope within which
the behavior is clothed. To do this successfully, the child has
to be literally englobed by therapy. It is our experience that
as these defenses and pleasure lunges are worked with, shak-
ened, loosened, and made less functional for the child by
repeated confrontations, sooner or later the material which

has been so defended against starts to appear, and many regressive wishes, thoughts, and acts take the place of what was originally a more defiant or pleasure-yielding but anti-social style of behavior. No small part of this involves a more or less vigorous control of the more overt acts on the theory that as the acting out is stopped, the underlying genetic-dy-namic material has greater opportunity to appear and be worked with. This approach is not only confined to gross antisocial acts; there is much neurotic behavior that can be so approached. For example, if a child wets his bed and then tries to hide the wet pajamas in the closet, it is possible that the bed-wetting itself is not available for direct interpretation or working with, but that the matter of his feeling as mani-fested by hiding his clothes can be taken up with him and discussed at some length, in the direction of altering this. Thus, the ego envelope within which the bed-wetting is clothed is worked with first. Such feelings and thoughts as he has about the bed-wetting itself will then gradually have a chance to appear and can, we hope, in time be worked with directly.

How these defenses are coped with, however, is a matter of considerable importance. If, for example, a child is re-proved for hiding his clothes and told with more or less sternness that this is not the way to handle wet clothes, that these things have to be put in the clothes hamper or given to the nurse, the chances of getting anything but increased defensiveness about the bed-wetting are very slight. On the other hand, a kindly and warmly accepting response to the entire situation with the assurance about lack of need for being embarrassed about this—that it is perfectly alright, that we do not punish or get angry at boys who wet their beds, and certainly he can go ahead and put his clothes in like anybody else—may provide a certain reassurance, but may not necessarily alter the situation much in the direction of understanding the bed-wetting; indeed, this type of reassurance may simply announce to the child that such pleasure seeking as may be hidden in this behavior is perfectly alright in this environment, and thus perpetuate the symptom. However, if the circumstances are spelled out for the child somewhat differently, perhaps first with a discussion of his need to avoid discovery and his inability to ask for help, and with some emphasis on the reasons for this, later with some explanation that bed-wetting has feelings hidden in it, feelings which are perhaps embarrassing, so that one hides the pajamas just as one hides the feelings, and finally the notion that the way to get help is to work with and talk about these feelings even if they are uncomfortable because that is what all of us are here for—to give help around such problems as this—in time, this approach might begin to move him in a therapeutic direction, one which comes to grips with whatever underlies the bed-wetting.

The complexity of this approach is not to be underestimated. There are many fine layers of defense and pleasure that have to be worked with in any given area of behavioral difficulty. It is the pleasure of what the child is doing *now*, or what he has just been doing that we have to point up, and the way he uses this behavior again and again to hide from what his problems really are. He acts the big bully on the one hand because it is fun to hurt and on the other because way down deep he is really afraid and this whole performance is to try to hide this both from himself and from us. All of this may have to be repeated again and again in a variety of ways by numerous persons in ad hoc situations and handling. If the tactics are properly undertaken, we will presently, as the frightened baby who was hidden behind the bully begins to show itself, be in the position of having to switch to ego-support techniques.

So much then for what I see as the two current areas of

major interest and development. One can hope that increasing refinements in ego psychology will in time lead to more specific techniques in both of these areas with increasing sureness of method and approach.

The question of psychotherapy so far has been avoided in this discussion; we come to it now. It is appropriate to reexamine the place of traditional psychotherapy within properly executed residential treatment. Generally speaking, youngsters in residence confront us primarily with the problem of massive ego weakness in some form and hence with a situation where the treatment response needs to be as massive. Can this best be achieved where patient and therapist meet in isolation and work problems out by themselves?

We have recently attempted two different approaches to this question at the National Institute of Mental Health. The first was the more classic in form. The therapist was a person apart from the residence proper to whose office the child was brought at fixed times for interviews that were scheduled, regular, and frequent. It is noteworthy that even in this setup a good deal of communication went on between the therapist and many persons in the child's environment, including the individual counselors. Indeed, therapists took a very active role in determining policy; they functioned in the role of consultants to the director of the cottage, and expressed their satisfactions or dissatisfactions about the youngster's program and how he was being handled. Occasionally, the counselor staff members felt that the pressures from the therapists were very intense and very uncomfortable, as well as diametrically opposed to the staff's own view of the child's needs. From their vantage point, therapists were occasionally quite perturbed by a failure of others to communicate some detail of the child's ward behavior, or by the failure of some communication *from* them, via whomever they spoke to about it, concerning what should be done with the child. Indeed, one

sometimes had the experience of their pointing to disturbances saying in effect, "I told you so," because something
they had advised was not noted or given adequate attention.
It was a not infrequent source of administrative difficulty to
integrate the activities of interested and active therapists and
an interested and active cottage staff.

On the other hand, we had an entirely different type of
operation going on in which the various youngsters involved
were worked with very actively by a staff headed by one ward
doctor. Both the staff and the patients were his, as it were,
to do with as he saw fit. He was called upon by the various
staff members to interview children in time of stress; he led
some of the children's group meetings, particularly those
centering around ad hoc behavioral issues; and he worked
consistently with the staff people around specific problems
raised by the interrelationship between these children and
the adults. From time to time, various youngsters would ask
him to take them to the playroom. They were familiar with
the fact that playrooms existed in the setting, although there
were no structured hours or regular appointments for any
of them there. Most interviews between this doctor and the
various children took place either in their own sleeping room
or in his ward office. These interviews were usually directed
toward some troublesome incidents of one sort or another,
or arose in connection with a chronic problem which had
been observed more and more clearly with the passage of
time and which had been decided upon at staff meeting as
an issue which should be worked on with this child. Superficially speaking, the material that emerged from many of
the interviews approximated in content what one would normally expect to find in psychotherapeutic interviews of the
more conventional kind. More generally, from the methodological point of view, it would seem that one is here accomplishing a type of "residential treatment" which is

strongly expressive in character, psychoanalytic in orientation, clearly built upon interviews with the children around matters of central importance to their development, and, withal, quite different from traditional psychoanalytic technique or a clinic's psychotherapy arrangements. Moreover, it should be emphasized that the ward doctor's interpretations and tactics did not remain his alone; all the staff were instructed in the action that was now to be taken toward a given child and the interpretations that needed to be stressed, so that the doctor's interview was the vanguard of a total staff technique of response. It was also part of our thinking that as a child's ego improved and became more competent, the need for an all-embracing therapy diminished accordingly, and the appropriateness of the normal analytic structure returned. When the child could handle many of his problems himself and could confine his vital difficulties to the therapy context, he was ready for more conventional therapy.

To summarize, we can observe several groups of environments: one which exists primarily to support therapy; another which emphasizes the development of good relationships with and imitation of the various staff members; and yet another which tends to use ego-support and ego-analysis practices as part of the milieu. The question of styles in residential therapy has been raised and a suggestion offered for an approach in which the roles of therapist and administrator are combined.

8

INTRODUCTION

Theory and Practice of Intensive Residential Treatment of Adolescents, by Donald B. Rinsley

The recent history of psychoanalysis has been marked by a turn toward clinical interest in severe disorders and, as a corollary, theoretical interest in issues of very early (preoedipal) development. This latter trend, represented by the work of Mahler, Kernberg, and Kohut in the United States and by the so-called "object relations theorists" (Guntrip, Fairbairn) and the Kleinians (Segal, Rosenfeld) in England, has been of natural interest to students of residential treatment, since most of the patients they deal with suffer from what Giovacchini (1979) has called "primitive mental states."

This growing tendency is clearly reflected in Rinsley's work. His conception of the therapeutic process in residential treatment is founded on a view of psychopathology that is rooted in object relations theory, a theory which emphasizes the pathogenic role of affective deprivation, early object losses, and pathological mourning processes (see Masterson and Rinsley, 1975; Masterson, 1978). Rinsley describes with great clarity an approach to treatment that addresses specific resistances and defensive operations, making use of interpretive and behavioral measures designed to deal with them. He is categorical in his insistence on the necessity for behavioral control of a closed unit, and of enforced separation from parents during the early phases of the treatment program. Both of these propositions are challenged in the papers of Erlich (Chapter 9) and Williams (Chapter 10), as well as by the work of Zinner and R. Shapiro (1972) and E. Shapiro (1978).

8

Theory and Practice of Intensive Residential Treatment of Adolescents

Donald B. Rinsley, M.D.

I am particularly pleased to address you under the auspices of the Institute of the Pennsylvania Hospital, first American hospital to open its doors to the sick. For I am by profession a hospital psychiatrist, a physician whose efforts are devoted to those whose mental sufferings are of such a nature and extent as to require the hospital ward in order to emerge from the dissembling limbo of their illness. It is not unfitting, moreover, that a hospital psychiatrist should address you at a particular point in the evolution of our discipline when we are beset with the polyglot claims of the so-called "third psychiatric revolution"—community mental health—some of whose advocates would assert that the proper goal of the mental hospital should be its own demise.[1]

I welcome further an opportunity to discuss with you my own special interest in the vast domain of psychiatry, the

Reprinted by permission from *Psychiatric Quarterly*, 42:611-638, 1968. New York: Human Sciences Press.

[1]For recent concise statements concerning the possible impact of the community mental health movement on the training and identity of the psychiatric clinician, see Kernberg (1968), Kubie (1968), and Wallerstein (1968).

adolescent who needs residential treatment, a subject as timely as the steadily decreasing mean age of our population
and the steadily burgeoning variety of problems that our
adolescent youth have come to pose for the society in which
we all hold membership. Finally, I bring to my discussion an
admitted psychoanalytic bias, a point of view descended from
Freud, vivified in the therapeutic contributions of the tradition of the so-called healing pedagogues, of Anna Freud
(1927, 1931, 1936), Federn (1926-1952), Aichhorn (1925,
1922-1948), Schwing (1954), and Sechehaye (1951, 1956),
and theoretically deepened in the writings of the so-called
British School of object relations, most notably those of Me-
lanie Klein (1950, 1961), Fairbairn (1954), and Guntrip,
(1961). The historical basis from which I shall take my departure includes the pioneering efforts of Simmel (1929) to
apply the insights of psychoanalysis to the treatment of hospital patients, extended in turn by the Menninger brothers
in Topeka (Menninger, 1936, 1937, 1939) and leavened by
the development of the child guidance movement in the
United States. Among the questions I propose to consider
are: What characteristics determine an individual's need for
residential, hospital, or inpatient treatment? What, in turn,
are the characteristics of the residential milieu that are conducive to lasting reorganization of the personality, and not
merely to those more superficial processes generally termed
"sealing over," "transference cure," or, more banally, "symptomatic dissimulation"? What is the natural history of the
hospital course of those patients who undergo the experience
of significant intrapsychic reorganization, as compared with
those who do not? Finally, what particular modifications of
the hospital setting are essential for optimal psychiatric treatment of the adolescent with the more severe forms of psychopathology?

THE "WEAK" EGO

As Simmel noted some 40 years ago (1929), individuals who by whatever route eventuate in the psychiatric hospital are regularly found to suffer from a variety of difficulties that together comprise the protean syndrome of ego weakness (Rinsley, 1968). We generally diagnose such persons as borderline or "as if" (Deutsch, 1942), or else append to them such labels as schizophrenic, psychotic, character neurotic ("psychopathic"), immature, impulse neurotic, polymorphous perverse, or infantile narcissistic (Gralnick, 1966). Careful genetic-dynamic study of these individuals reveals a variety of characteristics of the weak ego, including:

1. failure of normal repression;
2. persistence of primitive mechanisms of defense, with reliance on projection, introjection, regression, and denial;
3. impairment of the ego's synthetic function, leading to disruption of self-environment relations and dissemblement of perceptual, cognitive-ideational, affective, and motoric functions;
4. predominance of anxiety of the instinctual type;
5. lack of "basic trust";
6. pervasive impairment of object relations;
7. failure of sublimation of "raw" instinctual impulses;
8. persistence of primary-process thinking with reliance on transitivity, and gestural and word magic;
9. persistence of primary narcissism, associated with which are varying degrees of infantile megalomania;
10. serious difficulties with preoedipal and sexual identity.

The clinical manifestations of these underlying coping or

defense mechanisms include pervasive inability to trust, depression, impaired tolerance for frustration, failure to interpose thought between instinctual need and direct action aimed at relieving it, hence undue access of instinctual drives to motility; or else the individual's behavior, if not excessively action-oriented per se, seems otherwise peculiar, dissembled, or bizarre. As a result, there ensue various degrees of disruption of interpersonal communication and social disarticulation. As a consequence, in the majority of cases, others—the family, friends, and associates or representatives of the wider social community—bring the patient to the hospital. It is precisely in these cases in which one discovers the apparent lack of motivation for that nice cooperation between patient and therapeutic figure that classical psychoanalytic therapists put forth as a prime requisite for successful therapy, supposedly indicative of "lack of insight," hence illustrative of unsuitability for optimal reconstruction of the personality or "cure."

If reliance on the aforementioned coping mechanisms bespeaks the seriously ill adult, it more or less normally characterizes the intrapsychic organization of children, whence one calls it immature or puerile. Inasmuch as the clinical manifestations are in both instances similar, one refers to the seriously ill adult as immature or regressed, the latter from a presumably higher level of psychosexual function. Like the psychotic adult, the child, by virtue of the immaturity of his ego, will tend to act out. Deficient in self-objectification and in well-developed secondary-process or categorical ideation, which Piaget (Inhelder and Piaget, 1958) tells us develops only by early adolescence, the child will prove incapable of conceptualizing his need for treatment and the motivation of his prospective therapist to help him. Hence, if judged by the standards of the dynamically oriented therapist of the neurotic adult, the child will give the appearance of lack of motivation. Like the psychotic adult, the child normally, and the sick child overwhelmingly, must depend on the auxiliary adult egos who would treat him in the same fashion as his parents whom he would otherwise depend on for love, including protection, support, instruction, and the proper application of external controls for his actions. Hence, the intensity of the sick child's labile, direct parentifying transference to the prospective helping adult.[2]

The nature of this direct transference to treatment figures requires further elucidation. First, the life of the preadolescent or adolescent child is organized around the child's dependency on parental figures, whether the latter are natural parents or surrogates; hence, their teachers, coaches, scout leaders, and older siblings and peers come to be invested with needs, wishes, urges, and fantasies displaced from the primary parental objects, or, more properly, from the mental representations of the latter. This major aspect of childish transference assumes even more cogent significance for adolescents, one of whose major struggles involves powerful strivings toward emancipation from parental surrogates, leading in turn into pervasively ambivalent needs both to devalue and, paradoxically, to remain dependent on them. Thus, the normally labile transference of children becomes the more so among adolescents, replete as it is with further decathexis of parents, multiple anxieties over psychobiological experiences and functions, and substitute object-seeking, leading to the shifting bipolarity of instinctual drives and their affective derivatives so characteristic for the adolescent (Blos, 1941; A. Freud, 1958).

Second, the seriously ill adolescent suffers from oedipal fixations based, in turn, on traumata of a major degree earlier suffered at the hands of parents or equivalent surrogates.

[2]A cogent formulation of the significance of magical and parentifying expectations of the therapist is set forth by Rado (1956, 1962).

Hence, to the normal coping and defense mechanisms and identity struggles of adolescence are added, in these cases, a welter of cognitive, affective, and behavioral difficulties that are derived from very early insults to the archaic ego of the child. These, in turn, contribute to the patient's transference an added measure of ambivalence and lability, such that his treatment figures come to be invested with an extra measure of unneutralized instinct, of expectations and fear that represent the externalized vicissitudes of the patient's own internal object relations.

Third, adolescence is a period of life characterized in part by the individual's search for intimacy, by his efforts to bring his reservoir of infantile partial aims and his seeking of partial objects under the hegemony of genital primacy. His need for peer and adult models for identification in part witnesses various degrees of dynamic-genetic regression, with circular defusions and refusions of instincts and notable tendencies to reinstinctualize (Spiegel, 1951). Thus, reaggressivization and resexualization of previously autonomous ego functions contribute to the kaleidoscopic quality of the adolescent's self-seeking and object-seeking. Once again, these regressive tendencies are enormously accentuated among adolescents ill enough to require residential treatment, and they pose special problems for the adult treatment figures, whose countertransference is pulled hither and yon as a result of their needs both to enter and resist projective and introjective identifications with their young patients. These latter are wont to lead the adult figures into extremes of bipolar attitudes toward the management of the patient, which in turn reflect the bipolarity of the patient's own instinctual organization, namely, undue authoritarianism or undue permissiveness. In the former, one glimpses the elements of the new order therapies, exemplified in the writings of Szasz (1965), Glasser (1965), and Mowrer (1963a, 1963b), who emphasize behavioral conformity to accepted modes of conduct, or the assumption of responsibility by the patient, or who attempt to build in or strengthen the superego, as it were. In the latter, one glimpses a variety of antiauthoritarian reaction formations, which find expression in a congeries of laissez-faire, permissive approaches to the care of patients. These often involve the misapplication to adolescents of such varied modalities as classical psychoanalytic technique, therapeutic community, and child-centered methods based presumably on progressive educational views and organismic concepts that claim that, if left to themselves, children (including sick ones) will intuitively and spontaneously "actualize themselves," or will otherwise make the right decisions for themselves, much as laboratory rats will self-select appropriate diets.

The effect of overauthoritarianism is, of course, to preclude or forestall the patient's attempts to gain mastery by maintaining what amounts to an essentially megalomanic attitude toward the child and this, in turn, often reflects the adult's misguided efforts to defend against the infantile grandiose, narcissistic wishes that the child projects onto him. The effect of overpermissiveness is basically the same, for if the adult spuriously invests the child with adultomorphic powers, the child will inevitably misapply them, and hence will fail.

A fourth aspect of direct adolescent transference is of special importance in those cases in which the patient's fixations date from early infancy, prior to the inception of the normal mother-child symbiosis, which ordinarily flowers during the latter half of the first year of life. These adolescents, developmentally deviant from the very earliest postnatal period, comprise a group of patients whom Fliess (1961) would classify as autistic-presymbiotic—including the classical autistic children first described by Kanner (1943, 1949)—and whom Bender (1947, 1953, 1956) would classify as pseudodefective.

They are characterized by sweeping psychobiological deficiencies and dyssynchronies, and are not rarely mistakenly
supposed to have no object relationships. Careful clinical
study reveals, to the contrary, a pervasive, bizarre, fragmented autistic pseudocommunity, populated by a welter of
magical hallucinatory internal objects, the majority of which
are monstrous, terrifying, or "bad." The patient combines a
congeries of self- and object perceptions characterized by a
most intense fear and suspicion of others, and by a profound
degree of infantile megalomania specific for the stage of
primary narcissism; or else, one readily observes the persistence of the prenarcissistic condition to which Freud (1914)
referred as autoerotic, during which the various erogenous
zones pursue pleasure gain, as it were, mutually independently, without benefit of any degree of psychic organization.

Though individual psychotherapy is the cornerstone of the
treatment of such adolescents, the ward staff must wrestle
with the patient's exceedingly primitive introjective and projective defenses as the latter urgently seeks and yet is terrified
by and must massively resist fusion with them. In these more
primitive cases, the overall treatment pivots about the need
to build in, as it were, those "good objects," derived from the
patient's identification with the psychotherapist, which will,
it is hoped, serve as nuclei about which the earliest, most
archaic ego functions and representations will proceed to
crystallize. Thus, the milieu supports the individual treatment process, beset as the latter often is with innumerable
misunderstandings among the therapist and the other staff
members, which reflect the variable extent to which staff
members have become enmeshed in the patient's profuse use
of splitting defenses.

A fifth aspect of adolescent transference concerns the
child's defensive maneuvers with respect to the early object
losses, which are regular features of the history of the resi-

dential patient of this age. By the term "object loss," I refer to those situations in which key surrogate figures died, were lost through parental separation or divorce, or were in effect psychologically unavailable to the young child as a result of their own psychopathology. Early object loss leads the child into the persistent use of splitting, wherein the object loss is simultaneously and ambivalently both affirmed and denied (or, better, disavowed) by the ego (Freud, 1927, 1940). The splitting is, in these cases, associated with longstanding depression; the latter manifests itself in a wide variety of regressive symptoms so peculiar to children (Rinsley, 1965), in contrast to the classical depression of adults, a subject to which I shall later refer. As a result, the residential patient perceives adult treatment figures in terms of this background of loss, ambivalence, and splitting, and shows enhanced degrees of alternating anaclitic clinging and negativistic pseudo independence in respect to them. Thus, coupled with the patient's desperate need for objects is the fear that the objects he invests, hence on whom he comes to depend, will in the end desert him. Another way of viewing the patient's predicament would be to say that the patient despairs of object constancy, or is devoid of trust.

In such cases, the patient brings into play a congeries of restitutive efforts that center on a further regression to defenses of an introjective and projective nature, based, as is well known, on the mechanism of splitting. The lost object is reintrojected in order that its actual disappearance may be denied. But along with the reintrojected mental representation of the object are also reincorporated the welter of aggressive attributes that the child has previously projected into it, so that what is, as it were, taken in comprises in essence a hostile superego introject.[3] The clinical result is profound

[3] I use the term "superego introject" to refer to notably punitive, underpersonified or "unmetabolized" introjects of an archaic nature which have not become assimilated into the unconscious defenses of the ego. See Jacobson (1964) and Kernberg (1966).

guilt. Thus the patient feels that he has brought about the death of a natural parent, or parental separation or divorce, or has visited on his siblings a wide variety of insults and injuries; he feels himself to be "bad," which may mean destructive, homicidal, "crazy," stupid, and the like.

Much of the labile, kaleidoscopic, manipulative behavior of adolescent inpatients stems from the above. Their provocative alloplasticity, often called "transference splitting" or "transference diffusion," in part represents ambivalent efforts to work through the traumata associated with early object loss. The patient's guilt leaves him poignantly susceptible to the recurrent fear that intimacy with a love object will repel the latter, that his love destroys, that there is no real prospect for object constancy, hence that he is foredoomed to rejection and psychological starvation (Fairbairn, 1954). As a result, one witnesses the adolescent patient's abiding suspicion of adults, coupled with his peculiarly transilient efforts to extract from them proof of their love for him while he counterphobically acts in a manner to ward them off (Rinsley and Inge, 1961).

Some Axioms of Residential Treatment

The aforementioned characteristics of the transference of the adolescent residential patient are essential for an understanding of the child's immediate postadmission behavior. In part because of his intense struggle over dependency needs, the adolescent, who is often sensitively aware of his need for help, nonetheless can admit it only in the most obscure, oblique ways. As a result, he often seems unmotivated or resistant. The form and variety of the adolescent's resistances are described in greater detail below (see Rinsley and Inge, 1961). But the basic issue concerns the salient fact that inasmuch as early resistance behavior is heavily loaded with transference, the forms it assumes provide notable insight into the manner in which the patient has dealt with and attempted to regulate his relationships with key figures from his past, generally parents or equivalent surrogates, as these come to be expressed within the residential setting. Some learning theorists would perhaps say that the patient will perseverate in the use of outmoded, maladaptive, insufficiently drive-reducing adjustive techniques and that his illness in part expresses the narrowness of his coping hierarchy.

A first axiom of residential treatment would therefore hold that, to the degree to which the treatment setting otherwise tolerates or abets the patient's ongoing use of early transference resistances, their underlying significance will remain obscure, hence uninterpretable, and, further, that the patient will remain unengaged with the staff members. The obvious corollary to this axiom holds, therefore, that the residential milieu must provide controls for the patient's behavior, in some cases stringent ones, to preclude direct drive discharge through motility, and to rechannel it via intercalated processes, namely, thought and verbal communication. To this end, the closed ward is essential, for it alone provides the security of carefully titrated behavioral restrictions which must operate to force the patient back on and within himself.

A second axiom concerns the matter of the patient's contacts, both vis-à-vis and via correspondence, with members of his family. Inasmuch as the child's psychopathology develops within and in part gives expression to a skewed, pathological familial constellation, interruption of the hierarchy of pathogenic interactions among the patient and other family members must be effected as quickly as possible. In order to accomplish this with a minimum of serious trauma to all concerned, a concomitant psychiatric casework process is begun, within which the staff caseworker initiates the diagnostic study of the family, while simultaneously assisting the family to deal with the often profound anxieties that rapidly develop when a family member previously necessary for their repression or scotomatization has been removed. Often these anxieties propel the remaining parents and siblings into herculean, even bizarre efforts to undo their separation from the child, to so contaminate their contacts with him with double-binding communications as to decimate the patient's treatment by intimidating him into redoubling his resistance behavior. In some cases, the parents will attempt to bring attorneys, clergymen, interested friends, employers, public or political figures, other relatives, and a variety of other avuncular persons into the early diagnostic process, or may threaten litigation or even violence in eleventh-hour efforts to intimidate the staff into releasing the patient. Careful study of the family members' own early resistance maneuvers reveals that they both cover and convey a welter of terrifying fantasies, which become projected onto the treatment milieu in general and the figure of the caseworker in particular, and which they will attempt to communicate to the patient (Rinsley and Hall, 1962). Thus, the staff must have the necessary legal armamentarium with which to enforce, if need be, the parent-child separation and, during this early period of inception of treatment, must carefully regulate the patient's family visits and correspondence.

A third axiom of residential treatment concerns the use of specific restrictions of the patient's behavior, a matter of importance throughout the entire course of the patient's residence but of even greater significance during the early period of treatment. In connection with the matter of restrictions, I shall have recourse to the following relevant if oversimplified graphic representation (see Figure 1). W represents what one could call "useful psychological work," a term notoriously difficult to define, roughly analogous to the thermodynamic concept of free energy and to the psychological concept of goal- or task-oriented secondary-process thought and action;

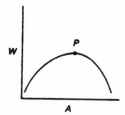

FIGURE 1

a key component of *W*, from our point of view, turns out to be related to the patient's ability to respond to verbal restraint or control from the staff members and to comprehend the significance of the interpretations they offer him. *A* denotes anxiety, in our cases predominantly of the instinctual type, whereas *P* denotes a critical point of inflection. That portion of the curve to the left of *P* we shall call the ascending limb, whereas that portion of the curve to the right of *P* we shall call the descending limb.

For individuals situated somewhere on the ascending limb of the work-anxiety curve, each increment of anxiety leads to a corresponding increment of psychological work; put more succinctly, one may say that under such circumstances, anxiety motivates. Similarly, in the case of an individual situated on the descending limb of the curve, further increments of anxiety yield corresponding decrements of work; we say, therefore, that under such circumstances, anxiety disorganizes.

Now it may be said that the overwhelming majority of residential patients undergo referral for admission because the level of their instinctual anxiety has propelled them onto the descending limb of the work-anxiety curve, past the point of inflection, *P*. This level of anxiety has, in turn, induced the well-known traumatic state of the ego, with more or less paralysis of autonomous ego functions and regression to the use of those primitive defenses or coping mechanisms to which I have already referred. As the traumatic state is known to result from breakdown of the defense mechanisms of the ego in the wake of relatively excessive endopsychic and/or external stimulation, the immediate therapeutic task resolves itself into efforts to limit incident stimuli. For this general purpose, we may use judicious dosages of ataraxic medication, or limit the patient's overstimulating peer interactions by restricting him to the ward or to his room; in some cases in which the patient finds himself beset by panic of a degree that has led to dissolution of his defenses against anxiety, a period of seclusion may be indicated (Charney, 1963).

The psychoanalyst would view such a program as justifiably analogous to the function of the infant's maternal surrogate figure as a stimulus barrier against both excessive exogenous stimulation and endogenous affectomotor storms (Bergman and Escalona, 1949; Masterson, 1968). Concomitantly, it promotes the patient's investment in the staff figures, whose early function amounts to protecting him while allowing a comfortable degree of regression to proceed apace. Most important, however, is relocation of the patient to a point somewhere on the ascending limb of the work-anxiety curve. So situated, he begins to reassume an increasing degree of self-control, to communicate more coherently with the staff, and to experience relief from the terrifying feelings of loss of control which have characterized his pretreatment state.

THE RESISTANCE PHASE OF RESIDENTIAL TREATMENT

As many authors have noted, the family member who comes to be identified as the patient emerges from a long-standing pathogenic manifold of familial intercommunications;[4] indeed, Zentner and Aponte (1970) have termed it

---

[4]For a concise review of major contributions to this exceedingly important area of psychiatric research, see Mishler and Waxler (1966).

the "amorphous family nexus." Many of these families are dissocial, alienated groups with varying degrees of effective social façade, whose membership is characterized by diffuse, shifting, interchangeable individual identities, multiple-binding communications, *pars pro toto* and *totum pro parte* roles, and superficially unpredictable lines of authority; thus they have been termed "skewed." Such families, or pseudofamilies, offer to their members a variety of protective gratifications, and the characteristic of the patient is his inability, for whatever reasons, to continue to use them; thus, the family appeals, with profound ambivalence, to the dreaded extrafamilial authorities or agencies for help, or else the patient is wrested from them despite their overt or covert protests. The purposes for which the help is sought are, of course, legion. The intricate if bizarre family nexus may be disintegrating, and the patient is selected out to communicate this. Or, one or more family members may perceive that the patient's continued presence in their midst threatens their composite existence; hence he must at least temporarily be expelled—though not rarely the patient may in fact be the least ill family member, and the burgeoning conflict between his own ineluctable urge for growth and the family's pathogenic pressures on him force him apart from them, by whatever means or route. Whatever the case, the family directly or otherwise carries its deviant member to the helping agency for its own purposes, which, in the case of families of severely ill adolescents, amount to a need either to get rid of him outright, or else to induce the agency to refurbish him so that he may once again assume his usual place, basically unaltered, within the family nexus.

The profound dislocation of the family's and the agency's respective expectations of the latter's functions of treatment contributes heavily to the wide spectrum of patient and family members' behavior which subserve the function of resistance to treatment. In the case of adolescent residential patients, the various resistance maneuvers subserve the need to preserve ongoing fusion or symbiotic ties, based in turn on the preoedipal fixations to which I have already referred. A particularly subtle manner in which the patient and the family will unconsciously conspire to accomplish refusion, described in detail by Zentner and Aponte (1970), is to behave in such ways as to attempt to incorporate the treatment structure into the family's nexus, to render the former into an arm of the latter, so to speak. Thus, the generalization common to the aforementioned axioms becomes: the major purpose of identifying, interpreting, and precluding the patient's and the parents' early resistance behavior is to precede refusion among them, hence to detach the patient from the pathogenic family nexus and to promote his engagement with the treatment staff. As already noted, the treatment facility must have at its disposal for this purpose, and be prepared to use fully and definitively, whatever legal means are available for those cases in which the family's and the patient's efforts to refuse assume herculean proportions.

The spectrum of the adolescent residential patient's resistance maneuvers, which ordinarily occupy a period of from six months to a year following admission, and the metaphorical communications they convey have been described elsewhere (Rinsley and Inge, 1961). I shall now briefly recapitulate them.

Identification with the aggressor. The patient in various ways attempts to imitate the adults' behavior in an as-if effort to ward off the latter. Included here are the well-known assistant doctor, assistant nurse, assistant aide, and related counterphobic efforts to scotomatize archaic instinctual urges which the patient has projected into the adult staff members.

Leveling. The patient attempts to make siblings or peers of the treatment figures. Leveling constitutes a rather more ad-

vanced variety of counterphobic maneuver than simple identification with the aggressor; certainly it displays a somewhat
greater use of intellectualization. Included under leveling are
the well-known buddy-buddy, pal, and we girls phenomena;
in addition, one notes the occasional adolescent inpatient
whose otherwise smooth pseudo reasonableness covers massive attempts to isolate affect and cover profuse use of projection; thus, intellectualized admissions or confessions of
illness (the famous adolescent copout), "Let's discuss things
as equals," and related maneuvers often signify leveling, the
more so during the resistance phase of treatment.

Flirtatiousness and seductiveness. The patient attempts to sex-
ualize the relationship with treatment figures. Techniques of
sexualization are legion, vary from the most subtle to the very
crude, generally have notably aggressive significance, and
allow notable insights into the adolescent's transference.
These maneuvers pose some of the knottiest countertransference problems that staff members must face; they are
particularly difficult in the case of the typical, all-American
boy and the genuinely physically attractive adolescent girl,
neither of whom, despite otherwise severe psychopathology,
looks sick.

Oversubmissiveness. Oversubmissiveness, obsequiousness, or
sycophantic behavior (including shuffling or the Uncle Tom
phenomenon common among black adolescents) comprise
yet another counterphobic maneuver.

Persistent avoidance. More frequent among the most seriously ill adolescents, persistent avoidance includes frank negativism, muteness, marked aboulia and apathy, seclusiveness,
sleepiness, disruptive efforts to provoke isolation, various
forms of seizure and dissociative phenomena (including self-
induced seizures in patients with epilepsy), absorption in daydreaming fantasy, and stubborn or persistent refusal to eat
(anorexia nervosa).

Scapegoatism includes such phenomena as denigration or vilification of ward peers ("He's stupid," "She's crazy," and so on), and efforts to manipulate wardmates into proxy roles by which the peer acts out for the subject (behind-the-scenes manipulator phenomenon); the purpose is to draw staff attention to others, hence away from oneself. The inverse or passive form of scapegoatism is also not infrequent: The patient actively or passively provokes verbal and/or physical assault from others—the personification of the injustice-collecting masochist; such an adolescent is invariably found to harbor a paranoid world view, perceives both peers and staff as hostile predators, and assuages depression through flagellation.

Outright rebelliousness. The major function of wildly disruptive ward behavior in part subserves the need to ward off closeness to staff figures by attempting to force them into unremitting efforts to provide simple and direct behavioral control; the underlying need for closeness is, however, glimpsed in the direct, physical staff-patient contact that the disruptive actions provoke. In many cases, outright rebelliousness represents a form of passive scapegoatism.

Transference diffusion. This is an exceedingly frequent and important resistance maneuver among hospitalized adolescents. It includes various forms of playing favorites, a wide spectrum of staff-splitting and manipulations of peers, gossiping and tale-carrying, aimed at keeping knowledge of oneself spread thinly enough to preclude any one of the treatment figures from obtaining a comprehensive view of oneself.

Somatization. Multiple bodily complaints serve to ward off staff attention to thoughts, feelings, fantasies, delusional preoccupations, and the like, as well as to communicate nonverbal material (body language). Careful analysis of the complaints will, however, often uncover the hidden (repressed) inner experiences.

Peer-Age caricaturing. Also called "out-typifying oneself," this consists in a variety of actions that seem to convey the patient's need to be viewed as a typical adolescent. The behavior ever so slightly exaggerates such things as dietary fads, emotional lability, popular idealizations, and the general excesses adults are wont to associate with typical adolescent behavior.

Clique formation. Seriously ill adolescents are incapable of generating normal teenage peer groups; the normal-appearing small groups they are prone to form on the ward are usually found to serve the need to share data about themselves with one another that never reach the treatment staff. Needless to say, such groups require the most assiduous scrutiny and staff regulation, particularly during the resistance phase of treatment, lest peer-peer relationships dilute or eliminate peer-staff relationships, which are, of course, essential for the individualized treatment each patient requires.

"Craziness" and pseudostupidity. The defensive function of disorganized ("crazy") behavior is to arrest, enthrall, or paralyze, hence to ward off the treatment figures. Similarly, the pseudostupid patient conveys the message, "I'm so stupid that you can't expect much from me (hence I can remain unengaged)."

Artistic pursuits. Included here are such varied activities as unsupervised autobiographical-novel and short-story writing, solitary drawing and game-playing, and premature diary-keeping; of particular relevance are complex or bizarre drawing and painting, and pseudoscientific preoccupations, such as electronic circuitry, graphic anatomical productions, and the like. Such pursuits have immense, if often autistic communicative significance; in many cases, they must be interrupted or interdicted, lest the patient remain immersed in them to the exclusion of consensual communication with treatment figures.

Elopement. Running away is a complex, overdetermined phenomenon, connected with all sorts of aggressive, erotic, rescue, and reunion fantasies. When it occurs, it obviously terminates therapeutic contact between the patient and the treatment staff.

SOME REMARKS ON PARENTAL RESISTANCE METAPHORS

As already noted, the patient's resistance behavior has enormous transference meaning; in addition, it expresses anguish over separation from his parents, or else from his fantasy constructs which serve as dereistic substitutes for them; at root, it conveys the expression of refusion or reunion fantasies. Concomitant with the flowering of the patient's resistances are those of the parents, whose fantasies are no less elaborate nor regressive than are the patient's. Careful study of the parents' fantasies during the resistance phase of their child's treatment discloses that they are, as expected, compounded of primitive aggressive and erotic wishes, that they are at root preoedipal, and that they are exceptionally prone toward displacement or projection onto the treatment staff and the physical characteristics of the hospital (transference to the hospital per se), in general, and onto the caseworker, in particular. The latter will in general develop only if the treatment structure precludes transmission of the parents' resistance messages to the patient.

Our own study of early parental resistance metaphors has led us to classify them as they in turn express (1) the parents' narcissistic or self-preoccupations, (2) the parents' view of the family's endogenous efforts to maintain its precarious equilibrium, and (3) the parents' particular ways of depersonifying the child, hence of attempting to put him to psychological use in ways that violate his own juvenile identity (Rinsley and Hall, 1962).

Insofar as the family is in various degrees dissocial, or in metastable equilibrium with extrafamilial objects and situations, revelation through whomever or by whatever means of the family members' idiosyncratic ways of maintaining the family group's pseudoequilibrium poses a severe threat to its perceived, ongoing integrity. Their overweening concern is that the child will "tell the family secrets," hence both their conscious and less than conscious efforts to admonish the patient against the development of trusting ties with the treatment staff. Thus is derived the patient's dilemma: If he acts on his nascent perception that the staff members can somehow be trusted, he courts disaster to his family, including loss of the parental figures; if he successfully resists treatment, he remains ill. Thus does the apparent paradox transpire that, from the child's point of view, getting well is worse than being sick, and a notable measure of the secondary gain of his illness lies in the preservation of his relationship with the parents and other members of his disordered family.

Rapid control of the patient's immediate postadmission behavior, regulation of contacts between parents and child, judicious use of ataraxic medications when indicated, and carefully graduated increments of privileges lead the adolescent to a point at which the aforementioned resistance maneuvers come into full expression. As these develop, they are dealt with in turn by appropriate further control of the patient's behavior, coupled with interpretations directed at their underlying transference significance. The major purpose of the latter, which we may consider to represent the inception of the resistance work proper, is threefold: First, it has the effect of reassuring the patient that separation from his family, in particular from his primary parental objects, will not prove disastrous to him or to them; second, it serves to stimulate the patient's curiosity about himself, to get him thinking about his past history and current behavior; third, it aims to promote the patient's early identification with staff members, thereby further detaching him from his symbiotic ties with his parent figures.

The patient's early identifications with staff figures, which find their inception during the resistance phase of treatment, are different from those he will later make with them. During the resistance phase, they assume the qualities of primitive superego introjects, and hence signify to the patient the operations of external surrogate egos which, like the "good" maternal objects of infancy, protect the archaic ego by limiting incident stimuli, curb self-injurious actions and, in part through the discipline they inculcate, provide reassuring nurturance. The resultant reduction of the patient's instinctual anxiety moves him gradually toward the ascending limb of the work-anxiety curve, and hence makes possible increasing increments of responsive, interpretive work by the patient, done increasingly, now, in collaboration with the adult treatment figures, and in particular with the psychiatrist.

Provided that the analogous resistance work is accomplished in the parents' casework process, it transpires that, in most cases within six to 12 months, the patient has developed sufficient trust in the staff and the parents sufficient trust in their casework process, which represents the treatment structure to them, that the parents begin in earnest to relinquish the patient to the staff's care. Thus, the definitive resolution of the well-known loyalty problem begins to appear. Parents and child have come to perceive that they may indeed exist without each other, the former in various ways communicating to the patient that he may work with the staff without fear of injury to himself or to them or of reprisal from them.

Resistance Behavior as Protest

Ongoing clinical study of the adolescent patient's and the parents' resistance metaphors led us to the conclusion that these metaphors, expressed both verbally and nonverbally, could be viewed as more than crudely analogous to the behavior of prematurely separated infants, which Bowlby (1960a, 1960b, 1961, 1962) has termed protest (Rinsley, 1965). Several factors seemed indeed to support the analogy. First, the adolescent's otherwise natural tendency to recapitulate, hence to work through, earlier oedipal and preoedipal conflicts appeared highly relevant; furthermore, such recapitulative working through is regressive, and fluctuating proneness to regression is a hallmark of the adolescent's struggle toward an eventually stable identity.

Second, as already noted, the patient's resistance metaphors seemed to convey a powerful need to undo the parent-child separation, hence to bring back the child's lost objects and to reinvolve them; thus, the resistance metaphors regularly tended to assume the quality of mourning.

Third, we recall that the persistent reliance on the defense mechanism of splitting regularly characterizes the mourning reactions of the child as he ambivalently reaffirms and disavows the object loss he feels called on to mourn. Persistent use of splitting likewise affirms the child's ongoing fixation at, or regression to, the early predepressive (paranoid-schizoid) position of infancy (M. Klein, 1950), which signals the use of part-object relations. Thus, the adolescent's redoubtable tendency to split or manipulate represents the clinical emergence of his use of introjective and projective techniques for regulating his good and bad part object relations. It comes as no surprise, therefore, that the fundamental psychological traumata on which the adolescent residential patient's illness is based occurred during the infantile years, in a majority of cases during the predepressive period prior to the inception of the second year of life, a fact that careful historical and psychodynamic study of our patients has almost invariably revealed.

Viewed from a genetic-dynamic standpoint, successful management of the resistance phase of residential treatment precludes the patient's use of splitting and guides him ineluctably toward entrance into what must be considered as later manifestations of the original depressive position. As these changes occur, the resistance phase of treatment draws to a close, and the patient enters the next arena of his treatment, the phase of definitive treatment which I have chosen to call the phase of introject work.

THE DEFINITIVE PHASE OF RESIDENTIAL TREATMENT: THE PHASE OF INTROJECT WORK

As Aichhorn (1925) originally taught us, successful treatment depends on the respective capacities of patient and therapist for mutual identification. Resolution of the resistance phase of residential treatment thus proceeds from the patient's ability to identify with the treatment figures who are charged with his care; in particular, it proceeds from the child's trusting ability to have internalized in significant measure the external controls for his behavior which the residential milieu has supplied to him. Thus is set in motion a complex congeries of processes of growth, common in the experience of the healthily developing child, but deficient in that of the child who reaches the adolescent years hobbled by psychopathology serious enough to prevent successful negotiation of the oral stage of psychosexual development ("I am"), and beginning entry into the anal stage ("I am separate and distinct; I can control and master"). It is my view, therefore, that an adequate, intensive residential treatment process comes to develop, within an admittedly compressed span of time, the basic attributes of a healthy child-rearing experience.

A major characteristic of all children is their early infantile omnipotence, a residue of middle to late orality. The healthily developing child comes normally to project his omnipotence into the figures of his parents, leading to a sweeping over-estimation of his loved parental objects.[5] The seriously ill child, essentially devoid of parental object constancy early in life, has found the normal projection of omnipotence impossible, hence has, in effect, clung to it. As the young child's omnipotence is comprised of primitive (raw) aggressive and erotic instincts, their projection into the residential treatment figures evokes the patient's fear that they will retaliate, injure, destroy, or absorb him, a fear that also in part accounts for his resistance to them. Thus does resolution of the resistance phase of treatment imply the treatment figures' acceptance of the patient's megalomanic projections into them, without acting on the primitive wishes associated with the projections, a situation that cements strongly the bonds of mutual trust between the patient and themselves.

As the patient begins, now, to part with the nucleus of bad internal objects, which have long comprised the roots of his psychopathology, he parts as well with what have been basic components of his early, pathological identity. The loss of these parts of the self induces him to mourn for them; and the two major components of his mourning are the emergence of depression and the appearance of regression, both of which are, of course, inextricably interrelated.

[5]There is considerable evidence in support of the view that the origin of belief in an omnipotent deity is derived from the parents' further displacement of the child's megalomanic projections into them. This displacement is in turn seen to result from the parents' need to ward off (deny) the child's projections, which threaten to reawaken in the parents their own repressed infantile megalomania.

Among adolescents, whether hospitalized or not, the emergence of depression heralds far more than the otherwise classical picture, combining as does the latter the subjectively felt loss of self-esteem, sadness, and various degrees of psychomotor retardation. Rather the depression in these cases is rife with splitting, and with denial or disavowal. Thus, the patient's mourning for the loss of his departing introjects conveys far more than the process of object removal (A. Katan, 1937), for the objects that proceed to be removed are, as it were, pejorative, and their loss is accompanied, in the case of residential patients, by the most profound ambivalence; thus, the mourning becomes pathological. Pathological mourning among adolescents is a protean process. It is accompanied by sweeping regression in all areas of psychological function—cognitive-ideational, affective, sensory-perceptual, and even motoric. The patient proceeds to assume a more primitive clinical appearance, which includes fluctuant clinging dependency, marked negativism, notable swings of mood, and unpredictability; of great importance are the experiences of depersonalization and estrangement (derealization); overt thought disorder may reappear, with classical associative loosening, tangentiality, syncretism, and concretism, and the occurrence of grandiose, self-referential, and nihilistic delusions. There occurs regressive reinstinctualization of bodily parts and functions, with all manner of somatic difficulties and, in some cases, frank somatic delusions. The patient now begins to speak of his "badness" and "evilness"; he talks of destructive wishes, and he berates himself for his past misdeeds, and for the harm he feels he has visited on others. His terrifying experiences may indeed be likened to the drainage of pus from a long-concealed abscess, as a necessary step in the healing of tissue that the purulent matter had previously infiltrated and split apart.

Our extended observations of the behavior of the adolescent who has entered this phase of residential treatment have led to the conclusion that it is, at root, analogous to Bowlby's so-called second stage of infantile mourning, which he has termed the stage of despair. Common to both are the protean complexities of the "impure" depression of children. Indeed, the phenomena classically grouped about the concept of depression per se may be wholly or in largest measure overshadowed by the multiple regressive signs that portend the onset of a period of undoubted disorganization of the weak ego so characteristic of the residential patient of this age (Rinsley, 1965).

The emergence of bad internal part objects and the concomitant introjection of good ones are of basic importance for the successful treatment to which the residential milieu is oriented. First, it strongly reinforces the patient's beginning awareness, during the resistance phase, that he and his parents are indeed capable of separate existence. Second, it moves the patient progressively from a condition of primary narcissism toward increasing self-objectification, which means enhanced ability to sense and test reality, and to exert mastery over endopsychic and external events. Third, it signals the patient's entrance into the later, depressive position of infancy, during which he begins to perceive that his aggression, whether innate or derived from the aggressive cathexes associated with his bad introjects, is incapable of destroying what he comes increasingly to experience as whole objects; thus he moves from part- to whole-object relations. Underlying the above are the processes characteristic of this second, or later, form of the adolescent residential patient's identifications with his treatment figures, namely, the gradual metabolization and depersonification of his introjects as these become assimilated to his self-representations, and hence become a part of his ego (Jacobson, 1964; Kernberg, 1966). Fifth, the identifications on which these critical processes and experiences are based have sweeping effects on the economic dispositions within the child's ego. They lead to defusion of instincts, with ensuing liberation of both aggressive and erotic energies for subsumption under the ego's synthetic function; thus, neutralized aggression comes increasingly to drive the defensive functions of the unconscious part of the ego, whereas libido comes increasingly to drive the ego's synthetic and perceptual functions, leading the ego toward increasing use of sublimations and growth of secondary autonomy (Hartmann, 1950; Rinsley, 1967b, 1968).

It will be evident in what I have said that, from the standpoint of the residential patient, there are two exceptionally critical junctures in the residential treatment process, successful management of which has an important influence on the prognosis of the child's residential experience. The first is, of course, successful conclusion of the resistance phase, with subsequent entry into the definitive phase. The second critical juncture comprises the staff's capacity to withstand the protean, regressive turn of events in the definitive phase. A most important resistance with which all must deal is, as expected, staff countertransference resistances to the often exasperatingly difficult regressive behavior of the patient as the exchange of introjects sets in in earnest. Staff members' efforts to bring the latter to a halt, whether by efforts to suppress it or through their own regressive identifications with the patient, must be precluded in largest measure if the patient is to work through his painful experience of mourning.[6]

The processes of mourning of the hospitalized adolescent ordinarily require the better part of another year of residential treatment, if not rather longer. As they proceed, and

[6]Hendrickson (1969), Hendrickson, Holmes, and Waggoner (1959), and Holmes (1964) have written cogently concerning transference-countertransference problems with adolescent inpatients.

as their associated regression begins to recede, the patient becomes ready for increasing reassociation with his family, the members of which he has begun to view as distinct from himself, as increasingly real objects, whose limitations he may allow himself to understand without remaining enmeshed in them. His enhanced internal controls, based on identification with the staff members who have signified his auxiliary egos, lead him to a gradual expansion of privileges; thus, with careful guidance, he assumes increasing responsibility for what he does. The time now approaches at which continued, full-time residential treatment becomes unnecessary and, depending on the circumstances of the individual case, the patient may be discharged to the day hospital, or to his own home, or to foster placement, in many instances to continue his psychiatric treatment on an outpatient basis for a variable future period of time.

Though my remarks have comprised but a bare outline of the natural history of the complex residential experience of the adolescent in full-time hospital treatment, they nonetheless permit several conclusions concerning adolescent psychopathology and reconstructive as distinguished from symptomatic treatment in the residential setting (Rinsley, 1963).

I have reference, at the outset, to the important contributions of Masterson (1967, 1968) regarding the etiological significance of adolescent turmoil, with which I am in thorough agreement. He concludes that this omnibus term makes reference to a wide spectrum of personality difficulties of more ominous significance than is usually recognized. As a result, the more ominous psychopathological phenomena to which adolescent turmoil refers are commonly viewed as little more than manifestations of transient situational or adjustment problems, frequent enough among adolescents, of relatively superficial importance, and hence in need of superficial handling or management. I believe that this situational view of adolescent turmoil stems from several readily identifiable factors. First, from a diagnostic standpoint, the criteria for recognition of classical (schizophrenic) thought disturbance, set forth by Bleuler (1911) and developed by numerous careful students of categorical ideation, are as applicable to adolescents as to adults; failure to apply these criteria in the careful study of the formal processes of the adolescent's thinking regularly leads to an underestimation of the degree of the patient's psychopathology. A second factor involves failure to recognize the stereotypical characteristics of the pseudoamorphous, skewed, psychotogenic family to which I have already briefly referred, within which the adolescent residential patient is regularly discovered to have grown up and to which his illness in part gives graphic and tragic expression.

Yet a third factor, basic to the foregoing, concerns the adult's not inconsiderable difficulty in recognizing any sort of major psychopathology in children. Such a difficulty is in direct proportion to the extent to which any given adult must repress or even deny the variety of his own subjective difficulties during that age that is personified in the patient he may be called upon to study. The well-known adult countertransference to the presumably noisome adolescent finds expression in a variety of approaches to his problems; these appear with regularity in the psychiatric literature and tragically too frequently in the attitudes of professional workers (Rinsley, 1967a). Thus, one finds problems of underdiagnosis, to which I have already referred; one finds statements to the effect that "adolescents cannot be analyzed"; one finds well-meaning programs in which seriously ill adolescents are treated on adult hospital wards, motivated in part by the need to pare institutional budgets, which leads to the placement of sick children with sick adults, and results

in endless prolongation of the adolescents' resistance maneuvers; one hears of short-term programs for adolescent
treatment, in which little or no effort is made to help the
patient and his parents to recognize and resolve the herculean problems of their mutual resistances toward separation.
Finally, one hears the view, appropriate to the needs of the
less seriously ill child, and thoroughly incorrect for the more
seriously ill one, that it is better not to sunder a family by
attempting to treat one of its members outside it. This view,
in fact, represents a failure to appreciate the dereistic, dissocial pseudo organization of those families who produce
severely ill children. For the child, whether adolescent or
younger, trapped within a profoundly disordered family
unit, sanguine efforts at outpatient treatment are in many
cases foredoomed to failure: The residual family members
will exert powerful pressures on the child to resist the therapist's "dangerous" ministrations, and the pressures will succeed because the looser therapeutic structure is unable to
cope with them. In such instances, the so-called community
mental health approach, which advocates "bringing the treatment to the family in its own setting," in fact proceeds to
transport the treatment to the very worst place for its inception and fruition.

SUMMARY

We may summarize, now, the basic goals of intensive residential treatment for the two major groups of severely ill
adolescents who require the full therapeutic services of the
inpatient milieu.

As already noted, the autistic-presymbiotic ("nuclear," or
process, schizophrenic) adolescent, who has failed to experience the normal mother-infant symbiosis, requires a therapeutic program oriented toward its inception. For such an
adolescent, the full residential setting provides a highly con

crete, compulsively styled, maximally predictable environment, as free as possible from peer-competitive experiences, and organized to provide comprehensive support for the one-to-one or individual therapeutic process that serves as its foundation. The goal of the latter process comprises catalysis for the crystallization of basic or archaic ego nuclei, and points toward establishment of the patient-therapist symbiosis which symbolizes the earlier symbiosis that the patient has failed to develop. Once established, the patient-therapist symbiosis requires extended efforts directed toward desymbiotization, which signals the inception of the patient's first genuine efforts at emancipation or individuation. (See Figure 2 for a diagram of the process.)

In the case of the autistic-presymbiotic adolescent, establishment and beginning resolution of the patient-therapist symbiosis occur during the resistance phase of treatment. During that period, the patient comes to reexperience and to begin to work through the transference psychosis; hence the enormously archaic experiences consequent on very early object loss. Among the various factors contributory to the exceptional difficulty of this work with autistic-presymbiotic adolescents, two emerge with special clarity: First, the patient's early resistances assume herculean proportions, as a

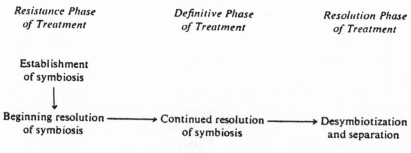

Figure 2

consequence of the terror that ensues whenever externalization of the bad internal objects threatens to occur; second, many such adolescents are products of thoroughly disorganized, fragmented pseudofamilies, or else have long since lost contact with parents or other family members. As a result, there is often little if anything in the way of concomitant casework treatment; hence the resistance phase of treatment is prolonged.

In the case of the symbiotic adolescent, essentially locked within a prolonged, unresolved mother-infant fusion relationship, the therapeutic goal comprises desymbiotization, with attendant emancipation and individuation. To this end, the predominant therapeutic work of the resistance phase of treatment is addressed to recognition, externalization, and interpretation of the adolescent's fantasies which center on reunion with and megalomanic control of family members, notably the parents, and especially the mother. As these occur, the residential program increasingly emphasizes progressive socialization, graduated expansion of privileges, peer-competitive participation, including residential school, occupational, and recreational therapy classes, and increased personal responsibility. Though individual psychotherapy may be prescribed, it is not considered essential for the symbiotic adolescent. (See Figure 3 for a diagram of the process.)

In keeping with the view that the psychoneurotic adolescent is rarely admitted into, nor long remains within, a carefully supervised residential setting, brief reference to the widespread problem of underdiagnosis of the severely ill adolescent is justifiable. (See Table 1.)

CONCLUSION

From the foregoing, one may distill the following generalizations concerning the intensive residential treatment of

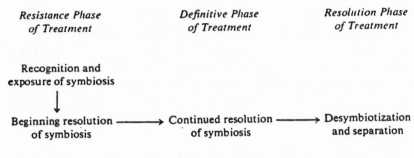

Figure 3

adolescents who demonstrate the more severe forms of psychopathology:

1. In the majority of such cases, physical or geographical separation of the patient from the remainder of his family members, notably his parents, is mandatory.

2. The patient should be admitted into a closed ward or cottage, within which careful scrutiny of, and application of appropriate controls for, his behavior become immediately operative.

3. A concomitant, dynamically oriented casework process with the patient's parents or with his responsible guardian surrogates should begin with his admission into residence.

4. Intensive psychiatric and parallel casework study of the patient and his family should begin coincident with his admission, utilizing the services of the full diagnostic team, including the admitting and ward psychiatrists, the clinical psychologist, the psychiatric social worker, the teacher of special education, and the ward or cottage nurse and aides or childcare workers. Though in a few instances the patient needs to resist the immediate postadmission study, the deepening intra- and interpersonal processes into which he feels himself to be plunged in most cases will be found to reassure him that those who are in charge of him are extremely in-

TABLE 1

RINSLEY'S TERMINOLOGY	EQUIVALENT DIAGNOSES	OFTEN MISDIAGNOSED
1. Autistic-presymbiotic psychosis of abolescence	Nuclear schizophrenia Process schizophrenia Childhood schizophrenia, pseudodefective type Schizophrenia, childhood type Schizophrenia, catatonic type (occasional) Schizophrenia, hebe-phrenic type (occasional) Kanner's syndrome (infantile autism) (rare) Atypicality	Mental retardation, moderate to severe Psychosis with: Organic cerebral impairment Mental retardation Chronic brain syndrome, owing to various causes Various syndromes of ego and developmental arrest
2. Symbiotic psychosis of adolescence	Reactive schizophrenia Childhood schizophrenia: Pseudoneurotic type Pseudopsychopathic type Schizophrenia, childhood type Schizophrenia, paranoid type Schizophrenia, chronic undifferentiated type Schizophrenia, catatonic type (occasional) Schizophrenia, hebephrenic type (occasional)	Adjustment reaction of adolescence Adolescent turmoil Neurosis (anxiety; phobic; hysterical; obsessive-compulsive; depressive, etc.) Various schizophreniform conditions Personality disorders, especially, schizoid, anti-social, dyssocial, delinquent inadequate School phobia (occasional) Various syndromes of ego and developmental arrest

terested in and concerned about him; hence, the diagnostic process becomes at once an integral part of his treatment.

5. The initial therapeutic task that faces the treatment personnel of the ward or cottage comprises the identification, recognition, control, and interpretation to the patient of those segments of his behavior that serve as resistance of warding-off devices, aimed at preserving the pathological symbiotic ties with his mental representations of parental surrogates. This early resistance work serves, in addition, to

uncover the nexus of pathological communications and object ties characteristic for the patient's family, in which the patient has heretofore been immersed.[7]

    6. Particular attention needs to be given to the adolescent's early communications, which convey a premature need to identify himself with staff members. Though one may discover much that augurs positively in such messages from the patient as "I like you," "I need your help," and "You are nice (handsome, beautiful, powerful)," naïve acceptance thereof as indicators of more profound ego identifications early in hospitalization is a grievous error. It bespeaks, in part, the adult's own difficulties in recognizing the patient's counterphobic use of the resistance aspect of early positive transference. It is significant that one recently reported inpatient program, in which much is allegedly made of such early

---

[7]In a recent book on adolescent residential treatment, Easson (1969) asserts that "open and direct staff interpretation" of the adolescent's nonverbal communications "would make the patient feel as if he had been stripped and his very integrity violated" (p. 35). Such a view stems from several misconceptions: (1) it fails to take account of the powerful resistance meanings of the adolescent inpatient's earlier postadmission nonverbal metaphors; (2) it therefore fails to conceptualize, and hence deal with, the innumerable phenomena common to the adolescent's resistance phase of hospitalization; (3) it profoundly underestimates the severely ill adolescent's capacity, not only to withstand, but to respond therapeutically, to early, vigorous interpretation of resistance behavior; (4) it confounds interpretation of resistance with violation of ego integrity, and hence tends actively to reinforce, through passivity, those very pathological defenses that most require interruption and rapid elimination; (5) it conveys a spurious, respect for the adolescent inpatient's fragile ego through what is, in effect, a hands-off policy toward communications of a peculiarly disturbing or primitive nature, thereby reinforcing the patient's inference that staff members are fearful of—and hence unable to listen to—the archaic self-experiences that frighten him so much; (6) such a view retards the essential process by which the patient's archaic nexus of communications may be translated into consensually valid ones, delays the formation of early identifications, and hence prolongs the resistance phase of treatment.

positive communications, actually "treats" adolescents for a maximum of six weeks (Abend, Kachalsky, and Greenberg, 1968).

7. It follows that the closed ward, with its endogenous security devices, provides the optimal setting for the inception and at least part of the work of the resistance phase of treatment. The closed ward also serves well as the locale for the more regressive experiences associated with the definitive phase of treatment, during which the work of exchange of introjects comes to the fore.

8. The residential staff must be prepared to recognize and deal with the ineluctable regressive changes that accompany the patient's entry into the definitive phase of treatment. During this period, ward or cottage staff require considerable help with their countertransference, lest they proceed into a variety of maneuvers aimed unconsciously at warding off or terminating the patient's regression. If this occurs, the treatment quickly founders.

9. It is necessary to restate the fact that adolescents who require residential treatment are products of families, the pathology of which involves ill-defined, diffuse lines of authority and variable blurring and shifting of the roles and identities of their members. Hence, sick adolescents do not belong on adult mental hospital wards with sick adults whose psychopathology mirrors the disabilities of the adolescents' own parental surrogates, a locale that abets the adolescents' ongoing immersion in the same sort of pathogenic experiences that contributed so heavily to their illnesses in the first place. The sick adolescent needs healthy adults, not sick ones, until such time as his treatment will have led him to extricate himself from them.

10. It must be remembered that psychiatric treatment in the general sense should constitute a growth experience for both the patient and for those who essay to treat him. The

residential treatment of the adolescent should point him toward the achievements of the latency period, during which the child makes otherwise notable strides toward the attainment of self-objectification, mastery, sublimation, growth of secondary autonomy, the beginnings of categorical ideation, and peer identification, which symbolize the further development of his identity as a person. Once this has set in in earnest, the patient begins once again to move toward synchrony of his overall level of psychological development and his chronological age. And with this, he reenters the arena of adolescence proper, to begin to struggle healthily with the numerous problems characteristic of this critical stage of his maturation.

9

INTRODUCTION

Growth Opportunities in the Hospital: Intensive Inpatient Treatment of Adolescents, by H. S. Erlich

In contrast to the predominantly theoretical expositions of Noshpitz and Rinsley on residential treatment, Erlich here sets forth in nuts-and-bolts terms the actual organization and mode of function of one such unit based in an Israeli psychiatric hospital. He describes in detail the interweaving of theoretical and practical considerations that have shaped the design and operation of his program within a particular cultural and geographic setting, each of which factor imposes its own constraints and suggests its own possibilities.

Erlich takes particular issue with Rinsley's insistence that a closed facility is necessary to provide the control and structure required by severely disturbed and delinquent adolescents. Perhaps in harmony with the Israeli ideal, the intense sense of community in Erlich's program appears to generate the needed structure, so that the unit can not only be open, but unstaffed at night. A family model permits the patient at once to separate from his family of origin and to achieve reintegration by way of nonpathological family-like interactions. This essentially sociotherapeutic modality is combined with intensive psychoanalytically oriented psychotherapy and other treatment methods to form a comprehensive program in which both the "transferential" and "reality" aspects of patient-staff interactions are carefully scrutinized and used as levers for change.

Given suitable resources, Erlich's eminently practical paper could well provide a model that might be replicated in other settings.

9

Growth Opportunities in the Hospital: Intensive Inpatient Treatment of Adolescents

H. S. Erlich, Ph.D.

The specialized treatment of adolescents in a residential or inpatient setting has not received the kind of attention and careful scrutiny in the literature that is commensurate with its growth. The few descriptions that do exist (Miller, 1957; Beckett, 1965) fall short of answering the numerous "how to" questions that one finds oneself bombarded with by practitioners in this field as soon as one is identified, for better or worse, with an ongoing, successfully functioning adolescent service. The following comments will similarly, and quite certainly, fail to satisfy these needs. I have nevertheless undertaken them in order to point out a few of the major underlying principles that guide our efforts. As usual in such circumstances, retrospection discloses that actual constraints and needs often foreshadow and even determine theoretical considerations. It is equally true, however, that the more successful moments in our daily practice are those that represent some happy marriage of theoretical positions

Reprinted by permission from the *Israel Annals of Psychiatry and Related Disciplines*, 14:173-183, 1976. Jerusalem: Ben-Zvi Printing.

and reality considerations, and that this maxim itself represents a major facet in working with our adolescent patients.

THE SETTING

Our adolescent service is a semi-autonomous ward in a psychiatric hospital situated some 15 kilometers out of Jerusalem, in a lovely setting of Judean hills pastoralia. Its U-shaped structure flanks an inner courtyard, and contains five rooms occupied by three patients each, a nurse's station, two staff offices, a small kitchen, and a large all-purpose room that serves multiple functions: group meetings, club room, mess hall, and classroom. Group life centers and revolves around this room which provides something along the lines of Redl's "Stube." This 15-bed ward is coeducational, the boys' rooms alternating with the girls'.

A brief description of the daily program consists of the following: Reveille is at seven, and patients are in charge of straightening their own rooms and morning exercise. Breakfast (like all the meals) is fetched from the hospital kitchen by the patients, who also distribute it, clean up, and wash dishes according to a rotation they determine and update. There are two daily therapeutic community meetings consisting of all the patients and staff: every morning at nine o'clock, and every afternoon at three (the time of change of shifts). The morning meeting lasts precisely half an hour, and the afternoon one 20 minutes. These, as well as all time boundaries, are strictly observed by staff.

The time from 9:30 to noon is devoted to work in various occupational therapy shops and centers. The main meal is at 12:30 (Israeli style) and a particular effort is made for all to eat simultaneously. There is then a one hour free or rest period, and from 1:30 to 3:00 the group, under the occupational therapist's guidance, works at some project on the ward. In the afternoons and evenings the counselors offer a variety of social, artistic, educational, and recreational clubs that are essentially voluntary. The evening meal is light, and the group may then participate in some hospital-wide program, or (once a week) go to town for a movie or other recreation. Bedtime is officially at 10 o'clock, but is not strictly enforced. The only provision is that those not sleeping do not disturb those who are.

We opted to have one nurse in charge and to base much of the work on a staff of counselors. These young men and women are recruited from among the psychology students at the university, are highly motivated, and selected with an eye toward their personal gifts and possible contribution to life on the ward. They function in a wide variety of roles, ranging from traditional nursing (distributing medication under guidance, washing patients) to occupational and recreational therapy (arts and crafts, drama, pantomime, newspapers, gardening, group outings, etc.). We found their personal involvement and investment in the work to be so great and intense that we limit them to one year's work period. They each work a total of three weekly shifts between the hours of seven a.m. and 10 p.m. There is no personnel on the ward at night, but one of the other hospital wards as well as the doctor on call are always available. It should be noted that in more than three years of this kind of operation we encountered virtually no nighttime problems. It is as though the patients "save" their acting-out behavior for the times the staff is around and can interact with them.

The ward sees its primary task as being an intensive treatment unit. In line with this, a variety of treatment modalities is offered. First, each patient is seen in intensive, individual, psychoanalytically oriented psychotherapy two or three times a week. Of equal importance is the sociotherapy (Edelson, 1970a, b). This finds expression in the therapeutic community program which has briefly been alluded to but will be elaborated upon below. This is certainly a pivotal and highly intensive aspect of the treatment program. In addition, psychopharmacological treatment is given to patients who require it; family therapy is done when and where indicated and possible, using a co-therapist approach (Klein and Erlich, 1975), and occupational and art therapy as mentioned briefly above.

Theoretical Considerations

One of the underpinnings of our setup and daily work is that theoretical knowledge and considerations are indispensable if we do not wish to find ourselves busy putting out brushfires and forever coping with emergencies. Theory thus provides for us the equivalent of what in psychoanalytic psychology is referred to as "psychic structure," i.e., the ongoing, cumulative, deeply rooted and integrated patterns that provide stability and continuity in our functioning, and prevent us from struggling with every situation as if it were entirely novel. Since the purpose of this presentation is primarily descriptive and empirical, no attempt will be made to review the by now fairly extensive body of knowledge and theory concerning adolescent development and psychopathology. Some of the concepts and principles that guide us must, however, be briefly elaborated here for the present context.

It is common knowledge that psychopathology during adolescence is extremely rich in variety and expression (A. Freud, 1958). Despite the confounding variability, however, the major foci of conflict, stress, and maladaptation are amenable to delimitation and definition. The intrapsychic problems arise, typically and expectedly, in one or a combination of the following areas: transformation and intensification of drives; new formations or deformations of ego processes and functions; conflicts around separation and individuation; and problems of identity and intimacy. In all these areas, the adolescent is never faced with *de novo* issues and conflicts; rather, they are always shaped and influenced by past developmental gains, deformities, and points of fixation. The adolescent struggle itself, however, provides a *new*, emergent, and frequently underestimated possibility of fixation and later regression. Life's stresses and pressures may, in later years, often force a partial regression to this stage of development, with corresponding reinstatement of behavioral, affective, and drive organizations more typical of adolescence than of earlier, well-recognized points of developmental fixation.

More important, perhaps, for the present discussion is the particular significance of adolescence as a period for potential cure or amelioration of earlier developmental difficulties (Sullivan, 1953; A. Freud, 1958). Such cure may be spontaneous in some cases, while in others it may follow successful therapeutic intervention. It is our expressed goal in our hospital work with adolescents to capitalize on this potential for change, and to maximize psychodynamic gains by means of our intensive psychotherapeutic intervention during this critical period of developmental upheaval. It is our hope, owing to the special impact of intervention at this period, that in many of the adolescents, though certainly not in all, our efforts will forestall or significantly ameliorate regressions at later critical points of the life cycle (Erikson, 1959). This may find expression in eliminating or appreciably modifying the need for massive psychiatric care and, in particular, for future hospitalizations.

The adolescent's need for identification figures is well known. This need is based on earlier identifications with parental figures and their introjected images. It is equally founded, however, on the adolescent's need for finding such figures safely outside the family sphere. The difficulties inherent in the successful integration of these two needs—to identify with one's parents and to establish safe distance and differentiation from them—are clearly reflected in the sometimes wild and outlandish ways in which some adolescents resolve this task. Indeed, it may be argued that the degree and extent of physical and/or psychological distance that the adolescent takes from his parents in his search for objects for identification, are one measure or index of his own psychopathology, as well as that of his family (Klein and Erlich, 1976).

There are actually four aspects of the parental "Gestalt" that may be discerned in this adolescent search. First, there is the *real*, actual parent. Second, there is the *internalized* or introjected image of this parent, usually couched in infantile levels of fantasy, affect, and meaning. Third, there is the *projected* image of the parent, as it finds expression in the adolescent's view of the world, particularly of those aspects of reality vis-à-vis which he is in a more childlike relationship. And fourth, there is the parental *function*, comprising those parental behaviors and roles to which the adolescent still needs to relate in his everyday dealings with reality, whether this takes place with his actual parents or surrogate figures.

The diversity and complexity of interaction among the parts that make up the parental "Gestalt" to which the adolescent must relate have numerous implications for those who deal with him in everyday life—parents, educators, counselors, or employers. Its most important implication, however, seems to be in the area of intensive psychotherapeutic work with adolescents. Here we can see that one of the great pitfalls, as well as potential boons, that we run into is his readiness and capacity for alternating between polarities of relating: He may regard his therapist as therapist, that is with full-blown transference manifestation, and alternately (sometimes simultaneously, just to make it more confusing) as a real adult who potentially may and can fulfill a parenting *function* toward him. The adolescent has the capacity for transferring onto the therapist, on one level, introjected parental images and patterns of expectation, and for relating to him as an adult who may teach, discipline, make demands, or give him rewards and satisfactions at another level. It is the tension and interplay between these two equally legitimate relational needs, between transferred experience and real, accruing experience with an adult, that makes psychotherapy with adolescents the uniquely exciting, rewarding, and challenging experience that it is. It is, in this sense, clearly demarcated from the treatment of children wherein the adult or parental role of the therapist is much more heavily "fused" with the transferential process. It is also different from psychotherapy with adults, in whom the transference needs usually outweigh the need for the "real" aspects of the therapist's person as a parenting figure.

We have geared all interactions and transactions on our adolescent ward to capitalize on this potential for dual or split-level relatedness. We invite our adolescent patients to interact and identify with the staff on both levels—the transferential and the realistic. We regard it as our responsibility to create and facilitate structures and processes that would assist them in teasing out and separating these levels. In what follows, I shall briefly outline a few principles that govern us and that help make this difficult task possible. The model underlying all these principles is clearly the psychotherapeutic one. These principles are designed to help discriminate the real from the transferred and the imagined, the personal from the other-personal, and the ego-syntonic and capable of introjection and identification from the ego-alien and rejected.

I. Principle of Volitional Admission

As stated, our ward is completely open and has no night-shift. These physical constraints in themselves would make the necessity of a strong and binding therapeutic contract fairly obvious. More fundamentally, however, we believe this to be a principle that must be observed in order to work meaningfully with adolescents. There is no way of, and even less point in, making an adolescent enter a psychotherapeutic atmosphere and setting against his will. We have discovered that if and when his motivation at admission is strongly negative, it is far preferable to turn him down and leave the door open for his return than to insist on his staying.

We interview every potential candidate in a joint staff interview. We consider this interview an important place for *two-way* acquaintance and for striking a treatment contract. Naturally, we learn a great deal about the prospective patient. But we also invite him immediately to learn a good deal about us and from us—in our manner, our principles and values, and our seriousness about our fidelity to them. We tell the prospective patient about the ward, and stress the daily routine, treatment procedures, cardinal rules, and the volitional nature of his admission. This is followed by a tour of the premises.

In order to stress the contractual and volitional nature of the admission, we almost never admit a patient on the same day of the interview. Instead we give him a date either to call us and announce his decision, or to come, if he declares his readiness. In this way an important lesson is learned: that matters between us are subject to negotiation, but are binding if agreed upon. This helps stress both our reality and that of the patient as a prospective partner. This procedure may eliminate certain kinds of patients, notably the most acutely psychotic ones. For these we advise brief hospitalization on a closed ward and reapplication for admission when there is remission of the more acute state.

II. PRINCIPLE OF SEPARATION AND REABSORPTION

A great many of the vicissitudes of adolescent turmoil are a function of the adolescent's need for separation from the family and individuation in terms of his own identity and course in life. Some authors have elaborated on the tie between the accomplishment of this task and various types of psychotherapy encountered in adolescence (Masterson, 1972). We see this need once again as part of a bipolarity. The other pole consists of the tremendous need of the adolescent to belong, to be absorbed as a part in a group of his peers, and in a different way, perhaps, in his family.

In light of this, the ward experience aims to provide outlets and growth opportunities in both directions. Our twice-daily therapeutic community meetings stress this point, in that they emphasize stringently and uncompromisingly each person's group membership and responsibility. Interpretations are most frequently given at the level of group process and group transference (Bion, 1961). At the same time, attention is given and occasionally focused on individual members. This is done not only in terms of their actual behavior, but also, and more importantly, in terms of their *potential* contribution to the group, which is always held out to them as a possible goal.

We see the therapeutic community as a family composed not of equals, but of people at many differing developmental stages and accomplishments (Klein and Erlich, 1970). As in a family, there is room and even a need to allow for this differentiation of roles and status. At the same time, the differentiation should not lead to ossification: Care must be taken to enable a certain amount of movement, both progressive and occasionally regressive, to take place. There are ample opportunities for this which cannot be elaborated here. The most telling effect, perhaps, of the family model in terms of the present context is that it provides quite elegantly and integratively for viewing the adolescent as being at the interface of two important needs: He may be seen as a person in his own right, differentiating out of the family's context, and he may be viewed as a family member, known by the quality and meaning of his membership in this specific group. In our daily work, the pendulum constantly swings back and forth between these points on the continuum.

The adolescent faces problems of individuation and separation most cogently and violently with his own family. Here our principle must provide for the creation and elaboration of a measure of distance and separation from the family, while taking into account the difficulty of such a transition. We do this, to some extent, by means of a rule: For the first two weeks after admission the new patient does not leave the hospital, nor does he receive visitors or even phone calls. During this period, he is "adopted" by an older member of the group, whose responsibility it is to instruct him in the various intricacies of normative behavior on the ward. Thus we emphasize his parting from his family and his temporary absorption by the ward family from which he will, in the course of time, continue his process of separation and individuation.

III. PRINCIPLE OF INTERDEPENDENCE OR SHARED RESPONSIBILITY

One of the areas in which the greatest amount of friction and psychopathology is frequently encountered in adolescence, especially at the level of presenting symptomatology, is that of conflicts with authority. Our family model provides for hierarchy and differentiation of roles, functions, responsibilities, and power. This differentiation exists not only within the staff group but also within the patient group. Yet the pressures towards peer group conformity strongly pull the adolescents to an unrealistic view and expectations of equality among themselves. One of the most sensitive and complicated points of the staff's work with the group, therefore, centers around the desimplification of these notions, in a direction that allows for recognition of the complexity of the group's differentiation.

Beyond the continuum of abilities and responsibilities, there is also a range of issues that lend themselves to various shades of an authoritarian/permissive stance. Issues arising on the ward must always be seen in terms of their own merits, as well as test cases challenging the fabric of group life and ward structure. Great sensitivity can and must be developed, by both patients and staff, in order to detect seemingly tangential but important underlying principles. One of these principles states that there are areas of ward life and function that are clearly the staff's responsibility and decision, and others that clearly belong to the patients' group. In addition, however, there are areas where the interests and responsibilities of both groups overlap. These are areas of interdependence the resolution of which requires that both groups cooperate. If the interdependent approach does not prevail, each group would be the loser in the long run.

Some illustrations are in order here: Admissions and discharges are entirely the staff's responsibility. The patients may recommend the removal of a certain member, and the staff is free to accept or reject the recommendation. A large measure of freedom is provided with regard to participation in activities, rising in the morning, doing one's turn at mealtime and cleanup. All these are certainly expectable behaviors that we see as belonging to the patient's group. Yet we feel free and even required to comment on and interpret flaws and lapses in the execution of these tasks. Such interpretation is usually in terms of a symptom of the state to the group, and not the individuals involved.

The interdependent approach finds its clearest expression

in two of our activities. First of all, in the therapeutic community meetings. Once again, these are binding and all are expected to participate; yet no effort is usually made to round up members. They are held responsible to come on their own, just as the staff does. There is a time limit of five minutes for lateness, after which patients are not allowed to come in. The meeting itself frequently deals with issues of patients-staff interaction and mutual expectations, along the lines of dependence on authority as against shared responsibility and autonomy.

The other activity that focuses on interdependent interaction is the Community Committee. This committee consists of three elected patients and two staff representatives. Its main function is the monitoring and guarding of norms and values underlying behavior on the ward. In addition to serving as a clearinghouse for general issues (e.g., experimentation with the time of reveille and the importance of activities that open the day), it summons individual patients in order to discuss with them their transgressions of ward rules and mete out punishment. The aim of such punishment is educational, not punitive, and the patients have readily internalized this approach. The measure used may vary a great deal, depending on the person and his state. Behavior that is understood as avoidance of the ward group, for instance (e.g., running away, preferring other wards, seclusion), will usually elicit some kind of token act that will symbolically bring the patient closer to the group. This in turn may vary from making an item in arts and crafts for the enhancement or utility of the common room, to being restricted to the ward or even one's room for a given period. Since the patients are in the majority on the committee, they can obviously outvote the staff. Though this has hardly ever happened, it emphasizes even more the need for interdependent action and sober, careful consideration of both speech and actual steps taken by both patients and staff. This may also be the source of the deep respect with which this committee is held by the group.

IV. PRINCIPLE OF ACTIVITY-PASSIVITY

The adolescent's struggle against his rising and changing drive constellation (Blos, 1962) frequently leaves him feeling helpless and passive. One of the major aims of a therapeutic program for adolescents must be the enhancement of the sense of ego autonomy (Shapiro, 1963, 1966). Much of the foregoing discussion bears out this point and will not be repeated here. Two points, however, must be made briefly. The first is that the activities program has as its specific aim this function, namely, to combat passivity in the face of inner and outer experience through the enhancement of competence and the active experience of the self, as engaged in various modalities and areas of work and creation.

The second issue has to do with passivity as expressed through regression. Here, of course, numerous issues are encountered in the area of clinical practice, management, and decision making. Applying the psychotherapeutic model once more, we regard a certain amount of regression as both inevitable and necessary in order to make progress, provided it can be delineated and contained within certain boundaries. In terms of the present context, we must understand the adolescent's need to turn what was experienced passively, as something that happens to him with little or no initiative, conscious direction, and competent mastery, into something he can experience actively, as belonging to him and of which he is author, and not merely object (Rapaport, 1953). The ward experience thus aims at providing selectively important opportunities for controlled or checked regression.

The adolescent group is an important partner in instituting and enduring such regressions. One aspect of the family model of differentiation within the group is related to this. It is quite possible for different group members to be at widely varying points in their own inner states and developmental trajectories. This must include the possibility of some regression. The group learns to tolerate this and even to be of help and assistance to the group member undergoing the regression. It should be pointed out, however, that we find this tolerance to be fairly limited in duration. Yet we see the tolerance for such regressions as an important aspect of life in the therapeutic community, in that one member is undergoing "regression in the service of the community" (Klein and Erlich, 1970), thereby enabling others to assume the role of the stronger and nurturing ones.

In summary, I have outlined some of the major theoretical and empirical underpinnings that form the guidelines of our work with the hospitalized adolescent. The foregoing discussion should have made it quite clear that while we certainly do not regard hospitalization as the treatment of choice in any or most cases of adolescent upheaval, it is equally true that we believe that the experience of hospitalization need not be a tragic trauma reserved for the severely psychotic adolescent only. Judiciously applied, and soundly grounded and structured in theory and psychotherapeutic approach, it can be a major and more complete healing experience for a much larger segment of the troubled adolescent population than hitherto realized.

PART III

Family Therapy

10

INTRODUCTION

Family Therapy: Its Role in Adolescent Psychiatry, by Frank S. Williams

Among those who have developed the use of family methods with adolescents, Williams has been preeminent in his flexibility and his lack of the doctrinaire stance that not infrequently appears in the writings of family therapists. In the paper that follows he outlines the developmental rationale for incorporating the treatment of the adolescent within a family nexus, suggests a number of clinical indications for doing so, and presents several convincing clinical vignettes. Williams particularly advocates family interviews as a routine feature of the evaluative process, and shows how they can reveal crucial aspects of pathogenic interactions that are unlikely to emerge in individual diagnostic interviews and the identification of which can contribute fruitfully to exploration in individual psychotherapy.

A further contribution to our knowledge of the role of family therapy in adolescence will be found in Chapter 18, where Liebman, Minuchin, and Baker describe their method of treatment for anorexia nervosa.

10

Family Therapy: Its Role in Adolescent Psychiatry

Frank S. Williams, M.D.

Much of the pioneer work in family therapy during the past 25 years has centered around the young schizophrenic adult, or the older schizophrenic adolescent and his family. During more recent years, the literature has included a growing number of reports of family therapy with the neurotically disturbed adolescent (Wynne, 1965; Williams, 1968; Brown, 1970; and Minuchin, 1971b). Though most psychiatrists recognize the interplay between an adolescent's intrapsychic conflicts and his family's interpersonal dynamics, there is disagreement among clinicians regarding the use of family therapy with adolescents.

Quite often, when child psychiatrists refer to family therapy with an adolescent, they mean that they actively involve the mother and father in the total treatment program (but separate from the adolescent's individual therapy). The family therapy that I shall be considering in this chapter, however, refers to a family interviewing technique that includes the adolescent and his parents seen together in the same

Reprinted by permission from *Adolescent Psychiatry*, 2:324-339, 1973. New York: Basic Books.

room with the psychotherapist.[1] Such family interviews may
be employed for one or two diagnostic evaluation sessions;
may occur in series over a period of several weeks or months
as part of an ongoing treatment program, which in turn may
include marital therapy for the parents and additional modalities, such as group or individual therapy for the adolescent; or may remain the primary or sole form of therapeutic
intervention with an adolescent and his family by means of
regular weekly family interviews over a period of many
months.

There is no doubt that a disturbed adolescent needs much
assistance in breaking his ambivalent family ties as he strives
for identity and independence. Some therapists feel this can
only be done by his developing a highly confidential one-to-
one relationship with an adult outside the family, his psychotherapist. Some psychotherapists are unique in their capacity to rise above ensuing familial resistances to the
establishment of such out-of-the-family relationships. They
are able to develop with the teenager a most powerful new
corrective relationship. However, I believe that in most situations the familial resistances will prevail, block, and overcome progress. As a child enters adolescence, these parental
resistances to his forward development can be quite severe.
For instance, at no time in a woman's life is her own identity
more threatened than at that point when her maternal role
must give way in light of her last child's adolescent maturity.
This is particularly so if her marriage is not a rewarding one.
Mothers at such points of personal crisis may unwittingly
hold onto their teenage sons and daughters, stifling their

[1]The major portion of the theoretical formulations and related clinical
studies described in this chapter represents experiences acquired by the
author during some 10 years of empirical clinical work in the field of
family therapy, along with others on the senior staff of the Cedars-Sinai
Department of Child Psychiatry, Los Angeles, California.

psychosocial growth. Seeing the adolescent together with his parents allows for a mutual working through of these resistances. Some of the questions raised by those who are reluctant to see the adolescent with his family include: Will family therapy help individuation or promote an even greater continued symbiosis? Will not such family meetings result in a break of confidentiality with the adolescent? The complex familial field that surrounds an adolescent often perplexes the clinician. This perplexity overwhelms many therapists to the point of avoiding working with adolescents and of adopting a stance of therapeutic nihilism. Some teachers avoid the perplexities by presenting students with an oversimplified exposure to adolescent psychiatry, primarily a one-to-one dyadic approach. Varing flexible and multitreatment techniques are not sufficiently introduced early enough in the student's or resident's training. Unfortunately, the reassurance that a beginning student attains from working in the one-to-one, easy to control, uncovering psychotherapeutic approach with adults often collapses when he faces an adolescent and the multiple forces within the family that he, the therapist, cannot control. I should like to suggest that therapists who feel in control while working exclusively in the dyadic one-to-one relationship with an adolescent actually have very little control, merely the illusion of it. Whittling away goes on behind the scenes in the form of overt and subtle sabotage within the family field.

I should like to discuss the indications for family therapy in adolescent psychiatry, both for assessment and for treatment. Attention will be paid to the most serious dilemma for the adolescent and his family, the age-old conflict between autonomy and individuation as it comes into conflict with dependency-control attachments, particularly in the next to impossible to treat symbiotic type family. The author encourages flexibility of approach within the total treatment program for the adolescent, a flexibility that includes therapeutically timed mixtures of one-to-one therapy and family treatment.

MAJOR CONFLICTS OF ADOLESCENCE

Before attending to indications and contraindications for family interviewing techniques, I should like to briefly review some of those major conflicts of adolescence for which families can either offer resolution or stifling perpetuation.

INDEPENDENCE VERSUS DEPENDENCY ATTACHMENTS

The adolescent, in his struggle to achieve freedom from his family, often threatens, within himself and his parents, very primitive fears of object loss and separation from symbiotic involvements. Brown (1969) indicated how the transactional field of the family is often used to reaffirm and preserve the internal infantile object constellation in an effort to ward off fantasied separation grief and anxiety. Minuchin (1971b) described how in working with very close-knit families the therapist must be aware of the powerful familial forces that impede maturity for the adolescent. He further stressed the need for clinicians to find effective ways of overcoming these forces.

Today, many adolescents attempt to solve their own intrapsychic and their family's problems over independence and dependency attachments by leaving home at an early age. Unfortunately, what often results from such attempts to jar loose from the family is a state of pseudomaturation. The underlying sense of weakness and object loss frequently persists and represents itself in a growing need for drugs and new attachments within hippie-type crash pads or communes (Williams, 1970). Such dependency attachments to peers —without the development of significant mutuality and intimacy—can result in a group of adolescents holding together like orphans in a storm, merely playing at the game of maturity. Some succeed in developing, in spite of the game; others fail and remain symbolically attached to their families, through the fantasied family objects in their new surrogate peer parents. In 1970 I described how adolescents in a hippie commune display an exquisite attempt to work through the attachment-autonomy conflict with the use of drugs. I offered examples in which the adolescent parent nurses his peer child back to health from a bad trip. At a later point, that same former child-patient becomes the mother and nurses his former peer parent back to health from a similar bad trip. Unfortunately, very little in the way of sustained day-to-day experiences in maintaining a role of growing leadership seems to occur.

RECRUDESCENCE OF OEDIPAL CONFLICTS

The sexual conflicts stirred up within the adolescent, by nature of his physical and psychosexual growth, often lead to the development of dramatic distancing mechanisms between parents and their sons and daughters. Mutual fears of fantasied hetero- and homosexual erotization of the parent-child relationships are often represented in extreme defensive hostile pushing-away maneuvers in some families. In others, the parents become overly involved in the sexuality of their sons and daughters. This may be reflected in either direct seductive contact, or in subtle cueing mechanisms, wherein a mother, for example, using the rationalization of instilling "a healthy wholesome attitude," overeducates her daughter about sex and elicits detailed descriptions from her young adolescent daughter of sexual fantasies and encounters.

The role of the parents and siblings in the reappearance of threatening incestuous fantasies in adolescence has received little emphasis in the literature. Family interviewing techniques offer opportunities to observe directly those subtle seductive stimuli from sisters and brothers, as well as from parents, usually not gleaned from sessions with the parents alone. The adolescent faced with symbolic or real incestuous provocation often finds it difficult to sublimate his feelings in the direction of nonsexual familial intimacy experiences. This is, in most families today, owing to a lack of experiences with intimate sharing of feelings between parent and child, after the initial maternal-infant symbiosis and parental-preschooler closeness. The adolescent is therefore trapped. He either leaves and looks for intimacy outside his home, or he remains within the family and suffers the fantasied and/or part reality threat of massive regression to those types of early oral and anal intimacy experiences he knew as a young child and as an infant. Should he choose to leave home, in an effort to seek love and intimacy, he has very little intimacy capacity with which to sustain himself. He often winds up substituting pseudosexual intimacies and the pseudointimacy of the hippie or drug scene.

INTEGRATION OF ANGRY AFFECT

In adolescence, significant real physical strength is available for the first time. Too, the capacity for calculation related to carrying out of crimes and physical harm is readily available. Adolescents are often frightened by their rage and destructive potential, particularly in relation to their parents. The rage often relates to inner struggles over autonomy and is projected onto the parents. Should the parents have intense problems regarding letting go, the projection, of course, becomes much easier to accomplish and more readily fixated. At other times, the teenager's rage represents a defense against emerging positive erotic feelings toward parents or siblings. Completely separating the adolescent's therapy from his family's therapy may parallel the negative effect of a teenager's premature leaving of home, as far as rage is concerned. When the adolescent leaves home (made easy today by the availability of hippie communes or crashpads, which will provide food and shelter), he does not have an opportunity to fight out certain rage-inducing conflicts with his parents and siblings. Fighting it out can help the adolescent test the extent and limitations of his own murderous rage in terms of potential action, as well as the extent and limitations of his parents' and siblings' murderous rage in terms of potential danger. Some adolescent peer groups maintain an ideology of love. The proclamation, "We love everyone, including the parents who hassle us!" may serve as a defense against the eruption of repressed or suppressed feelings of rage toward family members. Family therapy offers a safe and constructive setting in which to fight it out.

Much can be inferred regarding that portion of an adolescent's problem with angry affect which stems from familial relationships, by seeing parents in separate diagnostic or therapeutic sessions. Family interviews, however, which include the parents and adolescent together, offer an *in vivo* opportunity to determine whether the rage relates to defensive paranoid projection on the part of the adolescent, or to reality-oriented parental precipitants. Such a differential assessment helps in determining intrapsychic fixation and potential for the later handling of rage feelings once separation from the family does occur. Brown (1964) described an example of parental stimulation of inappropriate anger in a young teenage boy with self-destructive tendencies. In several interviews, which included the boy, his mother, father, and sister, a fascinating interplay between the boy's problem with inner controls and familial interpersonal relations was elicited. In part the therapist was able to observe how the father's avoidance of decisive discipline helped to perpetuate the youngster's problem with controls. He was also able to ob-

serve, within the nuances of the familial interactions, how
the father and son made a regressive alliance, a focal symbiosis, in which they both retreated from their phallically
feared mother and in which the father used his son both as
a retreat and as a symbolic expression of his own rage toward
his wife.

IDENTITY AND CAPACITY FOR INTIMACY

The adolescent's capacity for intimacy and his ego identity—his separateness—are affected by his family's attitude
toward his individuation. Some families with very powerful
familial identities display a wholesome working togetherness,
but unwittingly squelch the individual identities of the various
family members. Adolescents sometimes flee from such families in a desperate attempt to achieve a sense of individuality.
Once with a new family peer group, they are supersensitive
and on guard in relation to fears of their becoming possessed
and of losing separateness. A question pertinent to the field
of family therapy is, "Can an adolescent work through his
struggle between his desire for intimacy and his fear of loss
of individuation within the context of family therapy sessions,
or separate from his family, in a new, intimate, one-to-one
relationship with a therapist?" My own bias is in the direction
of a flexible combination of both modalities for adolescent
therapy. The family can often be helped to encourage the
teenager toward independent individuation; the teenager's
role in undermining that potential encouragement from his
parents is most observable and available for confrontation in
family meetings.

INDICATIONS FOR FAMILY THERAPY WITH ADOLESCENTS
ASSESSMENT

Regardless of the treatment modality eventually decided
on for an adolescent, family interviews during the diagnostic

phase help the therapist to understand the multitude of outer forces perpetuating and contributing to the adolescent's internal conflicts. Family interviews can be helpful during the initial workup, as well as at major points of resistance during an ongoing individual treatment. One or two initial diagnostic family interviews help the therapist with prognostic considerations. He is able to determine more accurately those factors in the family that will serve as major resistances to the uncovering work of one-to-one individual therapy with the adolescent. There are at times certain affects hidden within the adolescent related to past tragic family traumas. These affects may be continually held down via subtle parental cues in an effort to protect the parent from the pain of affective recall, memory, or expression. For example, a severely depressed 13-year-old boy was desperately in need of psychotherapy to help relieve him of self-destructive tendencies and his gloomy preoccupation with the hopelessness of failing peer relationships. Seeing the boy and mother in separate diagnostic sessions elicited historical material about the father's death several years earlier. Neither mother nor son showed the slightest affect while presenting the material about the father's sudden death. Mother's monotone presentation was noteworthy. When seeing the boy and mother together in a family interview, it was striking to note that whenever the boy attempted to discuss his feelings about his father's death, he immediately evoked from his mother a gentle but definitive prohibition against further ventilation. The boy's eyes would well up with tears as he would start to say with sadness that he "remembered when his father . . ."; the mother would immediately say something to the effect that "Your father was a good man and it isn't proper to talk about him." Even when it was apparent that the boy was about to say something positive about his father, the mother would again prohibit such expression by changing the subject or by indicating the potential hurt she would feel if one "dredged up the past." In this particular case, a series of family interviews was helpful in freeing the mother to give her son permission to uncover and ventilate his feelings of depression and rage about the loss of his father. One might have attempted to get this boy to reach the same point in individual therapy. I feel, however, that in so doing one could readily create new conflicts for the youngster, as he would have to struggle blindly with his conflict over loyalty to his own wish for relief and his mother's wish for continued burial of affects. Paul and Grosser (1965) described the values of uncovering such buried affects from the traumatic past during family interviews.

Diagnostic family interviews help to assess whether the intrapsychic distortions of the adolescent are firmly fixated and resistant to changes within the environment, or whether such distortions are still in a state of fluidity and primarily reinforced, daily, by parental cueing. I recently treated a 16-year-old girl with severe anorexia nervosa. The original diagnostic workup reflected some of the classical conflicts over fear of separation from mother and fear of her adult female sexual impulses. In individual diagnostic sessions, Marie tearfully told of how her wish to have a boyfriend and her dreams of sex with boys made her feel "trampy." She was openly anxious as she discussed her desire to eventually live away from home. In the parents' separate diagnostic history-taking interview, the mother convincingly indicated her own healthy approach toward sex, as far as her daughter was concerned, and stressed how she encouraged Marie to date and to learn about sex from both books and from questions put to the parents. In marked contrast to the tone of the individual sessions was one family interview, in which the question of Marie's dating and leaving home came up. As Marie's tears and anxiety level lessened, she began to talk of a boy she met at school who wanted to take her out. Marie's father blanched; her mother sat forward and said, "What do you know about him?" She then turned to me and said, "Doctor, we know that there are some nice boys, but my father was a policeman, you know, and I've learned about all the rapes and murders that go on, particularly with young girls; you never know what a boy is really like; he may just be putting on a friendly front!" The next day in an individual session with me, Marie appeared extremely frightened. She described how she had not eaten all day and how uncertain she felt about her feelings in relationship to boys and dating. This is a striking example of an observable direct influence by the parents on the unresolved autonomy and sexual conflicts of an adolescent.

When doing family interviewing, one has an opportunity to note such overt as well as certain subtle cueing mechanisms. At times mothers and fathers will discuss with seeming frankness their concerns about hetero- and homosexuality and will, at times, show zealous interest in their adolescent son's or daughter's sexual activities. The family therapist is in a position to see those cues that admonish or prematurely encourage sexual involvement. These cues are often missed in the more traditional diagnostic interview.

One has an excellent opportunity in family meetings to observe directly double-bind communications. For example, a 15-year-old boy lived alone with his divorced mother. In her initial individual intake session, the mother complained of her son's lack of friends; she wanted the clinic to "help him get out of his shell and make more meaningful friendships." In a diagnostic family meeting, the boy discussed his wish for friends, but added his concerns about his mother's loneliness. Mother broke into tears, saying, "I want you to go out, you need to be away from me, somehow I will survive; it is important for you to have your own life!" The boy was torn in that his mother had given him permission, but at the same time had indirectly indicated that she might die without him.

Family interviews during the diagnostic phase often elicit marital disharmony or potential disharmony which is covered up by the scapegoating of the problem teenager. Frequently, one of the siblings is the first to uncover the disharmony. Brown (1970), in his description of family therapy, indicated how family meetings can promote a readiness to deal with change in the marital relationship. He particularly noted how siblings who are not directly caught up in the pathological family dyads may move this process along. The scapegoated problem adolescent serves to ward off a threatened potential break in the family equilibrium should the parents' underlying hatred or intimacy deficit be brought to the surface. The designated teenage patient often loyally accepts his role as the sick one, though ashamed of it, in an effort to hold his parents and family together. In family meetings, one can observe the exquisite and precise timing of some of the shifting of attention to the teenager's problems, as the therapist or one of the family gets close to touching on the underlying marital conflict. A sibling may point out the lack of time mother and father spend together, or the lack of romantic feelings between the parents. Suddenly, and apparently out of context, the designated patient or one of the parents will draw attention to the adolescent's symptoms. In several family treatment situations, we have noted how symptom complexes such as aggressive behavior disorders, predelinquency, and poor school performance abate once the parents are able to ventilate their anxieties about the instability of their marriage. In these cases, the treatment of choice is often conjoint marital therapy without any therapy necessary for the adolescent.

In diagnostic family interviews one obtains a sense of whether a family will be of help in attempts to reverse an adolescent's intrapsychic distortions. In an interview with a 16-year-old boy with sleep problems, school failures, and a lack of friends, the youngster indicated severe conflicts regarding his wish to go to a nonparochial school. He feared his father, a long-time religious devotee, would condemn his wish to attend a coed school. He further feared that he would bear the brunt of peer ridicule if he wore his religious skullcap in a coed setting. The father, in a meeting with the boy and the therapist, shared his own mixed feelings about the matter, but convincingly encouraged the boy to go to a coed school and to remove his skullcap. It became clear that much of the work to be done in individual therapy would need to focus on the boy's underlying fears of sexuality, and that his father would probably be an ally, or at least not a sabotaging agent.

OVERCOMING RESISTANCES

In individual or group therapy, the clinician often faces what appears to be a major resistance to continuing treatment. Those of us who work a great deal with adolescents are all too familiar with the frequency of missed sessions, latenesses, and the boredom that often sets in, particularly at times when painful affects are expressed. As one gets close to a teenager's underlying struggles with sex or aggression, it is important to note whether an ensuing resistance is primarily motivated by the adolescent's anxieties or by the parents' discomfort with newly emerging affects and desires communicated at home.

Earlier, I mentioned Marie, a 16-year-old girl with anorexia nervosa. As Marie began to write letters to an 18-year-old, apparently healthy young man who liked her, she simultaneously reported dreams of having sexual intercourse with this young man and with older men. She suddenly began to miss sessions and indicated her wish to stop treatment. Interpreting the transference elements in her feelings did not dissuade her. She continued to express the feeling that we were wasting time and that she was not getting better fast enough. This was in spite of a 20-pound weight gain over a period of four and a half months. Seeing Marie together with her mother and father at this critical point in her treatment was quite revealing and helpful. The father kept looking at Marie with tearful, "basset hound" eyes, saying, "I don't mind that you don't want to go camping with me any more; if you are too busy writing to Marty, that's all right! I can always bury myself in work; I have to support you all and send you to college, so that you can see your boyfriend more anyway!" Mother, on the other hand, stated that she was very glad that Marie was now interested in dating, but quickly shifted the subject to an article that she had read in the paper about a coed girl being murdered in a parking lot. She added her convictions that the murderer must have been a sex deviant. It became apparent that the parents needed to be involved in either a parallel conjoint marital therapy or a total family therapy with Marie, to help them all separate out the parental fears and guilt-provoking affects from Marie's own psycho-sexual internal conflicts.

At times, passive young adolescent boys will be in individual therapy for many months, and will eventually become more assertive and aggressive, both verbally and physically. To the therapist's astonishment, they may suddenly be taken out of treatment by their parents, who are unable to tolerate their new expressions of anger. Seeing such adolescent boys and their parents together, at these moments of resistance, can elicit both the parental anxieties in response to the patient's aggression, as well as those ways in which the teenage boy may be unwittingly provoking his parents by an exaggerated display of his newfound power. An additional problem with such families, particularly in the case of the predelinquent adolescent, lies in confused communication patterns. There may be prohibition of direct expression of aggression at the same time that there is much subtle cuing from the parents provoking antisocial behavior. I recently (1967a) described how a predelinquent boy was attacked by his parents for investigating areas of the therapist's office that were obviously out of bounds, after they had cued his exploration with their own questions about the restricted area.

The value of seeing the family at these points of resistance is in seeing how the adolescent himself helps start or rekindle the familial anxiety patterns that then act to put down the threatening affects. For example, the adolescent beginning to struggle in individual therapy with his wish to separate from home may in family meetings continue to drop hints about his self-destructive potential once away from his parents. He might state: "Maybe I'd smoke a joint once in a while! Don't worry, I'll find a pad to sleep somewhere." The parents' anxieties are then reawakened in terms of their own reality separation and loss feelings, and in terms of fantasied distortions within them. These intrapsychic distortions may have to do with violence, loss of controls, self-destruction, annihilation, and death, all of which may seem imminent when one separates from parents.

CRISES IN FAMILIES

Series of family meetings aimed at opening up lines of communication can help an adolescent through major points of transitional crisis in a family's life. Crises can be particularly disruptive at points of significant separation, as in divorce, a move to a new neighborhood, a youngster's going away to school, hospitalization, or death. Very often the affects and anxieties that parents feel at times of major crises are repressed only to appear in exaggerated forms within their youngsters. Sudden school phobias or sudden aggressive predelinquent activities frequently occur on the threshold of a divorce or other imminent separation. Also, violent exacerbations of psychosomatic illnesses, such as ulcerative colitis or severe asthma, may occur in an adolescent following the death of a close grandparent or ambivalently loved sibling. Family meetings at such times of crisis allow for an equal sharing of the burden of affect experiences for every member of the family.

With encouragement and selective sharing of his own genuine affects, the therapist can serve as a model to the family for expression of a range of emotional feelings. He can help the family to express sadness and rage rather than let them dwell on positive sides of major transitional crises. Parents often emphasize the positive at such times both to reassure their youngsters and to keep repressed their own underlying potential for affect eruption regarding tragic separations.

In preparation for placement of an adolescent outside the home, either in a hospital or in a foster home setting, family meetings can be of great value in bolstering the potential success of the placement. Parents may mask unresolved guilts regarding certain wishes to get rid of a troublesome teenager by resisting a necessary placement. Too, the adolescent may struggle with guilt feelings about leaving his family behind, particularly if there is an unconscious or preconscious awareness of the marital discord that might erupt when the problem teenager is no longer the focus of concern. Such mutual guilts and anxieties, when openly discussed in a series of family meetings, are often worked through and seen in their proper perspective.

THE HOSPITALIZED ADOLESCENT

Schween and Gralnick (1965) and others, in their work with hospitalized patients, have during the past few years underlined the necessity for concomitant family therapy while treating the hospitalized patient. The hospitalized adolescent's family particularly needs a family interviewing approach for two reasons: (1) The teenage patient usually returns to the family. (2) Should the therapist see only the designated patient, he is not in a position to consistently deal with the familial resistances to change in the patient. These resistances usually manifest themselves after hospitalization, and alter the gains the adolescent has made by corrective relationships in the hospital milieu. Family meetings while the adolescent is hospitalized permit the therapist and patient to deal with familial, including sibling, resistances to change at every step of the adolescent's gain. The family sessions also help the therapist gauge the optimal therapeutic pace for his adolescent patient with which the family can keep step. This is most important when the plan is for the patient definitely to return to his original family environment.

Recently, a hospitalized, self-destructive, 17-year-old boy made frequent attempts to elope from the hospital, usually after visits from family members. Rather than discontinuing the visiting, family meetings were held on the ward with the patient, his divorced parents, his mother's fiancé, and his older sister. After several meetings, it became clear to all involved that the patient was acting out the entire family's ambivalence regarding the initial divorce, as well as the mother's imminent remarriage. The patient eventually communicated his loyalty conflicts and his wish for a closer relationship with his estranged father. In addition to the total family meetings, weekly father-son meetings were introduced. The elopement attempts soon subsided.

THE SYMBIOTIC FAMILY AND ADOLESCENT IDENTITY

For myself and many of my colleagues, the problem of the locked-in adolescent symbiosis has continued to present a major challenge and therapeutic dilemma. In viewing certain family symbioses, we note a precarious balance between the identity of the adolescent and the diffusion of that identity within the family—within the family identity, so to speak. In some families, a family identity is completely lacking; everyone truly "does his own thing." In others, however, the family identity may be so strong as to blot out individual uniqueness. In working with one such family, a professional vaudeville-type stage group, I readily sensed a wholesome family spirit as they discussed with warm feelings their group excitement and pleasures related to traveling around the country together performing as a musical team. However, it took much time and effort to pinpoint any individual, distinct personality differences for the various family members. The parents themselves, as well as the children, frequently confused each other's names, as did the therapist. In that particular family, as well as in one described by Minuchin (1971b), the teenager's autonomous identity was lost and submerged by the family's needs. In Minuchin's case, the boy's individuation broke through in the form of an idiosyncratic and life-defying self-starvation—in the symptoms of anorexia nervosa. In the stage family I treated, one of the teenage boy's identity erupted in the form of drug usage and antisocial aggressive acts. Minuchin utilized ongoing family therapy as the primary modality in his treatment. His successful approach to this problem of severe adolescent symbioses led me to reconsider some of my own earlier views (Williams, 1968). I had made a case for the contraindication of family therapy techniques in dealing with some symbiotic adolescents and cited some related negative therapeutic results. I suggested that such families often cooperated with a family treatment approach for long periods of time, just to stay together, paying ear service to but defeating therapeutic insight attempts. Minuchin, however, described a very active involvement by the family therapists in an effort to set up family tasks that highlight the family's internal power plays and eventually force a disruption of the family's pathological equilibrium. The problem with a passive approach to the locked-in symbiotic family may lie in the probability that the family's homeostatic power is truly stronger than most doctors' therapeutic powers. In the past, my own therapeutic bias regarding the symbiotic adolescent was in the direction of feeling that he desperately needed a separate one-to-one relationship, outside of his family, to encourage his individuation. I believed that in one-to-one therapy the therapist could demonstrate respect for the adolescent's autonomy, while offering the support necessary to incur trust of relationships outside the cloistered and somewhat paranoid symbiotic family. However, the results of long-term individual therapy with such adolescents, either in hospital or outpatient situations, are often minimal, as are some of the similarly long-term attempts with family therapy. Again, Minuchin emphasized the need for extensive activity by the therapist when working with such families. An example of a therapist-induced family task aimed at highlighting and breaking up control mechanisms within the family is seen in Minuchin's insistence that no one in the family was to eat as long as the anorexic boy would not eat. Since the youngster was already secretly in control of his entire family with the symptom of anorexia, and since the parents were already helpless, the family task merely brought to the surface and underscored that the boy was truly the despot. The despot interpretation, and family-fasting task, led to all kinds of severe familial disruptions. The therapist had to be available day and night during the ensuing crisis to move in and encourage forward movement and individuation at the point of crisis.

In certain families, teenage boys or girls "will not permit" their parents to go away without them to parties or on vacations. In exploring the value of family therapy and family

tasks with such families, I have insisted, after many sessions
of dealing with both the adolescent's and parents' resistances
to such individuation and freedom, that the parents go out.
My experiences in this regard are similar to those of Minuchin in relation to the essentiality of therapist availability for
crisis intervention. For example, when in response to the
parents' first weekend away a teenage boy crashes his car, or
a teenage girl makes a manipulative but dangerous suicide
attempt, the therapist has to be ready to continue to push for
the separation, while making himself and appropriate others
available to the adolescent for physical and emotional help.

For the present I feel that a combined approach that utilizes individual treatment, series of family meetings, and
major attention to encouraging peer relationships is necessary in dealing with the symbiotic adolescent and his family.

Conclusions

As therapists, but primarily as human beings, we like to
know our own roles and identity with a minimum of confusion. Psychotherapy with adolescents can be overwhelming
for the therapist because of complicating family forces, peer
crises, legal entanglements, the pressure for guidance, and
direct advice. We may wish the adolescent to go elsewhere.
On the other hand, we may handle our frustration by mag-
nifying the value of confidentiality and, with our adolescent
patient, "hide from the world." This unfortunate overem-
phasis on confidentiality can at times constrict the therapist's
diagnostic vision, as well as foreclose an opportunity to utilize
family interviewing techniques, a most helpful treatment
modality when working with adolescents.

Family therapy offers a means to overcome resistance to
an adolescent's psychosocial and psychosexual development.
For some adolescent problems the family approach should
be the primary therapeutic modality. In family sessions, the

therapist can offer a point of view and an attitude that embodies respect for the individuation of the adolescent, as well as respect for the family group and its identity. He can encourage communication of affects and the expression of feelings of intimacy in ways which do not threaten regression to infantile or erotic ties. My overall recommendation is geared toward a flexible approach, which includes family and individual therapy and which permits direct observation of those dynamic familial interpersonal forces impinging on the adolescent's psyche.

Flexibility of approach encompasses many considerations: When do we involve the entire family in a regular ongoing treatment? When do we utilize one or a series of meetings for diagnostic purposes? Will family therapy help individuation or promote continued symbioses in certain symbiotic families?

Teachers and students of adolescent psychiatry need much greater exposure to family techniques if we are to acquire significant clinical wisdom regarding these questions.

One can feel overwhelmed by the chaos of an adolescent's intrapsychic life. One can feel still further overwhelmed when seeing an adolescent together with his family, in the same room, over long periods of time. Nonetheless, I feel that we need to expose students of adolescent psychiatry to the reality of these interdigitating, overwhelming forces. More so than with any other age group, the psyche of the adolescent cannot be understood without appreciating the impinging and shifting pressures of the familial field.

11

INTRODUCTION

Indications and Contraindications for Family Therapy, by Daniel Offer and Evert Vanderstoep

The passage of the child through adolescence is frequently a period of major family stress. Anthony (1969) has described with clarity and wit the ways in which parents respond to the normal developmental events of their adolescent offspring's lives, while Leonard (1966), Esman (1982), and others have reviewed particular subsets of the family interactional processes that often characterize this phase.

Increasing attention has been directed in the past two decades to the total field of family relationships, its impact on the emergence of psychopathology in individual family members, and the potentiality for therapeutic intervention it affords. Today there exists a vast literature in this realm which it would be futile to attempt to summarize here. In their survey of the field, however, Offer and Vanderstoep provide not only such a summary, but also a useful classification of the range of family therapies and their theoretical foundations. With this introduction they offer a concise but cogent argument for the selective use of family therapy—or rather family-centered interventions—in certain types of adolescent problems. They also describe the reverse situation—a case

in which the family was treated through the individual patient. Their paper provides a broad conceptual background
for consideration of the family approach in adolescent psychiatry.

11

Indications and Contraindications for Family Therapy

Daniel Offer, M.D., and
Evert Vanderstoep, M.D.

The purpose of this chapter is to outline the indications
and contraindications for family therapy. We will review the
relevant literature and share our own clinical experiences in
treating families. We are limiting ourselves to the treatment
of families with two generations present. Our main interest
is in families where one generation is represented by adolescents (puberty to the end of high school) and the other
generation is composed of the parents of these children.

In order to condense a great deal of complex material, one
needs to develop a classification system. Practitioners of family therapy have been classified by Haley (1962), Haley and
Hoffman (1967), and Beels and Ferber (1969). We have developed yet another classification, based upon examination
of the literature on indications and contraindications for family therapy. Two distinct schools of thought emerge from the
literature: the psychoanalytical and the system analytical.
This classification may be useful in trying to understand the

Reprinted by permission from *Adolescent Psychiatry*, 3:249-262, 1974.
New York: Basic Books.

fundamental theoretical struggle in the field of family therapy.

REVIEW OF THE LITERATURE
THE PSYCHOANALYSTS

The following family therapists are selected to represent the psychoanalytic point of view: Ackerman (1966), Jackson (1959), Kramer (1970), Wynne (1965), and Williams (1967a). They hold to a nosological psychiatric classification system and conceptualize individuals and families along psychodynamic and psychopathologic points of view. For them, doing a diagnostic family interview enables the psychotherapist to diagnose psychopathological processes, and thus arrive at both family and individual diagnoses. With a diagnosis at hand, one can then select the most appropriate treatment or group of treatments. The nosological psychopathological point of view is natural to practitioners in the field of family therapy who are physicians. It employs the standard medical notion: disease—investigate—arrive at a diagnosis—select a proper treatment. There are very few nonphysicians in the field of family therapy who belong to this group.

For Jackson (1959), family interviewing is superior to collaborative work. More relevant data are gathered in family interviews, which enables the therapist to arrive at a better diagnosis. He distinguishes among four categories of families: (1) stable satisfactory; (2) unstable satisfactory; (3) unstable unsatisfactory; and (4) stable unsatisfactory. Families of the first category do not need therapy. He finds the unstable satisfactory category to be the one in which the best results are obtained from family therapy. In these families there is usually enough mutual regard between the spouses for the therapist to intervene directly. These people married because they were in love, and usually still are in love. The unstable unsatisfactory family comprises the largest bulk of severe psychopathology. In these families the nominal patient's recovery often poses a serious threat to the parents. There is only limited success in treating these families. Finally, in families of the stable unsatisfactory category, Jackson reports poor results. In a brief case report he describes a family session in which the nominal patient's brother, emboldened by his relationship to the therapist, tentatively offered some comments critical of his mother. The following morning the mother was taken to the hospital for an emergency cholecystectomy, and upon her return from the hospital the father was hospitalized for a coronary heart attack. In the midst of all this, the brother had an automobile accident in which he crashed into the rear of the car ahead. The family at this point decided they could no longer afford family therapy and placed the patient in a state hospital. Jackson's view was that treatment of the stable unsatisfactory family is a very risky undertaking.

Wynne (1965) states that he considers family therapy the treatment of choice under certain conditions. He feels that there are certain limitations intrinsic to family therapy, and other limitations which are imposed by external practical conditions. For exploratory family therapy a stable structured treatment setup is essential. An implied contraindication to family therapy is a situation in which a stable structured treatment setup is not possible. Family diagnosis—a necessary precursor to exploratory family therapy—may include home visits, psychological testing, and interviews with individual family members, and does not require a stable treatment structure. Family diagnosis is performed for the purpose of formulating a well-considered strategy. The general indications it offers for exploratory family therapy are for clarification and resolution of intrafamilial difficulties. In addition, family therapy provides a preferable approach to individual psychoanalytic or psychodynamic psychotherapies when a transference relationship cannot be established. Ideally, all family members should have a vital and continuing stake in the treatment. In order to set the stage for future possible family therapy, conjoint sessions are a necessary part of the initial evaluation. Wynne lists a number of psychiatric problems for which exploratory family therapy seems best suited:

Adolescent separation problems. The diagnostic problem here is whether the chief issue is an identity crisis or rebellious delinquent behavior. The problem is defined as an individual one if an identity conflict exists in the adolescent. However, for those adolescents who have failed to emerge from a symbiotic dependency relationship, exploratory family therapy is indicated.

The trading of dissociations. This involves an intricate network of perceptions about other family members and dissociations about one's own qualities. In this situation each family member projects a particular quality of feeling onto another family member.

Collective cognitive chaos and erratic distancing. These are families with schizophrenic members who manifest bizarre, disruptive threats and episodes. The members of these families suffer from a shared sense of being unable to reach one another on any feeling level. Each family member is painfully aware of his own need, and wishes for relatedness, but each feels that the others block intimacy. Some of the shared mechanisms for maintaining these exclusions have been described by Wynne under the headings of pseudomutuality and pseudohostility.

Amorphous communication. These families, mostly with a schizophrenic member, have an amorphous, vague, and distorted form of communication.

Wynne discusses several areas of skills that must be attained before one becomes a competent family therapist. By implication, he maintains that family therapy is contraindicated when a skilled family therapist is not available.

Kramer (1970, unpublished) provides a descriptive list of indications and contraindications for family therapy. He theorizes that there are two sets of problems: the intrapsychic and the interpersonal. One can distinguish between these two types, often just on the basis of the way the problem is presented to the therapist on the telephone. When it is presented as a difficulty the family is having with a certain member, or when the complaint is about trouble a family member is having with society, it is most likely an interpersonal problem, thus indicating family therapy. If the problem is presented in such terms as the unhappiness, shyness, or low self-esteem of a family member, it is likely to be intrapsychic and individual therapy will be indicated. However, Kramer recommends for several reasons that the evaluation be done with the family rather than with an individual. The first, of course, is to evaluate thoroughly if the problem is primarily intrapsychic or interpersonal, and decide if family therapy is the treatment of choice. Second, family evaluation provides a preparation for family interviews should they become necessary during the course of an individual treatment. Yet another important use of a series of family interviews would be preparation for psychoanalysis. Kramer believes that "the structuralizing and synthesizing effect of successful family therapy converts acting-out aspects of a character disorder into an internalized neurosis." He also recommends family therapy for helping families manage the care of a member who is severely physically or psychiatrically ill. A complete list of Kramer's indications and contraindications will be found in Table 1.

Shapiro (1967) stresses the importance of delineation, by which he means the image one person has of another. When these delineations are markedly inconsistent, exaggerated,

TABLE 1
Indications and Contraindications for Family Therapy

	Indications	Contraindications
Jackson	Unstable-satisfactory Unstable-unsatisfactory	Stable-unsatisfactory
Wynne	Adolescent separation problems	Some severe depressions
	Trading dissociations	Some severe masochistic states
	Collective cognitive chaos and erratic distancing	Acute schizophrenia
	Fixed distancing with eruptive threats	Lack of structured treatment setting
	Amorphous communication	Unavailability of skilled family therapist
Kramer	Majority of complaints interpersonal	Same therapist converting from individual to family therapy
	Conflict between family members and society	A firm decision to divorce
	Acute family crisis	Severe psychotic depression
	Families with poorly structured ego and chronically disturbed functioning	Hard core psychopathy
	Unsuccessful individual treatment	Chronic schizophrenic psychosis
	Supervision of one family member	One family member in intensive individual treatment
	Learning blocks in children	An older adolescent who is preoccupied with disengagement from the family
	Preparation for psychoanalysis	
Shapiro	Markedly inconsistent images of parents and adolescent of each other	
Howells	Necessary background for all therapies	Process schizophrenia

	Indications	Contraindications
Whitaker	Necessary background for all therapies	Unskilled family therapist; severe psychosomatic illness
Ackerman	A wide range of behavior disorders, especially: 1. Interpersonal conflicts that affect outcome of intrapsychic conflicts 2. Reducing secondary gains of emotional illness 3. Marital disturbances 4. Disturbances with relationship of children and adolescents 5. Acting out (delinquency, drug abuse, sexual promiscuity)	The process of a malignant, irreversible trend toward breakup of the family, which may mean that it is too late to reverse the process of fragmentation Dominance within the group of a concentrated focus of malignant, destructive motivation One parent who is afflicted with an organized progressive paranoid condition, or with incorrigible psychopathic destructiveness, or who is a confirmed criminal or pervert Parents, one or both, who are unable to be sufficiently honest; lying and deceitfulness that are deeply rooted in the group negate the potential usefulness of family therapy The existence of a certain kind of valid family secret The existence of an unyielding cultural, religious, or economic prejudice against this form of intervention The existence in some members of extremely rigid defenses which, if broken, might induce a psychosis, a psychosomatic crisis, or physical assault Finally, the presence of organic disease or other disablement of a progressive nature that precludes the participation of one or more members

and destructive in nature, family therapy is indicated in order to correct the family members' views of each other. Shapiro states, "The family session is an excellent situation in which to establish the actuality of the adolescent's maturation and the idiosyncratic and defensive aspects of the parents' response to it" (pp. 235-236).

Howells (personal communication) believes that a family orientation is a necessary background for all therapies. However, he has found family therapy unsuccessful and hence contraindicated in families with a member who suffers from "process schizophrenia." This diagnostic entity is more clearly defined in Europe than in the United States. Investigators like Friedman et al. (1965), Lidz, Fleck, and Cornelison (1965), and Wynne (1965) would probably disagree with Howell's statement.

Ackerman (1966) believes that family therapy should promote a sense of well-being, of getting rid of something from which a person is suffering. But, he believes, it is not enough to expunge the bad without being prepared to replace it with something better. Unless the patient is able to envision a new and better way of living, he will cling to his old ways. Families at any one time exhibit both health-maintaining and health-eroding forces. The balance shifts with time and the vicissitudes of life situations. Wellness or sickness are value concepts that reflect a way of life.

When a conflict cannot be adequately contained, it spills over into irrational acting out. On other occasions the control of the conflict fails and leads to progressive disorganization in family relations. Prejudicial scapegoating is a result of conflicts being misperceived and hence uncontained and unresolved.

In evaluating families, Ackerman stresses that we must keep in mind the goals of psychotherapy. They are to remove disabling symptoms, to strengthen the patient's personality, to enable the person to realize his potential by capitalizing on his resources, and to help him become an efficient, productive, and happy human being. The method is influenced by many factors: (1) personal expectations of the patient; (2) orientation of the psychotherapist toward his role; (3) group influences surrounding the patient; and (4) group influences surrounding the therapist.

Family therapy can appropriately be applied to a wide range of behavior disorders. It can be useful in the treatment of neurosis, psychosis, and character disorders, especially those that show acting out, but it must be flexibly accommodated to the specific and unique features of each of these conditions. It is especially helpful in those conditions in which the current interpersonal struggles of the family potentially affect the outcome of individual coping with intrapsychic conflicts. Family therapy is also uniquely effective with marital disorders and with disturbances involving the relationship of children and adolescents with the family.

THE SYSTEM ANALYSTS

The system analysts are usually nonmedical practitioners who view people in distress as individuals who are part of a system, and believe that considerations of nosology and psychopathology are a potential interference with the most helpful response. Such a response can only occur when the two systems engage each other in a most open and flexible way. Unterberger (personal communication) believes that discussion of when and when not to do family therapy can be an externalization of the therapist's question of himself: "What am I willing to do and what do I not want to do?" To say that a family is unfit for family therapy because they are unmotivated may mean that they will not come to the office. In that event, home visits are in order. To say that the inability to convene a full family session is a contraindication may miss critical issues for that family. When a therapist takes the time and energy to convene the family network, he accomplishes a considerable amount of therapeutic work in the process. Clear statements about what we want to accomplish with a family, shared with a family, often pave the way to effective interventions with "untreatable" families.

In the system analysts' view, everyone, therapist and patient alike, is limited by the developmental level of his current system. Good therapy takes place when patients are fortunate enough to encounter a system in which the participants can accomplish mutual growth. Hence, all concerns about disease and psychopathology become irrelevant. The only important thing is the potential for mutual evolution and change in the two intermeshing systems. A well-known expositor of this view is Whitaker (1968). A good deal of the thrust of Whitaker's work can be described by his term "the growing edge." He believes that the most crucial factor in indications for family therapy is the presence of a skilled family therapist. Respect for the power of the two-generation system has prompted Whitaker to insist that family therapy be done by two therapists, but cotherapy is only possible where the therapists respect each other. He also asserts, as do most system analysts and psychoanalysts, that one should never schedule interviews at the outset of treatment with less than the entire family in attendance.

Haley (1971) has some of the strongest words to say on the matter of indications and contraindications for family therapy. He clearly states that he believes it is a "nonquestion." According to Haley, the more experienced family therapist will appear puzzled, since he finds defining any kind of therapy a way of intervening with a family. Psychopathology is redefined as a relationship problem, and the unit of diagnosis and treatment is no longer the individual but the family. Explorations of the genetic background of unsatisfactory patterns can be safely dispensed with, since they are a bore to the patients and a waste of time. Psychodynamics may be interesting to the therapist, but are not useful to people in distress. Understanding of one's interpersonal operations is not helpful because what is needed is "change," and understanding does not produce change. Different interpersonal operations, with their own feedback and redundancies, must be established for therapy to take place. The agent of change is change itself.

Haley discusses contraindications for family therapy when he describes the disquieting effect upon the standard outpatient clinic of the introduction of family therapy methods. Several reasons are advanced for this effect. The usual existing hierarchy will be disrupted, inasmuch as most staff members will only be students in family therapy, hence changing the old division of who does and knows more than whom. This can develop to a point at which the lower-paid professional staff are more skilled than the higher-paid staff. The other disquieting aspect of the introduction of family therapy methods is that it requires abandonment of cherished theoretical systems and their replacement by interpersonal theories. In addition, the emphasis on diagnosis and evaluation, which, according to Haley, is a device to deal with the therapist's anxiety, has to be replaced with an action-oriented point of view in which experienced therapists share an awareness that much can be accomplished with active intervention. The primary concern in evaluation becomes the nature of the family's response to intervention by that particular therapist or cotherapy team. When a family meets the therapist, their systems are interacting, and progress is a product of these interactions.

McGregor (personal communication) states that family therapy is indicated when the family can be convened, and not indicated when the family cannot be convened.

The system analysts do believe that many helpful forces can be brought to bear on the family system in distress. Behavioral modification techniques, individual psychotherapies, and group psychotherapies all find their place in a natural evolution from the base of the naturally occurring system—the family. In summary, the system analysts regard discussion of indications and contraindications as not meaningful or germane to principal therapy issues. For them, the only possible approach to distress is attending to the family system.

THE FAMILY IN PSYCHOTHERAPY

Psychotherapeutic interventions involving the family as a system are of recent origin. Freud (1909) recognized early that the relationship between generations is of utmost importance for the mental health of the child. In the case of Little Hans, he treated the child through the father, although he did not see the child himself. Later, in the child guidance movement in the United States, the team approach was instituted in which a family was treated in the clinic, but never together in the same room. The child had his own therapist, as did the parents. It was not until shortly after World War II that investigators began seeing the family as a psychosocial unit with its own aims, problems, psychopathology, and coping devices. It was felt then that if the unit was treated together—at the same time, and by the same therapist—the changes which would take place through therapy would affect the family as a whole. Thus, if the family changed its style of adaptations and the nature of the relationship among its members, a new homeostasis would develop. Roles would change and an opportunity for new experiences could appear. The stereotyped and rigid relationships between generations would be lessened, hence giving rise to a potential for growth through learning. Open and flowing communications were seen as an essential ingredient for the functioning of a relatively healthy family.

We do not intend in this chapter to explore the difficult question of the characteristics of a normal or healthy family. Like medicine in general and psychiatry in particular, it is easier to describe the characteristics of a disturbed family. For the purposes of this chapter, a disturbed family is defined as one which has come to the psychotherapist and has asked for help. The family can be self-referred, referred by a friend, or by another professional. They can have a nominal patient often defined as the "scapegoat" (Bell and Vogel, 1960), or they can feel that they have a family problem.

As often happens with relatively new psychotherapeutic techniques, schools or movements may develop. Adherents of the new school extol the virtues of the technique, find its leaders charismatic, and have the tendency to dump other forms of treatment. This overreaction to the appearance of a perfectly valid new technique has the tendency to: (1) make enemies of adherents of the old schools who have not tried the new method but are suspicious of the excessive claims made; (2) encourage the practitioners of the new school to overextend themselves and try to cure all mental illness with their new approach; and (3) lead to inevitable disappointments in patients and psychotherapists alike.

We believe that the field of family therapy has now reached the stage at which we can begin to take a sober look at both the achievements and the failures of this particular approach. We have chosen family therapy as a technique with adolescents because this is a period during the life span of the individual when intergenerational conflicts are expected to arise. It might be helpful to work out such problems with the total family; however, this approach also creates special problems.

It has been our experience that, in general, we can divide adolescents into three groups (regardless of their diagnosis):

The individual. The adolescent who states emphatically that he has a personal problem for which he seeks help and under no circumstances does he want to be in a room with parents.

The individual as part of the family. The adolescent who states that he will come into treatment only if his whole family comes because they have a family problem.

The individual as part of the group. Lately we have seen a number of adolescents who claim to have peer group problems and want to be treated only in group therapy.

The parents can, of course, also be divided into the three groups. These groups do not necessarily correspond with those which, theoretically, could benefit from family therapy, but it is important that the therapist take into account the initial bias of the patient. A charismatic therapist can often convince the patient to try another approach; it depends on the depth of the patient's conviction.

At times the specific belief system or cultural environment precludes the use of family therapy. For example, one of us recently saw a 15-year-old acting-out adolescent girl for evaluation. There was much discontent between the parents. The mother was depressed and the father readily admitted to having extramarital affairs. The girl had run away from home on numerous occasions, had acted out sexually, was angry, and did poorly in school. She admitted that she needed psychotherapy, but absolutely refused to be seen together with her parents. Here the therapist has a relatively simple choice; he begins by seeing her in individual psychotherapy or refers her to another therapist.

We would like to stress another form of distortion which often may affect the therapist. A therapist in a community begins to be known for his expertise in working with a particular set of problems or special kinds of patients. If his field is family therapy, he would tend to get referrals from colleagues, other mental health professionals, and former patients which coincide with his major interest. The initial screening has already been done for him. When he meets with the family for an evaluation he finds that the majority belong to the third group of patients—those who want to work as a family. In the past five years over 60 percent of the adolescents between the ages of 13 and 17 who were referred to us by colleagues or other mental health professionals came specifically for family therapy. A therapist in this position might get the erroneous impression that most adolescents are amenable to or interested in family therapy. This is not the case. One of us has recently moved his private office to a new location where his interests in family therapy were not known. The first four teenagers that he saw have all had family therapy in the past and stated that under no circumstances will they try it again!

We do not believe that there is any single type of psychotherapeutic technique which is applicable to most adolescent problems. Many variables have to be considered, including the value system of the patients. For the relatively healthy adolescent, most psychotherapeutic methods used by an expert will prove helpful. For the very disturbed, most psychotherapeutic techniques are inadequate. A firmly developed therapeutic alliance based on a positive initial impression (likability factor) is often more important than the type of intervention used.

We disagree with those who say that failure to convene the family is a demonstration of the therapist's lack of commitment to family therapy. At times failure to convene a family may indicate a problem in the therapist's commitment. However, the following case vignette is offered to illustrate that family therapy is not always possible, even though clearly indicated, and that to be effective we had to operate like Bowen (1966), treating the family through one member.

The therapist met this patient when she was 18 years old. She had had previous treatment with a series of therapists, including an experience with family therapy. In each case the therapy was aborted either because the therapist couldn't stand the patient or the patient couldn't stand the therapist. However, she liked the present therapist from the beginning, and the therapist liked her, though he found her very trying. The therapist struggled alone with her and her parents for six months, recognized that he needed help, and introduced a cotherapist. No amount of documentation of the complementarity of the family members' moods and behavior could persuade this family to meet as a family. The therapists did browbeat the parents into agreeing to meet with them every third week, and they did so for 18 months. However, the only recorded effect of such interviews was that the parents fought more for a few days following each interview. The interviews with the parents did provide the therapists with a backlog of experience and enabled them to speak with the daughter about her parents from a position of experience.

Over several years of treatment, the strong symbiotic tie between mother and daughter and the strong support that father gave to daughter in order to enable her to tolerate a life of sacrificing everything for her mother have gradually been unraveled and loosened. The process of treatment is so far very encouraging, in that serious suicide attempts are a thing of the past, and the daughter has been able to achieve a measure of calm and some satisfaction and joy in her life. She has not as yet achieved independence from her parents.

This case demonstrates that the therapist needs to be flexible and work with a family when feasible and appropriate, but not withdraw when one part of the system refuses to go on. The family may not always cooperate with family therapy, particularly if the parents are threatened by the potential improvement in their child without concomitant benefits for themselves. Although family interviews were resisted in this case, the family was treated in absentia.

It is important to select the functional social subsystem for participation in family therapy. This functional social subsystem may, but does not necessarily, correspond to the legal definition of the family. Unavailability of one or more members of a defined functional social subsystem may well be a contraindication to family therapy. A necessary condition for exploratory family therapy is the stability of the membership that meets with the therapists.

A further consideration when making a recommendation for family therapy is the phase in the psychotherapeutic process. There may come a time in exploratory family therapy when individual therapy should supplant the family therapy, or family therapy may be contraindicated initially because of prominent intrapsychic problems that need to be dealt with first. Some depressed or severely masochistic individuals, who soak up all the blame for family difficulties, need a period of individual therapy before family therapy can actually be started. In families with an acutely schizophrenic member who is still in panic and has not yet established a relationship with a therapist, family therapy is contraindicated. Such patients may be unable to tolerate the complexities of family interviews. In these situations, it may be best to delay family interviews for a month or two until the psychotic individual has developed some trust in the therapist and the panic has diminished.

There are a number of psychological routes from childhood to adulthood. One type of normal, middle-class suburban adolescent goes through adolescence with relatively few overt conflicts (Offer, 1969). His general behavior does not conflict with the parents' values, and his rebellion, which occurs in early adolescence, is in the service of emancipation and separation from the parents. The disturbed adolescent may have a variety of psychodynamics which stem from different intrapsychic conflicts. There is nothing, however, which disturbs parents, teachers, law enforcement officers, and society in general as much as an acting-out adolescent. The behavior of the acting-out adolescent may represent itself in promiscuity, drug abuse, delinquency, perversion, vandalism, or violence. These adolescents are seen as spiteful, angry, negativistic, solemn, narcissistic, egotistic, and unconcerned with their fellow man. At times they possess enough insight to know that they have problems. They often want help, but find it hard to ward off impulses when they are with their peers. It is for these adolescents that family therapy can be particularly helpful. The therapy shows the teenager and his family (parents and siblings) that the acting out has meaning and is not performed in isolation, but rather is in response to verbal and nonverbal cues from other members of the family. The family discussion may demonstrate clearly that the behavioral response of one of the teenagers reflects tension in the whole family system. When the acting-out behavior stops, other parts of the family frequently show overt conflict; for example, marital disharmony between the father and mother may not come to the surface until the acting out has stopped. Even more dramatically, the parents, together or separately, stimulate the acting out of their child in order to have an external problem with which to deal. In our experience, acting-out behavior can be interrupted most dramatically by family therapy.

Recently, one of us saw a 15-year-old boy who was referred because of behavioral problems in the home and in school, because there was evidence of active sexual play between him and his eight-year-old sister. The parents have had a poor relationship. The boy did not want psychotherapy. Only after a number of family sessions, at which it was pointed out to the entire family that they had a "family problem," did the boy consent to come for help. It was not long before the family realized that there was considerable similarity among the boy's acting out, the mother's seductive behavior, and the father's solemn, depressed, and withdrawn attitude. Symptom relief came relatively fast (after three months). Tension in the family was reduced and the family was able to function on a higher level of integration. With the improvement of communication, understanding between the generations became possible.

Conclusions

In reviewing the relevant literature on the indications and contraindications for family therapy, we discovered and described two major groupings of practitioners and their approaches. The psychoanalysts essentially utilize the medical model, which emphasizes diagnosis and attempts to select the proper treatment: individual, family, or group. These therapists evaluate indications and contraindications as they revolve around a determination of the quality of intrapersonal struggle versus interpersonal conflict. The group called the system analysts are usually nonmedical practitioners who view people in distress as part of a system, and believe that considerations of nosology and psychopathology interfere with the open and flexible response necessary for both patients and therapist.

The field of family therapy has reached the stage at which it can be evaluated in an objective manner concerning its usefulness. Family therapy is a valuable technique with adolescents because adolescence is a period when intergenerational conflicts are expected to arise, and therefore work with the total family may be indicated. However, no one type of psychotherapeutic technique is applicable to all adolescent problems, and development of a therapeutic alliance based on positive initial impression may be more important than the type of intervention.

PART IV

Group Therapy

12

INTRODUCTION

Group Psychotherapy with a Mixed Group of Adolescents, by Nathan W. Ackerman

In principle, group therapy would seem to be an ideal technique for the treatment of adolescents. Given their natural propensity to form and communicate in groups of peers, the discomfort many of them experience in one-to-one relations with adults, and their tendency to use the peer group as a source of emotional support, one would expect adolescents to take favorably to the group situation.

As a result, group therapy has, since its conception by Slavson (1945), been used by many therapists as either an adjunct to individual treatment or as the primary modality. This has been particularly the case in settings where groups are naturally available—i.e., in psychiatric hospital units, residential treatment centers, and reformatories.

Ackerman's was one of the earliest reports of experience with the outpatient treatment of adolescents in groups. A restless experimenter, as evidenced by his later pioneering work in the field of family therapy (1958, 1966), he was one of the first to undertake work with mixed male-female groups, a practice frowned on by some who feared that sexual excitation would interfere with group process. Ackerman found, on the contrary, that the sexes complemented each other in such groups, and that the mixture promoted the expression of crucial conflicts. And, well before some other students of the field, Ackerman recognized that adolescence involved something more than the recapitulation of oedipal conflicts (see Blos, 1979b). In many ways, too, Ackerman's emphasis on the adolescent's sense of incompleteness of self-image and on the therapeutic effort to promote its consolidation prefigures some important current trends (e.g., Kernberg, 1975; Kohut, 1977) in psychoanalytic thinking on narcissism and "the psychology of the self."

12

Group Psychotherapy with a Mixed Group of Adolescents

Nathan W. Ackerman, M.D.

The most striking aspect, by far, in the behavior of adolescents in group therapy is their yearning to complete their incomplete selves. They simply do not feel whole, and from this feeling arises a painful tension. Very transparent, indeed, is their effort to extract selectively from their group experience that which they lack, so that they may win approval, and in their own eyes more closely approximate their ideal image of themselves. This striving holds for male and female alike, though on a different plane, and toward different goals. Such behavior is clearly a phase of the adolescents' extensive preoccupation with self in an era of development in which they must all too rapidly accommodate both to the critical growth changes occurring within themselves, and to the rigorous requirements which society imposes upon youths about to take their place in the community as adult men and women. During this phase, one observes their extraordinary sensitiveness to other persons' judgments of their worth, their constant concern with proving adequacy, their

Reprinted by permission from the *International Journal of Group Psychotherapy*, 5:249-260, 1955. New York: International Universities Press.

profound sense of vulnerability to criticism and attack from without. They are caught between the twin horns of conformity and defiance. It is small wonder that they show such trigger-edge irritability.

In this crucial period of maturation, these young people display tender skins, but nowhere does one see their rawness, sensitiveness, and need to prove themselves more vividly than in the relations between the sexes. The drama of male and female, each coming into their own, is intense. The awareness of each other is acute. Each stands poised, hyperalert, and vigilant, prepared to react with lightning rapidity to the other's slightest move. The feeling of incompleteness and the need of each other is strong, but being immature, and lacking the sure movements of the more experienced adults, they approach each other in gingerly fashion, each waiting for the other to make the first move, each seeking to feel out the ill-defined dangers of proximity, and ready at a moment's notice to leap to their own defense or retreat. They need each other, but fear and mistrust each other. The craving to complete themselves in the other is clear, but the fear of betrayal, and the fear of losing oneself in the other are equally intense. The elemental urge for union is tempered by the fear of injury through domination. They yearn to uncover themselves but do not dare. Unnamed dangers loom large, so they run for cover. The desire to exhibit themselves turns into a fear of exposure, and exaggerated hiding. Because of insecurity, confusion, fright, and the frantic flight to self-defense, the basic urge of the one sex toward the other turns into a battle of the sexes on a grand scale. The ambivalence is conspicuous and dramatic. The struggle of the sexes becomes waged in a domination-submission frame. In this struggle, all too frequently, safety is sought in protective alliances with members of the same sex. The drama is fierce, dangerous, deadly serious, but thrilling.

This description gives some of the emotional coloring of interaction between the sexes in an adolescent therapy group. Feelings are not merely verbally expressed; they are intensely lived out in the permissive atmosphere of a therapy group of this sort. Obviously, the experience is not without some risk, but with understanding, caution, and appropriate channeling of expression, the risk can be reduced to a minimum.

Two related dynamic trends stand out sharply: the adolescent's reactions to shifting images of self, propelled from within by the physiological processes of maturation, and from without by the demands of the outside world. On the one hand, they must accommodate to the pressures of sexual need, to changes in physique and appearance; on the other hand, they must accommodate to what others expect of them. In this last respect, they are influenced in two ways: by their beliefs as to what the opposite sex wants of them, and what members of the same sex, particularly those whom they admire and wish to emulate, expect of them. The adolescent personality is squeezed between these several conflicting pressures. This is the pivot around which much of the therapeutic interaction in the group proceeds. On this stage of conflict are reflected the confusions and anxieties relating to sexual identity, the feelings of inferiority associated with awareness of physical difference, the compensating aggressive reactions to anxiety. On this stage, too, emerge responses of guilt and shame, guilt deriving particularly from conflicted sexual temptation and aggressive impulses, and shame deriving from exhibitionistic urges, preoccupation with shortcomings, and failure to live up to the idealized image of self. In this connection, the dread of ridicule and humiliation is often intense.

Again and again, conflict with parental authority intrudes on the scene, literally loaded with the ambivalent emotions of unresolved dependence, the urge to demonstrate self-sufficiency, and the apprehension of one or another form of castration. It is not true, however, that the stage of adolescent conflict represents purely the reactivation of unresolved oedipal conflict. What one observes actually is a reactivation of all significant previous levels of conflict, oedipal and preoedipal as well. Clearly dramatized here are the deep formative influences of the "oral" and "anal" levels of personality on the later emerging genital conflicts. Equally transparent are the patterns of defense mobilized against guilt and anxiety deriving from these conflicts.

The therapeutic group provides a social testing ground for the distorted, inappropriate perceptions of self, and relations with others, deriving from all the stages of maturation. On this testing ground, the adolescent has the opportunity gradually to put his confusion to one side and achieve some dependable, stable clarity in his personal identity.

For some 10 years, I have observed the reactions of adolescents of both sexes in weekly group-therapeutic sessions. Originally, each of these patients was clinically known to me. All of them entered individual psychotherapy, some with myself, others with other therapists to whom these patients were referred. The weekly group experience was conceived as a supplement to individual therapy, not as an independent therapy on its own. The role of group therapist was mainly assumed by myself, though the therapists treating other members of the group individually were regularly present. They were themselves active participants, shared with me the responsibility of conducting the proceedings, and in my absence, took over fully the role of group therapist. In this sense, the other therapists in the group were closely identified with me and served as auxiliary therapists. Usually there were three, sometimes four therapists present, both male and female. Not infrequently, too, we had some "visiting firemen," psychiatrists and caseworkers who wished to observe the proceedings. At such times, the patients learned to accept them into the group freely and with a minimum of anxiety. As a whole, the group evolved a rather free, mobile, fluid character, of which this casual attitude toward visiting professionals was but one feature.

For the patients, attendance was voluntary. Fees covered a broad range, and were often waived. The emotional connotations of fees for professional service did not play a prominent role. The personal atmosphere was informal, intimate; the business aspect of the relationship was reduced to a minimum. Though attendance was purely voluntary, with some few exceptions, the patients came with great regularity. No pressure was applied with regard to occasional absences, no demands for explanation were made, no stimulus for self-justification was offered. Attendance was accepted at face value as an indicator of the presence of incentive and the wish to participate. When absences occurred, they usually turned out to have been unavoidable, and often the patient spontaneously expressed regret at having missed the pleasure of the session. The group was inconstant in size and composition. In numbers, it varied from five to six to as many as 18. The optimum size for effective participation seemed to be roughly eight to 10. The age range was also wide, from 16 to 23, with occasional exceptions reaching up to 27 years. Also, a special influence was injected into the experience when now and then a married person entered the group, or a member changed status from single to married. When this happened, the group was fluid enough to welcome the participation of the spouse. From time to time old patients left, new ones were added. Not infrequently, group members invited personal friends to visit once or twice, who were usually freely accepted into the group. The exceptions to this usually occurred when the visitor was arrogant or held himself defensively aloof; this generally stirred up resentment.

Diagnostically, all categories of personality and types of emotional disturbance were included with the exception of frank psychoses. In the case of neurotic characters with a strong propensity for "acting out," particularly the exhibitionistic personalities, there seemed ordinarily to be no special problem. The group patterns spontaneously imposed restraint on these characters, and seemed to exercise a salutary effect. If the grandiose and exhibitionistic tendencies were intense and strongly pathological and the group after a time proved not to be too congenial, such persons usually left of their own accord. Apart from clinical diagnosis, the main criteria for admission were confused attitudes concerning social and sexual adaptation and the individual therapist's judgment that the patient was emotionally ready for, and would profit from, group experience. This judgment was usually mutually agreed upon by patient and therapist, after a variable length of preparation in individual therapy. I emphasize here that improvement in individual therapy was conceived in part as preparation for group experience, because many of these adolescents were seriously ill at the time of initial examination. In making this comment, I am aware that for some categories of disturbance, the opposite principle may hold, namely, that group therapy can be considered as an emotional preparation for individual therapy.

Of immediate interest are the varied types of response patients displayed when the therapist discussed with them, in individual sessions, the possibility of entering the group. They were distinctly of two types, fear and recoil, or an instantaneous burst of enthusiasm, a "raring to go" attitude. The first type of reaction was by far the more common, the latter relatively infrequent. In the first response, one observed initially fright, dread of exposure, attack, and ridicule. The patients seemed dominated by their anticipatory fantasies of the aggressive dangers lurking in such an exposed experience. Obviously, the intensity of this initial reaction derives from projection of their own aggressive impulses. They reacted at first with a strong urge to retreat. In anxiety-ridden personalities, this is easy to understand if we remember that the individual therapeutic relationship provides a safe haven, that the patient is offered immunity against retaliation by the therapist. In the group, there is no such immunity, no guarantee of protection from aggression. The situation is an exposed one. The patient must take his chances. Generally, after a period of time and continued discussion of the opportunities in group interaction, the initial apprehension and urge to retreat subside, and anticipatory fantasies of pleasure become stronger. Spontaneously, the patient's inner urge to seek out gratifications of personal need in the group asserts itself and soon the patient expresses willingness to try the group, though often with a sense of insecurity and with continued reservations.

At the other pole are those rarer individuals who burst with delight at the anticipation of group experience, who indulge pleasant fantasies of a grand and glorious landing in the group, creating a "wow" of an impression, smearing the landscape, so to speak, with their superiority, sophistication, and irresistable attraction. These are the adolescents with a strong push to impress others with their superior attributes, with their sexual finesse, and triumphs. These are the aggressive, impulsive exhibitionists, who hide their anxiety behind their competitive aggressive drive. I have found, though, barring the extreme types, the psychopathic or near psychotic, that the group is a useful instrumentality for taming these bold ones.

Between these two extremes, the acutely frightened adolescent and the grandiose exhibitionist, one finds every intermediate type. Most usually, the reaction to the suggestion of group therapy is a strangely ambivalent one; the effect is to whet the appetite for direct gratification of personal need in the group, while at the same time the excitement of temptation is sobered by the stirring of anxiety connected with anticipatory fantasies of exposure, betrayal, and humiliation. One possible contributing factor to this reaction may derive from certain components of transference; the patient extends from the individual therapist to the group his repressed hope of getting direct gratification of sexual need, his guilt, fear of punishment, and urge to retreat. In certain instances, the mere suggestion of group therapy energizes in the individual therapeutic experience a working through of specific problems hitherto undisclosed. For example, certain specific fantasies of punishment for sexual transgression may remain mainly repressed for a time in individual therapy, due to the special kind of protection the individual therapist provides his patient. In the group, this artificial immunity is removed. In this sense, the very anticipation of group therapy holds some potential for enhancing the value of individual sessions. The transfer of influence from the one therapeutic situation to the other moves in both directions, however; the proceedings in the individual sessions often give concrete substance to the problems the patient struggles to solve in the group; the effect of group experience activates useful work in the individual sessions. In my judgment, an arrangement for concomitant individual and group therapy is of specific value in that it holds this rich potential of mutual fertilization of the proceedings in the two therapeutic situations.

I should like now to convey something of the concrete quality of the behavior of these adolescents in a group session. Typically, at the outset, there are some rapid, casual banterings as people get seated, and the seating arrangement is of great emotional significance. Who sits next to whom and why? Sometimes there is a dramatic parting of the sexes, in that all the males seat themselves together, on one side, and all the females on the other. This is a specific sign of sexual tension. It means awareness that someone is "making a play" for someone else; the someone else plays "hard to get" and there is suspense in the air as to whether the gamble will win. At other times, there is conspicuous recognition that a particular boy seats himself next to a particular girl and this excites admiration, envy, competitive maneuvering, and barbed jokes. A rival tries to steal the play. All the excitement becomes suppressed, however, just as soon as the therapist takes his place and indicates readiness for the session to begin. There is typically a hushed silence, a silence that speaks eloquently of the air laden with the tension of suspense. The question is, Who will make the first move to expose himself, or will the therapist "pick on someone"? Facial expressions either light up or suddenly go blank; the members peer penetratingly at one another. Occasionally, a particular adolescent stares at the ceiling conspicuously or averts his gaze. This last is an indicator of his urge to reveal himself. He wants to be the center, he wants to be looked at; yet he is afraid. The struggle is between the urge to show oneself and the fear of getting "out on a limb." The danger of hurtful consequences of exposure seems ever present. Now and then, the struggle as to who will make the first move becomes crystallized in the battle between the sexes. The mutual suspicion of the two sexes is striking. The boys shove the girls into the open, the girls shove the boys. They tease each other. The males are particularly sensitive about their adequacy, imagining that every girl wants an athletic hero, a superman. The girls make flip remarks about the boys' masculinity, thus covering their own anxiety about femaleness. Each wants the other to uncover, each wants to see and be seen, but fears being hurt in the process. The issue is: Which urge will prove the stronger, to "undress," figuratively speaking, or keep safe behind one's coverings?

Sooner or later, the tension cracks, some one opens up. The initial suspense subsides, and the group gets down to work. The discussion gathers its own momentum. The problems these patients toss into the hopper of group interaction center on several main subject matters: personal fears and incapacities, conflict with parental authority, conflict concerning sex, aggressive competition, and attitudes toward future plans. Whatever the subject matter, the members of the group are "all ears," listening with rapt attention, envious of the person holding the center of the stage, but constrained by a sense of fair play, and inhibiting the urge to usurp the speaker's position lest they be accused of wanting to "hog the show"; though, with true ambivalence, if offered "the floor," they will often demur. Despite these rivalrous feelings, a high level of camaraderie evolves which insures a fair "sharing of the cheese." When the picture is added up, there is little "hogging"; the group morale is of high quality; everyone has a chance.

In a typical instance, the adolescent hides his anxieties by couching his problem initially in circumstantial or social terms, playing down and obscuring the specific psychological content of the problem. The influence of the therapist, and the group members follow his example, is to challenge the patient's incentive for a more sincere, more honest, and deeper level of revelation of the personal and psychological core of his problems. The first task, then, is to strip away the protective garb and achieve a clear, straightforward definition of the problem, articulated and revealed in personal terms. At this juncture some members of the group may immediately be tempted to exploit one patient's personal exposure for purposes of attack. The greater the personal anxiety, the greater the temptation to seize this channel for the release of hostility. Should this happen, however, the therapist and the morale of the group act as restraining influences. Frequently, the opposite occurs; the patient engaged in personal revelation, instead of being subjected to attack, is pleasantly surprised and rewarded by a show of support and encouragement, often from unexpected quarters in the group. This emotional support is of great moment in facilitating increasing candor of expression. In any case, the problem is battered back and forth in the group. Other members are stimulated to disclose similar problems, and, bit by bit, the emotional content of the problem becomes more precisely and nudely revealed.

The therapist's contribution can be defined in several facets. Words as words are anathema. It is not "talk, talk, and more talk," since conversation can and is used so deftly to hide rather than reveal, but rather the effort to reach behind words to the genuine affect which is being experienced.

I am reminded here of the famous reflection on the nature of conversation by Nietzsche. He related how two people, on meeting each other for the first time as complete strangers, have an instantaneous impression of each other, before each has had opportunity to utter a word. As soon as conversation is initiated, the initial impressions the one person has of the other become progressively modified. Each thinks the very first impression must have been completely wrong. Nietzsche says that the first impression was exactly right and the subsequent ones wrong, and that the conversation which ensued served merely the purpose of deceiving the listener.

It is somewhat in this spirit that an effort is made in the group to reach behind mere talk to genuine feelings. The technique for accomplishing this is to be intensely attentive to nonverbal patterns of behavior, facial expressions, body posturings, quick shifts in the motor behavior of patients as they react to the stimuli of group interaction processes. At the same time, the therapist with calculated intention ignores and sidesteps the kind of talk which is mere talk. The ther-

apist's spirit in reaching out for genuine emotional communication is contagious, affects the attitudes of group
members, and the push for more honest self-revelation is
accelerated. The therapist's emphasis on the theme, "the
body talks," carries over to the group; not only the therapist
but patients as well search out the nonverbal emotional communications concealed in the spontaneous posturings of patients. The therapist does this sometimes by interpreting an
obvious expressional attitude in a given adolescent, or by
arousing the curiosity of the entire group as to its meaning.
For example, an 18-year-old boy is greeted in the conventional manner. Asked how he is, the quick reply is "fine." But
his face is like a wet blanket, frozen, hang-dog. This is immediately challenged. Or another boy, the same age, is talking, but isn't saying anything. His words are mumbled, they
run into one another, as if he were rolling potatoes inside
his mouth. Someone calls out challengingly, "Tight ass, don't
you want to give us anything?"

Four-letter words are used freely and casually, not to show
off or defy social conventions, but rather because intense
affects are often associatively tied to them; by comparison,
the more polite, conventional terms seem feeble, because the
significant emotions have been stripped away from them.
When on occasion an adolescent uses four-letter words with
the obvious motive of exhibiting his sophistication or in order
to shock other members, he is quickly told off. Gradually,
the members of the group become conditioned to a code
which promotes frank self-revelation, minus rationalizations,
alibis, and other self-protective dressing. Tolerance for this
can be and is learned. The anxiety connected with exposure
progressively lessens.

Of particular importance in the group atmosphere is the
shedding of conventional social hypocrisies. Adolescents de-
test polite dishonesties, and are genuinely grateful for a

group experience in which they can shrug off the unpleasant burdens of conventionally sanctioned patterns of deception in social relations. It is a comfort for these adolescents to be relieved of the silent compulsion toward "good manners" and conformity with other aspects of hypocritical morality which prevail in adult society. It is of significant cathartic value, and it adds something to their strength and dignity to be accepted for their real selves, rather than for their conformity. The group develops a morality of its own, in many respects a superior one. The members begin to feel the group as their own creation, built uniquely for their own needs. They feel understood, and they accommodate to their increasing recognition that the group is special, that it has standards distinct from those of the wider community, that elemental honesty in human relations in the group pays off, and that the group serves its function of lessening anxiety and sharpening the clarity of their images of themselves as young males and females.

Once the ice is cracked in terms of dissolving initial inhibitions of the group participants, the process rapidly warms up and begins to move thick and fast. There is an ebb and flow of tension, a rapid shift in the level of participation, and in the level of excitation of the group. Sometimes there is a quick rush of the aggressive members to "undress" the more retiring ones, thus hiding their own anxieties. Some of the boys, as well as the girls, though anxious, like being "undressed." Passive, shy, coy, they seem to say with their bodies, "Come and get me." The spontaneous interaction between passive and active members is heated and intense. Either mechanism, passivity or aggressiveness may be exploited for self-protection.

A characteristic worthy of mention is the remarkable tolerance of individual idiosyncrasies shown by group members. There is much joking, teasing, bantering, flirting, a great deal of "laughing with," and almost no "laughing at." All too tangible is the evidence of empathy with the underlying fear and suffering of other members. If one member seems wounded, another rises quickly to his defense. In this way, they parentify each other. Sometimes, the group may sense an unusually strong fear of the therapist on the part of a particular member. The group responds by "ganging up" on the therapist. They offer each other protection against unwarranted incursion by parental authority. On the other hand, in other circumstances, they will turn to the therapist for refuge against the attacks of others. These trends reflect, in my opinion, the tendency of the members to identify with each other, with the group aims, and with the therapist.

There is a further value to the therapist's effort to bring nonverbal aspects of patient behavior into the open. An alert awareness to the motor reactions of patients, facial and bodily posturings, provides concrete clues to particular sexual conflicts, anxieties, feelings of inferiority and shame connected with certain physical features of the patient's personality. The deliberate intention here is to exploit these clues for a ventilation of specific disturbances in self-image, so profoundly shaped both by the physiological processes of maturation and social experience. A female participant yawns at the very moment when a male points a personal, sexual comment her way. The escape motive in the yawn is interpreted. Another female is silently angry because she feels neglected; the attention of a boy she likes is moving toward another girl. She has a blank facial expression, but is agitatedly tearing a piece of paper in her hand. The therapist arouses the group's curiosity concerning this act. A girl repeatedly brings flame to her cigarette lighter and promptly blows it out. She is intensely castrative toward boys. The implications of her gestures are discussed.

Such episodes as these provide quick leads to disturbed

inner images of self, and the associated conflicts. The urges connected with these conflicts, sexual, aggressive, or the effort to compensate feelings of guilt, shame, and inferiority, are freely ventilated. In the course of this experience, there is opportunity to expand awareness of discrepancies between the way the adolescent sees himself and the way others in the group see him, and also opportunity to understand better the discrepancies between one image of self and another as they shift over time. This is reality testing.

The interaction processes of the group lend themselves effectively to the purpose of pointing out the distortions in the patient's interpretation of both self and the group reality. It is this phenomenon which has impelled me to attempt a formulation of the dynamic relations of individual personality to group role. Access to personality in the group is partial, not total. The level of access achieved is the dynamic content of the patient's role adaptation in the group, to the self-image projected into the group at a particular time and under particular interpersonal circumstances. Role phenomena are conditioned by temporal and situational factors as well as by the propensities of the individual personality. As these temporal and situational factors change, so does the patient's role adaptation. It is therefore possible through group interaction processes to achieve therapeutic access to a series of integrative levels of personality functioning depending on the vicissitudes of role adaptation.

I have tentatively formulated the following criteria for examining the dynamic correlation of individual personality and role: the aim or goal of the individual, his perception of surrounding reality in terms of the prevailing interpersonal processes, the image of self projected into the group role, the techniques of emotional control of the interaction with the group, the pattern of pursuit of gratification of personal need, the related conflicts with special reference to discrepancies between conscious and unconscious components, and the defense patterns mobilized against anxiety. With knowledge of the attributes of individual personality, and the use of such criteria, it is possible to define the dynamics of role function. The implementation of such concepts may be helpful in the effort to trace the specific mechanisms of group-therapeutic influence.

Thus far my comments have been mainly descriptive. Now some additional comments concerning dynamics. I take as my starting point for a discernment of what is unique in group therapy the processes of social participation. Starting here, it is possible to move back and trace the interrelation of the events of social participation with the intrapsychic structure of the individual, and also to move in the opposite direction, tracing the interrelations of social participation with the group entity as a social system. I believe this is a logical approach, since the phenomena of social participation are intermediate between the individual and the social system. In order to understand the dynamics of group therapy, it is necessary to take the components of the therapeutic process basic to all forms of psychotherapy and discern their pattern of operation in the social situation which is structured in a therapeutic group. I conceive the common denominators of all forms of psychotherapy to be mainly the following: the establishment of an emotional relationship between patient and therapist, with a continuous process of interchange between them, the emotional support the patient derives from this relationship, the release of pent-up feeling and conflicted urges, the processes of reality testing, which bring a diminution of anxiety and guilt and create conditions favorable to a progressive modification toward reality of the patients' interpretation of experience.

All these partial processes, overlapping and interacting, point their merged effects toward a more correct perception of self and relations with others, and thus make possible a more realistic and healthier adaptation. Now let us agree on a few terms relevant to these processes. Transference is the projection into the experience of interaction with the other person of a set of unreal expectations. Resistance is self-protection against those forms of exposure of self which seem to threaten injury. Defense is the counteraction of anxiety generated within.

If we translate these partial phenomena into the context of an adolescent therapy group, what do we see? The therapist is the recognized leader. He personifies the therapeutic objectives of the group and organizes the processes of group interaction toward the realization of these objectives. But he is a participant as well as an observer; he has face-to-face relations with his patients. He is a real person, he must reveal himself along with his patients. He is less of an omnipotent figure. At the same time, he shares the therapeutic functions with the other members of the group. Patients occupy the dual and alternating roles of patient and therapist. As a result of this special feature, patients in the group react to images of other persons which represent a fusion of elements of the identity of other patients and the therapist. The function of support is shared by group members and therapist. Emotional release is energized by the process of multiple interacting relationships. The clash of real and unreal images takes place on the broad stage of these multiple relationships. Transference emotions are not projected exclusively on the therapist, but are divided between patients and therapist. Sometimes, the components of transference are dissociated, certain components moving to the therapist, others moving toward other patients. Patterns of resistance and defense are shaped, not only by the intrapsychic makeup of the individual, but by the perceptions of support and threatened exposure the patient builds of the group proceedings. The vicissitudes of conflict, guilt, and anxiety will vary accordingly. It is easy to see that the special social structuring of the group, as contrasted with psychoanalytic individual therapy, commands an altered view of the role of the partial processes of therapy.

The psychotherapist must modify his techniques accordingly. To carry out his role effectively it is incumbent upon him to have disciplined knowledge at three levels: the group as a social system, with a specific social structuring of its own; the processes of emotional integration of an individual into the group, which involves the dynamic relations of personality and group role; and the intrapsychic mechanisms of individual personality.

13

INTRODUCTION

Indications and Contraindications for Adolescent Group Psychotherapy, by Irving H. Berkovitz and Max Sugar

It gradually became evident to practitioners that group treatment with adolescents poses particular problems that differ from those encountered in such work with adults and that, as with individual therapy, the specific developmental characteristics of adolescence stamp their mark on the therapeutic process. Kraft's (1968) comprehensive review of the literature on adolescent group therapy spelled out many of the issues raised by the early experimenters and catalogued the range of settings, approaches, and methods of group composition that had been attempted. Of particular note was his summary of evaluative studies which, at the time of writing, were unable to offer more than anecdotal evidence of substantial therapeutic efficacy. This remains, of course, the situation that obtains with most forms of psychotherapy today, and represents one of the major challenges that confronts the field in the immediate future.

Berkovitz and Sugar, though claiming only to review the indications and contraindications for group treatment, actually provide an up-to-date survey of the field, bringing Kraft's review to the present. Their paper abstracts the experience of the major students and practitioners in the field,

347

highlighting the wide scope of their efforts to apply group methods to clinical problems. They conclude that the indications are broad and the contraindications few; they are able, however, to present little more in the way of solid outcome data than Kraft could find almost 10 years earlier.

13

Indications and Contraindications for Adolescent Group Psychotherapy

Irving H. Berkovitz, M.D., and Max Sugar, M.D.

Essential to determining indications for any form of therapy for adolescents is a concept of the developmental tasks of adolescence. The concept held by the authors includes (1) emancipation from parental attachments; (2) development of satisfying and self-realizing peer attachments, with ability to love and appreciate the worth of others as well as oneself; (3) an endurable and sustaining sense of identity in the familial, social, sexual, and work-creative areas; and (4) a flexible set of hopes and life goals for the future.

In addition, in deciding the need for therapy for an adolescent, one has to keep in mind that suffering in adolescents is often registered first by the immediate objects, i.e., the persons in the social system around the teenager: the family, the caretakers, the individual's social network, or the legal system. In this age group it is important to keep in mind that the boundaries between the normal and the abnormal are shifting, often fluid, and frequently a matter of judgment.

Reprinted by permission from *The Adolescent in Group and Family Therapy*, ed. M. Sugar, pp. 3-26, 1975. New York: Brunner/Mazel.

Of significance are the manner in which the individual copes with problems and the way the social system reacts.

If the adolescent needs treatment for other than a transient personal or situational crisis, individual therapy, group, or family therapy, or a combination of these may be considered. In some instances, family therapy which includes several siblings offers the opportunity for periods of discussion which can resemble and provide the values of a group therapy experience within the family session. In many cases the choice among these three major types of therapy is, indeed, a practical one related mostly to the circumstances of the individual teenager, his family's acceptance or finances, or the persons (individual or agency) providing the treatment. Each of these three major types of therapy provides unique advantages, benefits, and complications. Frequently, there is value in periods of alternation or simultaneous use of all three.

The recommendation of group therapy for the adolescent depends to a great extent on the availability of a suitable adolescent group. Unfortunately, a dearth of therapeutically oriented groups prevails in most communities. Many teenage groups, available in free clinics, schools, churches, or clubs, with or without therapeutic orientation, can provide therapeutic and growth values.

In this chapter we will present some of our ideas and what many practitioners have written about the special usefulness of group therapy, with or without the concurrent presence of the other types of treatment. Indications in the inpatient as well as outpatient settings will be considered.

Small groups allow exposure of typical behavioral patterns leading to a decrease in feelings of isolation and of being peculiar, with a rise in self-esteem. Concomitantly, they foster new ways of dealing with situations, along with an evaluation of techniques in use.

A prime advantage of group therapy to many teenagers

is the feeling of protection vis-à-vis the adult therapist. The opportunity to rap with peers seems less associated with being ill (at first) and safer from possible adult domination. Many teenagers are curious upon first learning of group therapy as to the nature of the discussions and the possibility of making new friends. Of course, in some adolescents, especially those who fear peer relationships, an opposite reaction may prevail. The youngster's distrust of adults, beginning with parents, usually makes the peer group especially acceptable at this stage of development.

Group therapy has special value in engaging the adolescent in therapy, as noted by Peck and Bellsmith (1954), who state:

> A properly selected group will expose the patient's characteristic distortions as they appear in the interaction between himself and certain members of the group. Since he is also capable of entering into relatively healthy relationships with certain other members of the group, he is able more easily to examine and work through his relationship distortion, because he is supported by the reassuring reality of his healthy social ties within the group [p. 65].

> It soon became apparent that a number of the children who had appeared passive in individual sessions rapidly became surprisingly active in the group setting [p. 67].

Buxbaum (1945) describes the violent swings from rebellion to submission that occur in adolescent groups. She feels that both processes are of equal importance for the adolescent's development since breaking away encourages independence and increases identification with the leader, while being submissive to peer approval gives him an opportunity to satisfy dependency needs in a setting where he retains control of when to terminate this role. Giving the adolescent a chance both to submit and revolt alternately is one of the characteristics, according to Buxbaum, which particularly makes the group indispensable for the adolescent. This is especially exemplified in group therapy with delinquent adolescents, detailed later in the chapter.

Group therapy may be especially indicated currently, since the "do-your-own-thing" ethos of the 1960's and '70's often encourages some teenagers to prolong a normal narcissistic orientation. Rather than learning empathy or understanding, for some teenagers manipulation or disregard of others may become more prevalent. Group therapy, experienced even briefly, may afford an opportunity to open the individual's mind to fuller appreciation of, and, it is to be hoped, reduction of, blocks to warm, honest, nonexploitative relationships with others. The group experiences available in "normal settings," that is, schools, clubs, or churches, may often provide the same benefit. One has to beware, in some, however, of an emphasis on group comfort, or sometimes of traumatic interpersonal encounters, instead of a slower, more gradual, and tolerable pace of coming to know oneself and the other person. Josselyn (1972) cautions of some dangers in ill-timed or too pressing a group experience.

This presentation of the values in adolescent group therapy does not signify that the group is rigidly the treatment of choice for all teenagers, with or without concurrent individual or family sessions. There are many examples of individual therapy in which the adolescent has developed a corrective child-adult experience that has allowed for repair of previous maturational lags and/or various symptoms. However, even in these cases, as helpful as the individual treatment may have been, a social practice arena often may have been of added value in deepening and consolidating the therapy. In many individuals (not only the very schizoid) one may encourage, suggest, and even arrange for extratherapeutic group experiences and opportunities, such as recreational clubs and other groups, but without successful involvement developing. An adolescent therapy group, on the other hand, provides this opportunity intrinsic to the therapy itself, with the excellent possibility that blocks to learning from, and sharing with, peers may be pointed out more effectively.

Group therapy, skillfully handled, with attention to psychodynamic considerations, may be useful to many neurotic, antisocial, or psychotic teenagers. It may suffice as the only therapeutic experience in many mildly disturbed youngsters, but more disturbed individuals may well need the added assistance of individual and family therapy as well. The use of individual, family, or group therapy concurrently by the same therapist deserves more detailed discussion than can be given here. A communication gap may occur when two therapists are involved. However, an equally significant resistance can occur even with the single therapist when the teenager tries to avoid involvement in the individual or group relation by pitting one against the other (Brackelmanns and Berkovitz, 1972).

Relevant questions in this discussion, therefore, would be: Which teenagers are appropriate for group therapy? At which stage of individual or family therapy should group therapy be recommended? What benefit can be expected from group therapy? Or what detriment? What is the best method of recommending or preparing the individual teenager for group therapy? Which group and therapist should one choose for the particular adolescent? Some possible answers to some of these questions will be suggested in this chapter.

Some have tried, usually in the treatment of adults, to determine criteria by which to predict gain from group therapy and the most productive composition of a group (Yalom,

1970). Criteria are yet to be similarly described for adolescent group therapy. While there is rarely the ideal group, some individuals may do better in one type of group than in another, and with one particular group therapist than with another. Moreover, indications for group therapy must also include some thought about the effect of the individual on the group, since unplanned entry and premature termination will hurt or impede the group as well as the individual.

The degree of indication for recommending group psychotherapy to any teenager may be crudely quantified into absolute, relative, or minimal degrees. Under absolute degree of indication, we would consider those youngsters so well defended against therapeutic relationships that only in a peer group or network group (Sugar, 1972) can there be any significant confrontation, introspection, or interaction with therapist or peers.

Minimal degree of indication would include the teenager who relates to the adult therapist fairly well. He may defy or withhold at times, but to a manageable degree, a degree which does not prevent growth or understanding. This category of young person has meaningful group associations in some areas of his life. In many ways this adolescent's individual therapy is already proceeding beneficially, and the degree of psychological impairment may well be minimal.

The category of relative indication for group psychotherapy would be somewhere between the previous two categories. In this case, experiencing group therapy would help add greater here-and-now evidence, from interpersonal application, of changes or understanding arrived at in the one-to-one therapeutic relationship. At times, even relationship problems not previously known may be uncovered.

Once a practitioner has decided that group therapy may be useful for a teenager, the next step is to obtain agreement from the youngster for this treatment plan. If he has come requesting group therapy, as some do, there is little problem. When the teenager has been so poorly prepared for group therapy or any therapy by the parents and therapist that he denies any need for therapy, it is best not to embark on group therapy. The parental messages to him need to be examined and if the parents are mostly for the youngster being in therapy, then a preparatory period of individual therapy should be the next step. Thus he may gain some comfort with the therapist which could prepare him for the group experience. Some youngsters have such negative, suspicious feelings and expectations of getting hurt (through rejection or other painful methods) that they reject individual therapy automatically. Then group therapy may offer them an opportunity for dealing with these feelings as well as give them a possibly corrective experience.

> Members may initially come to the group under pressure; but if the group is to form and become a viable entity, members must come to feel this sense of belonging and to accept their part in the group and some responsibility for it. Thus, consent is ultimately crucial. Members come for some common purpose; but they also have their separate needs, their hidden agendas, and there will be struggles to reconcile these in the group and pressure for members to conform to the demands of the group as a whole and to reach agreement [MacLennan and Felsenfeld, 1968, p. 7].

Entry into group therapy indicates a wish by the teenager and therapist for several mutually desired changes:

> (1) a greater enabling of interdependent autonomy; this would include emancipation from disabling attachments to parental demands and expectations but allow for a respectful appreciation of and reconciliation with posi-

tive qualities of parents and other adults; (2) reduction (but not crippling) of childhood narcissism, so that there is greater ability to respond to the worth of other individuals, beginning with peers; (3) enhancing appreciation for personal creative energies, so that a sustaining life goal and zest for what is available in living become more stable features in the personality; (4) a greater sense of sureness of self, in terms of familial, sexual, and social identity, with a minimum of arrogance and rigidity [Berkovitz, 1972, p. 6].

Fried (1956) aims at developing a "self-servicing ego" to replace the "parent servicing ego."

GROUPS IN OUTPATIENT SETTINGS

There are many types of outpatient groups. One type, conducted primarily in the office or clinic setting, emphasizes such features as mainly weekly sessions, primarily verbalized confrontation of behavior, description of feelings, interpretation, and increased intellectual-emotional understanding.

Brackelmanns and Berkovitz (1972), discussing this type of group, consider as positive indications two types of resistance to forming an alliance with the therapist:

The first of these is represented by the youngster who passively accepts his fate and allows himself to be carried back and forth to the office but refuses any involvement. There was an example of a thirteen-year-old boy who offered no overt resistance to coming to treatment but, upon arrival, sat silently for the entire time. More often than not, he appeared drowsy or fell asleep. The second form of response, more common in girls than in boys, is a more open hostile rebellion to treatment. This type of young adolescent is full of promises of failure, feelings of distrust, threats of termination, and raw insults, both personal and professional, which are directed at the therapist . . . [p. 37].

Two relative *contraindications* to group psychotherapy are overt psychosis and severe narcissism or nonempathy. The latter is an interesting problem which the group and therapist find difficult to deal with. This patient tends to be very verbal and preoccupied with himself and his own problems and has little genuine concern for other people. He angers the group, but they find it hard to control him because of their own narcissism, their concerns about being critical and being criticized, and the way in which this patient transmits an aura of being fragile and helpless. An attack on him (or her) results in the attacker's feeling guilty. It has been very helpful to have this type of patient also in individual psychotherapy, and to educate him in group conduct with emphasis on developing his skills toward greater empathy and more effective interpersonal interaction . . . [p. 38].

The therapist must consider the danger of *mixing nonacting out adolescents with acting out adolescents*. It is possible that the young person, as he makes separation from his family and engages with the peer group, will identify with acting out adolescent behavior in order to gain acceptance. In addition to this process, the group often provides a sanctioning body with the tendency to encourage certain kinds of acting out behavior in order to deal with feelings [p. 40].

Several other contraindications need additional consideration. The youngster who refuses, but whose refusal is symptomatic of anxiety (about exposure or other matters), should not come into the group until it is clear that this anxiety has been managed suitably so that he has some positive feelings about entering the group. Sometimes, when this is not considered, the youngster may abruptly break off treatment, or may seemingly act out in some other way. But this may be due to the therapist's not handling adequately the youngster's extreme anxiety. In one such case, the youngster, aged 13, needed his father to intervene and decide that group therapy would interfere with the son's other activities. By that time the therapist had a clearer picture of the situation and he agreed to continue only with individual therapy, whereby the anxiety was managed suitably.

Another type of contraindication is illustrated in the case of a young man of 19 who requested group therapy after he had heard about it from his friend. He was not accepted for group therapy because he was impulsive, unstable, irregular in appearing for individual sessions, and tangential in all his relationships, including that with the therapist. It was uncertain if he could attend the sessions regularly enough to become constructively involved. He might well have hurt the other members through disruption, and not have gained anything for himself as well.

Teicher (1966) feels from his work with groups of disturbed adolescents from economically and emotionally deprived walks of life that the therapist could focus on:

(1) helping in the group process with the presenting problems of the youths—problems which prevented them in many instances from dealing with the psychological work of adolescence; and (2) helping with the psychological work of adolescence, although in many of them this could proceed if they were freed sufficiently of pathological defenses and constricting, inhibiting anxieties [p. 21].

The previous authors, while recognizing the importance

of individual development, would probably define as a prime indication for group therapy facilitating the development of self in *the social context.*

Many groups do not emphasize as strongly an interpretative therapeutic focus. Braverman (1966) describes a fascinating use of group discussion as a *facilitative* adjunct to individual casework therapy in an outpatient clinic. The lounge was open two nights per week for three hours each night, and the adolescents who had individual interviews on those nights were invited to drop in before or after individual sessions. A casual light atmosphere was encouraged, so they could just sit around and talk, or play games. This group was felt to help alleviate anxieties at the outset of treatment, and provide support in coping with varied everyday problems such as homework, parental controls, relationships with the opposite sex, or spending money. Braverman feels that the group provided "useful, humane ego support" to allow for sustained individual treatment. This may have been confirmed by the finding that only one teenager left individual treatment.

A very different group of adolescents, aged 13 to 15, most of whose parents were on welfare, were at times given carfare, excuses from school, food, play equipment, and occasional trips (Stranahan, Schwartzman, and Atkin, 1957). After this treatment of their deprivation, the boys were able to identify with the therapists, function better in school and in the community, and want individual therapy. Stebbins (1972) responded to a need and met with a group of black teenagers in a housing project. She arrives at the following helpful insights:

1. Adolescents who are completely unaware of the process known as "therapy" can learn the "patient" role as easily as many other people involved in psychother-

apy. For those youngsters whose emotional problems are compounded by reality problems, it is better to curtail this. It is not advisable to encourage ventilation and insight production as the sole purpose for group activity. It is more rewarding for both adolescent and therapist to place primary emphasis on action *resulting* from an intrapsychic focus. There can also be some experiential, recreational, social, and informational values to groups for teenagers.

2. Not always, but many times, in a minority community, the peer group or the neighborhood group is a stronger group than the family group. This peer group then becomes a more natural group with which to work. In this way, the individual appears to be more able to satisfy his needs and build the skills he lacks. The transition of these skills to other groups and to nongroup life situations appears to be facilitated by working with whatever group is natural.

3. Privacy and closure are especially important in working with youths whose day-to-day lives bring them in constant contact with each other. For psychotherapy to have any value or to be respected at all as a helping process, it must allow for this privacy.

4. A therapist offering help to a group of oppressed adolescents must have more to offer than his clinical skills. Commonality of background, lifestyle, or mode of communication helps greatly. As one human being who has some realistic perception of the pitfalls encountered by other human beings, you must offer something for these young men and women to hold onto. You must extend yourself, your time, and your mind. This increases greatly your chances of receiving reciprocal sincerity [Stebbins, 1972, pp. 132-133].

MacLennan (1967) has long been an ardent advocate of the values of this type of group conducted in the indigenous setting. Sugar (1975) uses a somewhat related approach in dealing with a high school crisis.

DELINQUENT ADOLESCENTS IN OUTPATIENT GROUPS

In other outpatient settings, the teenagers are more severely delinquent, angry, and uncooperative. Again, approaches can vary between the more therapeutically oriented interpretive-mode therapy group to the more indigenous discussion-style activity group. In the situation of delinquent youth, indications and contraindications for group techniques vary with the type of delinquent being served. Redl (1966) describes four types of delinquency usually encountered: (1) delinquency as a defense in basically healthy individuals; (2) delinquency in adolescent acute-growth confusional states; (3) delinquencies on a neurotic basis; and (4) delinquency based on deformities of the psychical system. Indications and style of group can vary further, depending on whether the setting is outpatient, institutional, or residential.

In an outpatient group of delinquent boys, aged 14 to 17, Jacobs and Christ (1967) developed three guiding principles for treatment of this type of group: (1) providing outlets for tension reduction; (2) formal structuring; and (3) flexible setting of limits.

In two groups of delinquent adolescents, the fortuitous availability of the group as a forum helped avoid imminent physical combat in the streets (Rachman, 1969; O'Shea, 1972).

Furthermore, group therapy has been seen to deepen and maintain the involvement of these action-oriented youngsters in examination of action and feeling (Peck and Bellsmith, 1954). Their follow-up indicated that "of all the adolescents placed in groups after failure in individual therapy, about 60 percent achieved varying degrees of improvement" (p. 68).

While most groups meet weekly, some therapists make a special point of the need to meet more often (Franklin and Nottage, 1969). These authors report that by treating

> seriously disturbed delinquents in psychoanalytic group therapy five times a week, where direct focus on personality exploration is explicit and consistently maintained from the outset, it is possible to involve them successfully in deeply meaningful and highly productive understanding of themselves [p. 165].

They claim that adolescents considered untreatable by others were helped in this type of group experience.

Heacock (1966) urges that

> . . . in our experience, the most important tool the therapist has is the strong positive transference. The therapist must have a tolerance for lateness and absences but must apply consistently firm pressure to get the patient to change this behavior. He must work generally in the framework of a very positive transference constantly reaching out by phone, mail, telegrams, or home visits [pp. 42-43].

He lists as not suited for his type of group therapy

> the acting-out boy whose antisocial behavior is not nearly as severe as that of the other boys. He is made too anxious by the discussions and behavior of the rest of the group.
>
> Another unsuitable type is the severely delinquent and hyperactive boy who "acts in" during the sessions. His disruptive behavior spreads to the others who are quite

responsive to this, and so therapy becomes impossible. Suggestible patients who are easily led should be eliminated, as they are frequently stimulated to more acting out by the therapy. Often these are borderline mental defectives. Boys presenting overt homosexual behavior are also unsuitable [p. 41].

Positive reinforcement techniques, along with group discussion, are used by some. Pascal, Cottrell, and Baugh (1967) recount the use of videotapes with five boys, aged 12 to 18, who were referred from juvenile court, charged with offenses from petty larceny to attempted murder.

James, Osborn, and Oetting (1967) conducted a reinforcement type of "self-concept" group for 14 girls aged 13 to 17. These girls had been "runaways, court cases, and school dropouts. Three were potentially suicidal, rebellious, and acting out sexually" (p. 377). The group's focus was

on charm and grooming, while selected female leaders provided role models. Discussion was like group therapy. Draw-a-person tests and check lists showed changes suggesting greater feminine identification, less hostility to authority, and greater openness to criticism after 12 weeks [p. 377].

The authors feel "it was not threatening, as group therapy might have been, but the group leader was able to carry discussion into areas that would have been considered in group therapy" (p. 377).

INDICATIONS AND CONTRAINDICATIONS FOR ADOLESCENT GROUP THERAPY IN HOSPITALS

A necessary question, when one considers the hospital setting, is the indication or contraindication of the previously detailed types of small groups with adolescents alongside the variety of group experiences offered in a therapeutic hospital milieu. In some large public hospitals with less abundant therapeutic facilities, the small group may have a more special therapeutic indication (Powdermaker and Frank, 1953).

Rinsley (1972) makes several important points with respect to the pertinence of the small group experience in the hospital milieu.

> A . . . consideration has to do with the timing of the prescription for the adolescent inpatient's inclusion in a therapeutic group, which is closely linked to whether the adolescent is yet immersed in the "resistance phase" of his treatment, or has passed beyond it, made therapeutic identifications with the ward or cottage staff members, hence has begun to perceive the residential setting as potentially helpful to him.
>
> In numerous cases, initiation of formal group psychotherapy while the adolescent continues actively or covertly to resist the therapeutic milieu as a whole simply intensifies the resistances, spreads them out, as it were, and abets the adolescent's use of splitting defenses, now carried over, in addition, to the "group." By the same token, attentively conducted and properly structured groups which meet directly in the patients' living areas serve to minimize the clinical-administrative splits which adolescents so readily exploit from fear of self-revelation, hence may actually supply motivation for treatment.
>
> A . . . matter concerns the use of group psychotherapy in the residential setting in conjunction with ongoing individual psychotherapy. Despite his artful and often stentorian resistances against "closeness," the adolescent inpatient, like his otherwise healthy brother in the community, struggles mightily with the problems and at-

tainment of intimacy. As he works on object removal and proceeds to devalue parents and their transference equivalents from anxiety over the prospect of regressive re-fusion with them, he nonetheless assiduously pursues closeness as prefatory to the capacity for later, mature object relations. In part for these reasons, group treatment without concomitant or parallel individual treatment proves inadequate for the adolescent inpatient, both as an opportunity for working through problems with object removal and as a means of exploring and resolving highly delicate, personal issues which are exceedingly difficult if not impossible to express within the peer group. [pp. 234-235].

Blaustein and Wolff (1972) find that after three months of conducting a small group of teenagers on a mixed (adolescent and adult) ward in a large general hospital

there was a distinct decrease in friction between adolescents and staff and adolescents and adult patients. From the experience with our adolescent group thus far, we are impressed by this form of treatment as a way of reaching teenagers. The stresses experienced by the adolescent patient in the intimacy of a one-to-one relationship seem to diminish within the group. Intensity is diffused, demands on the individual patient are fewer, and therefore, there is less need to defy for the sake of defiance. The result seems to be that dependency needs may be revealed and dealt with in a growth-producing way. There is the possibility of learning to talk intimately without use of drugs as a crutch, admitting to enjoyment of the spotlight, along with learning to share it, and talking openly with authority figures in a mutually respectful way [p. 189].

In another small hospital, an adolescent group served ther-

apeutically, but also as an administrative program development unit (Grold, 1972). Group discussions included discipline
and suggestions for change in program, e.g., the buying of
an old car for teenage boys to work on, setting up cooking
and sewing for the girls, setting up dances, etc. There was
a "dramatic lessening of destructive behavior. Testing of the
limits of the staff advisors continued, but to a considerably
lessened degree" (p. 194). Moadel (1970) gives an account
of successful use of a group therapy program on a female
adolescent ward.

Group discussions are seen to have a value in an occupational therapy activities program as well (Mack and Barnum,
1966): ". . . the group meetings deepened greatly the meaning and therapeutic impact of the hospital experience" and
resulted "in the development of close object ties with the
leader and one another, in greater cohesion on the ward"
(p. 461).

INDICATIONS FOR ADOLESCENT GROUP PSYCHOTHERAPY IN RESIDENTIAL SETTINGS

In residential settings designed usually for delinquent teenagers or those with family problems which require placement,
still other uses of group therapy have been depicted. Again,
the question regarding the therapeutic contribution of small-
group psychotherapy alongside other treatment modalities
in the setting must be considered. Redl (Redl and Wineman,
1957; Redl, 1966) has written extensively on this approach.

In a series of three articles, Persons and associates (Persons,
1966, 1967; Persons and Pepinsky, 1966) highlight the therapeutic values of group therapy with individual psychotherapy in reducing recidivism of incarcerated delinquents.
The occurrence of negative transference in group is associated with positive therapeutic benefit by Truax (1971), who
feels that "it may be that the occurrence of negative feelings

towards the therapist as an authority figure leads to some resolution" of difficulty in relating to authority figures (p. 136).

Evans (1966), carrying on analytic group therapy at government-approved schools in England, concluded that in the group setting

> . . . Most of the delinquents are increasingly able to look at difficulties, tolerate anxiety, and not run away from their problems. They have been able to modify their aggressive outbursts and use their aggression more constructively [p. 195].

A therapy group in a probation department girls' residential treatment center underwent dramatic changes when the group, having previously met in the therapists' office, assembled instead in the girls' living unit (Pottharst and Gabriel, 1972). Rinsley (1972) stresses this point also.

The fact that the previous groups met five times per week undoubtedly added to a more significant therapeutic impact. Elias (1968) depicts a five-days-per-week program in a residential setting for delinquent boys (Highfields) termed "guided group interaction." Attendance was not compulsory. The group leader often played "a relatively active part." The total program and type of delinquent boys undoubtedly were critical factors, in addition to the groups, but "after one year of freedom in the community only 16.5 percent of the Highfields boys, as compared with 48.9 percent of the boys from the state reformatory, engaged in new delinquencies" (p. 290).

In contrast to this frequency, Wolk and Reid (1964) claim to demonstrate that changes occur when inmates in detention are offered group psychotherapy for only eight weeks, meeting twice per week for one and a half hours, a total of 16 sessions.

Fortunately, some authors attempted more structured evaluation of group psychotherapy in the residential setting. Taylor (1967), in a girls' borstal in New Zealand, conducted a rigorous experiment

> . . . using (1) three comparable control groups of 11 borstal girls, (2) an experimental variable of group psychotherapy over 40 weekly sessions of one and three-quarters hour each, (3) an adequate range of pretherapy and posttherapy measures, including introspective reports, rating scales, objective, reliable, and valid personality tests, and social action effects, and (4) a follow-up period.
>
> The results established that the borstal girls demonstrated improvement in the absence of treatment, more improvement with the moderate treatment of group counseling, and most improvement from group psychotherapy. The differential rate of improvement in the three groups indicates that neither a placebo effect nor spontaneous remission was an important factor in the results [p. 177].

> At the end of the experiment, the Experimental Group members were less radical, less criminal in attitudes and behavior, and more outgoing, reflective, and interdependent. They expressed guilt for their behavior and had positive attitudes toward the borstal and probation officers. The Experimental Group was, in fact, released before the other two groups, but the difference was not statistically significant [p. 174].

In residential settings with a less delinquent population, other changes were noted. In one such setting (Mordock, Ellis, and Greenstone, 1969), adolescent and preadolescent boys with "learning difficulties concomitant with emotional disturbances" (p. 511), when involved in small groups (six or seven members), "improved their interpersonal relationships to a greater degree than did those in individual therapy, particularly their work-oriented relationships" (p. 517).

In a voluntary child placement agency, groups were useful for maturing sexual attitudes (Berkovitz, Chikahisa, Lee, and Murasaki, 1966). Group therapy was initiated originally as a way of increasing therapeutic contact with children who had not been successfully reached in previous individual case-work relationships.

GROUP THERAPY WITH SPECIAL POPULATIONS OF ADOLESCENTS

PREGNANT TEENAGERS

Adolescent pregnancy, especially among the unwed, will involve characerological factors, as well as important identity issues. Therefore, group experience with these girls often needs to extend beyond the period of pregnancy alone. One group for girls aged 13 to 16 continued for a year and a half, though all the girls had delivered after four months of group therapy.

> A combination of group therapy and group counseling, orientation, and education was used, not only with the patient, but with her mother as well. The goal with the parent was educative, geared toward helping resolve antagonisms and hostilities in the family of the patient. Group treatment with the girls demonstrated the need of oral gratification for these emotionally deprived patients [Kaufmann and Deutsch, 1967, p. 319].

Barclay (1969) did not involve parents but narrates a two-year group experience in which "the sense of frustration and hopelessness appreciably diminished as mutual support developed in the group meetings and outside" (p. 384). After the two years, all except two (of the nine) were involved in work, training, or continuing education.

Even in obstetrical clinics, primigravid adolescents respond better to health education programs when in peer groups, after they feel like part of the group (Barnard, 1970). Visits made to members who had delivered their babies, and to the delivery room, helped further to reduce fear about impending delivery.

DRUG-ABUSING ADOLESCENTS

Use and abuse of marijuana, barbiturates, psychedelics, psychoactive drugs, and heroin may occasion entry into treatment before or after legal intervention. Methadone projects often include group discussion. In office, school, or clinic groups many of these youngsters have found some new understanding of self, leading to a change in patterns of chemical usage, as well as occasional personality change.

In more severe cases, group therapy, with or without individual or family therapy, may not appreciably alter the self-destructive use of these substances (see Bartlett, 1975). A more totally involving community structure which can bring about self-knowledge and new lifestyles is necessary. Youngsters involved in moderate drug use who live in stable, caring families may at times find benefit in the outpatient group, individual, or family approaches previously described (Brackelmanns and Berkovitz, 1972). Slagle and Silver (1972) point out the value of an involving group experience for depressed drug users in a clinic.

To meet the needs of the more disturbed youngsters, many communal living arrangements have been established. Many of these include intense, small-group interactions (Casriel, 1963; Shelly and Bassin, 1965; Levitt, 1968) which differ in each setting. At Daytop Village one of the principal methods for "achieving self-image and behavioral change" is three-time-a-week group encounter therapy.

> Many professionals are abashed and frightened by the fierceness of the attack therapy. But Dr. Lewis Yablonsky, research consultant to Synanon, after his first 25 sessions, found that the group "attack" was an act of love in which was entwined the assumption: "If we did not care about you or have concern for you, we would not bother to point out something that might reduce your psychic pain or clarify something for you that might save your life" [Bassin, 1968, p. 52].

When communal settings are not available, hospital settings are used. Here the small therapy group has particular usefulness. As some "addicts" expressed it:

> "Alone in hospital you forget what you are in for, but in an addicts' group other addicts don't allow you to forget!"
>
> It was felt that "mixed" arrangements would help particularly in preventing girls from becoming too difficult with each other, and such groups should have a preponderance of boys . . . the majority prefer a heterogeneous mixing with non-drug-dependent patients, and with very rare exceptions dislike mixing with other "mental" patients, preferring alcoholics despite all their grievances against them. . . . "Addicts must learn there are other people in the world, with similar problems, who are able to overcome them, people who are experienced and mature and who work." Living with non-addicts "brings you down to earth, helps you cope with problems, teaches you tolerance . . . you didn't realize before how irresponsible you were" [Glatt, 1967, p. 519].

However, the results are not clearly positive in all approaches for the problems of youngsters who abuse drugs, as Bartlett (1975) describes.

OBESE ADOLESCENTS

The literature describing group therapy for obese adolescents is meager. With this oral control problem, just as with drug abuse and alcoholism, group methods need to include a wider social context. With obesity this may be residential camp, weight-reducing programs, or hospitals.

In one program, 11 adolescents were hospitalized in a children's chronic-disease hospital for six weeks and then followed for a year.

> The inpatient phase consisted of an intensive program including group and individual therapy, recreation, exercise, dietary education, etc. During the outpatient phase, the groups were seen at monthly intervals. The parents were involved during the entire program.
>
> At the end of the program, three patients were still below their admission weight, three were holding their weights steady, and the remaining five had gained weight [Stanley et al., 1968, p. 207].

On the other hand, when the treatment program is less aggressive, the group may be useful as an adjunct to the program. In an adolescent medical clinic, it was reported that

> While group work . . . appeared to produce an improvement in appearance and in the attitudes toward obesity, we could not show it to be any more effective than individual treatment in achieving long-term weight loss. Group therapy did provide an opportunity for socialization and for handling other conflicts [Hammar, Campbell, and Woolley, 1971, p. 51].

ADOLESCENTS IN FOSTER HOMES AND WELFARE PROGRAMS

Children in foster homes have usually undergone a loss of family, deliberately or inadvertently. Engagement with other children in the foster home or with foster parents may be blocked by conscious or unconscious hostility, depression, and other factors.

> The climate of the group, which lends itself to the development of self-confidence in the adolescent and trust in the leader, has definite carryover into life. Through the groups, many adolescent foster children are now able to handle some of their unresolved feelings concerning their natural parents and, as a result, have better relations with their foster parents [Carter, 1968, p. 27].

Outpatient groups have proved useful in one department of public welfare in *avoiding placement in a foster home.* Eight nondelinquent teenagers attended weekly for one hour, in two groups, one for those under 15 and one for those older.

> They have served as an alternative to placement. The sessions provide a means of diagnosing the quality of an adolescent's peer and authority relationships as well as other aspects of his functioning.
> These meetings have accomplished what they set out to do: provide an ego-building experience and help the members move on to other constructive social outlets [Riegel, 1968, p. 418].

ADOLESCENT RETARDATES

The degree of impairment of teenage retardates is of significant importance, as much or more so as in group procedures with neurotic, delinquent, or other adolescents.

> One . . . finds reports of groups composed of individuals who have nothing in common other than the fact

that they have been subsumed under a societal role definition, "retarded." . . . There have been situations in which delinquent retardates, culturally deprived retardates, mongoloids, brain-damaged youngsters, and so on have constituted a poorly composed group [Borenzweig, 1970, p. 178].

Participation in a group work program has been reported as increasing the verbal capacities of moderately and mildly retarded adolescents (Rafel and Stockhammer, 1961). With mildly retarded, hyperactive, behaviorally disturbed adolescent and young adult girls, group therapy helped 37 of 56 to move from being inmates on a closed ward to learning a repertoire of behaviors that facilitated their return to community living (Fine and Dawson, 1964).

Most of the group therapy or group work described in the literature occurred in workshops or institutions. Some outpatient groups have been reported in conjunction with school classes for the educable mentally retarded. As in the case of the psychotic, delinquent, obese, or drug-abusing teenager, the retardate often has to be treated in a therapeutic community setting, which involves training and socialization, as well as small group therapy. Consequently, the same issues arise, namely, the role of small group therapy in the wider therapeutic context.

In workshops for mildly retarded adolescents (IQ 50-70), Bellis and Sklar (1969) feel that the "group experience of the shop is a stress situation in itself" (p. 21). In one workshop, "mildly and moderately retarded trainees made excellent use of group process . . ." (Rosen and Rosen, 1969, p. 52). The small group provided (1) a reference point for change in the lives of the trainees, allowing support of peers to help in renouncing previous "dysfunctional patterns of behavior"; (2) a forum for reality testing; (3) a place to receive encouragement from peers; as well as (4) facilitation of a new set of values and attitudes compatible with the wider society. Rosen and Rosen found role playing especially useful in this regard. After six months they observed that "the therapist no longer played an active role," and concerns raised moved into the area of interpersonal relationships. The more retarded members of the group became more participatory and verbal.

In institutions, more disturbed and lower-IQ retardates may be involved. In this setting, Sternlicht (1966) states, "Activity and other nonverbal techniques are the method of choice in the group psychotherapeutic treatment of delinquent adolescent retardates" (p. 93). Miezio (1967), in working with groups of perhaps less delinquent retardates, affirms gains similar to those described for nonretarded adolescents. Groups were able to

> enhance social awareness, elevate self-concept, diminish egocentricity, improve impulse control, externalize aggression, and develop appropriate sublimations. Sexual identity problems were explored and clarified. Separation from home and family, the dominant theme in all of their lives, was, to some extent, worked through and accepted [p. 326].

In another institution, after 67 sessions over eight months,

> the utilization of moderately structured directive group counseling methods helped to realize the goals of the project: the reduction of acting out behavior, the increase of educational and/or work placement functioning to a higher level, and the further integration and acceptance by the patients of their assets within their own life situation [Rotman and Golburgh, 1967, p. 13].

Psychodrama was used by Pankratz and Buchan (1966) in

treating retarded delinquents in a hospital setting and they conclude that the director should be manipulative and directive. Begab (1962) raises a critical note in general about the use of group work with retardates:

Actually, some of the "group" programs currently in effect are lacking many of the elements inherent in the group process. There is little, if any, interaction between the members and a common purpose or problem does not emerge. The members look to the group leader rather than to each other for the fulfillment of certain needs. In the absence of this necessary interdependence, communication is slow to develop and the individual's role in the group is poorly defined. When these conditions prevail and group dynamics are relatively inoperative, the true value of the group experience is lost. Group sanctions do not emerge, social controls are minimized, and there is little impact on the behavior, attitudes, and values of members [p. 7].

Rather than constituting a rejection of the indication of group methods for these teenagers, the criticism offered by Begab seems to underline the need for a special directive, leader-oriented element in groups of retardates. Bigman (1961) states that the worker must be the central person because severely retarded young adults do not have the social or task skills necessary for interdependent participation with other members of the group. Borenzweig (1970) also confirms that "even those groups of retardates that appeared to have little structure, interdependence between members, impact on the individual retardate, or concern with problems external to the group" had the power to exert a beneficial effect upon the retardate (p. 180). The individuals were changing without significant change in group structures in the process.

Summary

The variety and array of different formats and settings within which groups of adolescents gather or are brought together for new understanding are indeed impressive. A few simple generalities to describe the themes and indications are certainly inadequate.

Some of the indications for groups for adolescents can be listed as follows:

1. to support assistance from and confrontation with peers;
2. to provide a miniature real-life situation for study and change of behavior;
3. to stimulate new ways of dealing with situations and developing new skills of human relations;
4. to stimulate new concepts of self and new models of identification;
5. to feel less isolated;
6. to provide a feeling of protection from the adult while undergoing changes;
7. as a bind to therapy to help maintain continued self-examination;
8. to allow the swings of rebellion or submission which will encourage independence and identification with the leader;
9. to uncover relationship problems not evident in individual therapy.

In some settings, indications may include the above or may also include special indications related to the needs of the particular population being served or particular setting; for example, hospitals, residential centers, or detention centers for delinquent teenagers.

Contraindications are few and involve primarily the exclusion of an adolescent who is too deviant from the rest of the particular group. This is determined by the therapeutic needs of the individual, the goals and the availability of a suitable group in which the youngster is not an isolate. This is not a precisely determinable relationship and often is a matter of judgment, or trial and error. Some teenagers categorized as "narcissistic" may require individual therapy to help them make a successful relation in a group. Youngsters with deficient controls may benefit from individual and family therapy as outpatients, but group therapy may be inadvisable due to potential excess group contagion or stimulation leading to disorganization.

14

INTRODUCTION

Transference, Resistance and Communication Problems in Adolescent Psychotherapy Groups, by Irving Schulman

As in individual therapy, so in group treatment special technical modifications are required to meet the phase-specific needs of adolescent patients. The two pillars of psychoanalytic therapy—transference and resistance—both manifest themselves in ways different from those seen in the treatment of adults, and the therapist's expectations of the treatment process must take these divergences into account.

It is to these unique features of adolescent group therapy that Schulman addresses himself in the next paper. Most importantly, he considers the particular nuances of group structure and interpretive style required to deal with the adolescent's narcissistic vulnerability, his sensitivities regarding sexual issues, his orientation to the present, and his tendency toward action rather than reflection as a preferred mode of tension reduction. Schulman's approach is highly practical; he brings to the consideration of technique an extensive experience with a wide range of adolescent groups.

379

14

Transference, Resistance and Communication Problems in Adolescent Psychotherapy Groups

Irving Schulman, Ph.D.

The problems encountered in psychotherapy with emotionally disturbed adolescents tend to be exaggerations of the
attitudes and reactions that *normal* youngsters of this age
show during this difficult period of adjustment. The struggle
which the adolescent goes through to establish his identity,
coupled with his extreme sensitivity to evidence of failure,
immaturity, and dependency, prompts the therapist to modify the psychotherapy technique that he would ordinarily
employ in treating adults. Actually, one finds that the preferred psychotherapy approach with adolescents is one aimed
at character synthesis through an integration of reasonable
defenses rather than the more intensive therapy of a deeper
analytic nature (Gitelson, 1948; Josselyn, 1952).

In stressing character synthesis, it is not implied that the
therapist does not aim toward helping the adolescent gain
some understanding of his defenses and emotional conflicts.
However, in attempting this, one must always keep in mind

Reprinted by permission from the *International Journal of Group Psychotherapy*, 9:496-503, 1959. New York: International Universities Press.

the extreme sensitivity of the disturbed adolescent, his intolerance of anxiety, and his need for emotional support. Since the adolescent ego is still coping with the process of integration, and since the disturbed adolescent has particular difficulty in developing constructive interpersonal relationships, it generally proves unwise to attack the remnants of his existing defenses in the hope that his deeper emotional conflicts will be resolved (Gitelson, 1948; Josselyn, 1952). One usually finds that an analytic approach leads to increased anxiety and in some instances pushes the youngster into withdrawal, aggressiveness, or sexual acting out. The discontinuation of treatment by many adolescents is frequently the result of an anxiety-provoking therapeutic approach. In considering psychotherapy for the adolescent, one must also keep in mind the impact upon the ego of newly developed biological drives, the frequent reactivation of infantile conflicts during puberty, and the increased pressure from adults and peer groups for social and personal interaction (A. Freud, 1936; Josselyn, 1952). These unconscious and reality factors have a particularly stressful impact upon the disturbed adolescent since they magnify his discomfort immensely, and thereby interfere with emotional maturation. The ease with which the troubled adolescent's anxiety interferes with his everyday relationships leads him to react quite positively to psychotherapy which is aimed at anxiety reduction.

Considering the many problems which adolescents present in individual psychotherapy, one might question what value group psychotherapy would have with these youngsters. Would it not follow that the group situation would prove too threatening to the adolescent with emotional problems? Actually, one frequently finds that the idea of entering a psychotherapy group proves upsetting to the adolescent. However, with a reasonable degree of assertive and supportive attitude by the therapist, most adolescents will agree to enter a group for a trial period. The significant factor during this important introductory phase is whether the therapist himself feels that the adolescent will be uncomfortable in a group. If this is so, the discomfort is usually transmitted to the patient whose anxiety and distress may be intensified in anticipation of the experience.

In contrast to the initial resistance to group psychotherapy, we find that most adolescents integrate themselves rather quickly once they enter a group. This can be attributed to the supportive aspects of a group therapy situation, and, more specifically, to the fact that it is comforting to learn that others of similar age also have difficult emotional problems.

Some of the initial difficulty one may encounter in setting up and maintaining a psychotherapy group for adolescents is often related to the circumstances which usually surround the referral of these youngsters to an outpatient clinic. Referral often follows a particular crisis such as an alarming sexual experience, stealing, aggression, or sudden school failure. The threat which the adolescent feels when there is this sudden focus on his problems increases those existing anxieties related to being nonconforming, or to a fear of loss of control, and may, in turn, intensify his anticipations of being punished. Despite the intensification of anxiety, the therapeutic process with the adolescent may very likely be characterized by a rapid decrease of anxiety, which often is seen to wane with the speed with which it developed. Frequently, one finds that a manipulation of the environment, together with a supportive attitude by the therapist, reduces anxiety sufficiently so that the motivation to continue treatment is lost. This frequent development poses an important problem when considering the period of therapeutic contact at which an adolescent should enter a group. If a youngster goes through a period of successful individual therapy and is then considered for a group, an important motivating factor—his anxiety—may be absent. I have found that the most desirable time to enter most adolescents in a group is at the beginning phase of therapy, when anxiety and concern about the outcome of the therapeutic contact are still present.

The groups from which the conclusions in this paper were drawn have been homogeneously female, homogeneously male, as well as mixed groups. The age of the members ranged from 13 through 17 years; there were eight in a group, with the groups usually meeting once a week. The mixed groups had both a male and a female therapist present at each session. The first groups carried were homogeneous in regard to sex and personality type. I have found since that this proves less desirable than having a sexually mixed group composed of adolescents with many different personality problems. The reasons for this will be discussed in a later section of this paper.

Schizophrenics and severely psychopathic adolescents were excluded from the mixed groups, the schizophrenic youngsters because the group experience may stimulate feelings and fantasies which could threaten the schizophrenic's weak defenses, and the psychopathic adolescents because of their intolerance for an interacting, goal-directed experience. The therapist may find it necessary to require extremely manipulative, aggressive adolescents to leave a group after a trial period if he finds that the intense resistances in this type of youngster cannot be dealt with quickly. If this is not done, the therapist might be faced with a group that is moving toward disintegration, stimulated by the destructive influence of the severely dissocial youngster.

When comparing adult psychotherapy groups with those made up of adolescents, one finds that adults assume increasing personal responsibility for carrying out the therapy in a group. The degree of interaction in adult groups tends to reflect the degree of emotional involvement of the members; consequently, the therapist can anticipate that this interaction will lead to positive movement. When an adult group is moving well, the therapist may often limit himself to interpreting resistances and examining transference manifestations as they occur between members of the group or between the group members and himself. In contrast to this, one finds it necessary to be cautious in handling transference material with adolescents. This is particularly true as it applies to the transference among members of the group. The intense hostile components of the sibling problem which one frequently finds in disturbed adolescents can be exceedingly threatening if exposed abruptly in a group.

Another factor which encourages discretion regarding this type of interpretation is the difficulty that adolescents have in dealing with the abstract concept that conflictual feelings stimulated by earlier life relationships may really be the stimulus for current feelings in the group. In fact, the transitional affective and integrative state experienced during adolescence makes the clear-cut definition of "feelings" quite uncertain. Thus, if the therapist interprets hostility between two members in a group and attempts to examine these feelings in terms of sibling relationships, both adolescents in the group may regard these feelings on a personal basis, related more to the current group interaction. Because of the antagonism which might be created between members of the group, the therapist should keep this type of interpretation at a minimum and, in fact, avoid these interpretations during the earlier group sessions.

Most adolescents seem to have greater tolerance for expressing negative feelings toward the therapist in group psychotherapy than toward peers. Actually, the expression of negative feelings tends to be more common in group therapy than in individual therapy. This appears to stem from the fact that there is "group support" and consequently one might feel less personal threat. Similarly, tolerance for accepting interpretations of these feelings in a group is somewhat greater than in individual therapy. Contrary to one's expectations, I have found that the possibility for handling sexual problems in adolescents is enhanced in a mixed group. This applies to homosexual as well as heterosexual problems. It appears to be related to the reality situation in a mixed group which discourages the "horsing around" about sex which one often encounters in homogeneous groups. The reality of both sexes being present limits the degree to which one can engage in discussions about fantasied sexual experiences. Another factor may be the strong supportive element that is created by the recognition in the members that both sexes have sexual problems. I have noted spontaneous discussions arising in mixed groups regarding concern about sexual identity and adequacy—something which is rarely encountered in a group composed of adolescents of one sex.

It is generally recognized that the neurotic adolescent has difficulty in handling sexual feelings in therapy. Therefore, it is quite important to approach this problem with considerable sensitivity, particularly when confronted with the adolescent's sexual feelings for the therapist. In view of the frequent intensification of conflictual oedipal feelings during early adolescence, interpretations of sexualized transference toward the therapist can easily arouse intense guilt in girls and equally intense castration anxiety or homosexual panic in boys. The presence of both male and female therapists in these groups helps to allay anxieties in those youngsters who may be in extreme conflict with only one parent, and often serves to reduce guilt, since it can deter the development of a strong sexualized relationship with one of the therapists.

If we think of transference in the classic sense, that is, the distortion of the current interpersonal relationship in therapy by reacting to one's infantile emotional needs, and then examine the quality of transference in adolescent groups, we find few gross exacerbations of these infantile feelings. However, one does find a continuous low level of transference reaction which one would actually expect in view of the reactivation of infantile conflicts during puberty and the ever-present struggle to ward off gross expression of these feelings. By recognizing this, the therapist soon learns that he cannot expect the adolescent to deal with the transference in the same way as an adult.

In view of the lability of the disturbed adolescent's feelings, his ego limitations, his constant fear of retaliation and scorn from peers, and his easily aroused anxiety, one finds that the therapist has to take a more active role in these groups. One of the major contributions to a rapid disintegration of many adolescent groups is the adoption of a passive attitude by the group therapist. If the therapist maintains reasonable control of the group situation, he will usually reduce anxieties caused by the adolescent's feelings of uncertainty and insecurity and will also encourage the development of a closer dependency relationship, which is frequently desirable in therapy (Gitelson, 1948).

One of the important problems to keep in mind when carrying a mixed adolescent group is the possibility of sexual acting out among group members. This would be particularly true in a mixed group of adolescent delinquents, since most delinquent girls are adjudged so because of their promiscuity. This has not presented much of a problem in the groups with various personality types since many of these youngsters present unusually exaggerated superego development. Despite this, it is particularly important for the therapist carrying a mixed group to be aware of countertransference attitudes which might stimulate sexual acting out among group members. The presence of two therapists tends to act as a control, especially if they feel free to evaluate one another's approach.

In group psychotherapy with both adults and adolescents, resistances may be expressed in the form of group resistances, such as prolonged silences, group aggression, etc., or may take the form of the classic character resistances, such as obsessive talking, tangential thinking, persistent denial, undoing, etc. One usually finds in adult groups that the interpretation of resistances, together with the encouragement to bring forth associations, not only overcomes the current resistance but also leads to the expression of important conflictual material. In adolescent groups, interpretations of this type may not unbind the resistance. In fact, they seem frequently to intensify it. Many adolescents take interpretations of resistance as personal criticism. If this feeling grows, it may lead to group members banding together in a hostile attempt to control the situation. In order to avoid chronic resistances from developing in adolescent groups, it is important for the therapist to be more active than he would ordinarily be with adults. In most instances, the therapist would not call on a specific member of an adult group to express himself about a particular matter. However, in adolescent groups, this is often found necessary.

Regarding the overall problem of the adolescent's resistance to therapy, one finds it necessary to lend considerable ego support whenever one makes interpretations which stress the presence of resistances. Due to the adolescent's need to defy authority, one expects a good deal of resistance in group therapy and, in fact, if it is not encountered, it should be of some concern to the therapist. One reason for excluding schizophrenic adolescents from psychotherapy groups is related directly to this problem. In the schizophrenic, defective repression and the quick dissolution of defense diminishes resistance, often resulting in an outpouring of unconscious material which is emotionally out of tune with the feelings that neurotic adolescents can tolerate.

Concerning communication in adult groups, one finds that progress is enhanced when each member can draw on his associative thoughts. If the group therapist inquires about the thoughts of each member, it is possible to observe and deal with a variety of idiosyncratic feelings. It is also possible, at times, to demonstrate the common thread in divergent associations. In adolescent groups, it is extremely difficult to get members to produce associative thoughts. Free association plays little part in any psychotherapy with adolescents (Gitelson, 1948; Josselyn, 1952; Schulman, 1956). This is readily understandable in view of the state of emotional development during adolescence. The adolescent's constant attempts to flee from himself, his fear of perceiving threatening infantile conflicts, and the ease with which intense anxiety besieges him, all explain his unwillingness to produce associations which might harbor threatening emotional components. Herein lies one of the greatest limitations in group psychotherapy with adolescents. If a group therapist persists in searching for associative ideas, it may lead to negativism and antagonism in the adolescent. Prodding for associations tends to stimulate anxiety in the adolescent, who is led to sit in fearful anticipation that he might be asked what his thoughts are.

In the adolescent a good deal of affect is expressed on a motor basis. Anxiety is often handled by the adolescent through active manipulation of the group situation. It is important for the therapist to concern himself with these physical expressions of anxiety since these provide a route to emotional conflicts. Despite the value that might exist in interpreting the physical manifestations of emotional conflict, it is important for the therapist to maintain control of overt aggression in adolescent groups. Regardless of how aggression is expressed—in kicking under the table, throwing things, walking around, etc., it can lead quickly to a disintegration of the group.

It has been my impression that the adolescent's ability to articulate his problem is somewhat enhanced in mixed groups. This may, in part, be due to the lesser degree of physical acting out in mixed groups. Physical acting out is frequently regarded as a means of limiting ideational development or subsequent verbal expression.

The handling of symbolic material in adolescent groups poses an interesting problem. It presents, in extremely cogent fashion, the intolerance that the neurotic adolescent has for interpretations which are not bound to reality. For example, one frequently finds that by attempting to interpret symbolic dream material, one may get one of the following reactions. When the symbolism deals with hostile or sexual feelings toward the therapist, it produces intense anxiety which, in turn, results in withdrawal or aggressive acting out; when the symbolism expresses feelings about relationships outside the group therapy situation, the reaction of the adolescent is frequently that of indifference, disinterest, or evasion. In view of this it proves best not to attempt symbolic interpretations with adolescents who tend to avoid concentrating on the more basic disturbing feelings.

To summarize, our group therapy program with adolescents has clearly demonstrated that a modification of approach is required if therapy is to prove helpful. Actually, the goals of treatment are limited by the fact that the adolescent is in a transitional phase of development which in itself imposes considerable threat to his ego. The limitations of therapy with this group may not be in keeping with the therapist's conception of dynamic or intensive group therapy. If this is so, then it is bound to lead to a disappointing experience for both child and therapist.

If the therapist familiarizes himself with the nature of adolescent transference and recognizes the inherently intense resistance of the adolescent to accept and deal with his problems, one can see positive, albeit limited, results in group psychotherapy. Foremost in the mind of the therapist should be the matter of anxiety reduction, which often permits the adolescent to integrate and solidify his defenses. This can best be accomplished by clearly discerning the areas of greatest conflict in each adolescent in the group and then approaching these with sensitivity, lending both support and reassurance to an uncertain ego. Generally speaking, the therapeutic handling of adolescent problems is best accomplished in the context of current reality relationships, which the adolescent perceives as his only pertinent struggle.

PART V

Behavior Therapy

15

INTRODUCTION

Operant Conditioning in a Comprehensive Treatment Program for Adolescents, by Paul Lehrer, Lawrence Schiff, and Anton Kris

The use of behavior therapy, based on the principles of learning theory adumbrated by Wolpe (1958), Rachman (1959), and others, has found an increasing place in the treatment of children and adolescents in recent years. Werry and Wollersheim (1967) have described some of its specific applications, and Blom (1972) and Wachtel (1977) have attempted to map out the areas of overlap between behavior modification approaches and those of psychoanalytic psychology. Some of the polarization that characterized the views of early proponents has diminished in the later literature; Lazarus (1971), for instance, gives explicit recognition to the role of transference factors in the efficacy he claims for his modified operant techniques.

Though simple reward/punishment methods have been traditionally used to promote learning and/or modify specific symptoms thought to be undesirable (e.g., enuresis), the conceptualization of their integration into a comprehensive multimodal approach has lagged, perhaps because of difficulties in collaboration between practitioners of divergent theoretical orientations. Lehrer, Schiff, and Kris present in this paper a substantial effort in this direction, describing some of the ways in which operant conditioning by means of a token economy served to facilitate more traditional psychotherapies and to promote growth through largely nonverbal means. The incorporation of the parents into the overall treatment process was a crucial ingredient; parents learned new and better ways of influencing their children's behavior.

The "Project Re-ed" program of Nicholas Hobbs (1966) represents another significant application of behavioral principles to the treatment of disturbed young people. This psychoeducationally based approach, which incorporates, though is not limited to, operant reinforcement techniques, has been used primarily with latency-age children, but has been extended in recent years to adolescents as well. Unfortunately, this phase of the work has not as yet been published.

Yet another application of behavior therapy is described in the paper by Halmi, Powers, and Cunningham (Chapter 19) on the treatment of anorexia nervosa.

15

Operant Conditioning in a Comprehensive Treatment Program for Adolescents

Paul Lehrer, Ph.D.,
Lawrence Schiff, Ph.D.,
and Anton Kris, M.D.

Operant techniques, based upon the results of laboratory experimentation on the systematic application of reward and punishment (Honig, 1966), have been gaining increasingly wider application in psychiatric settings during the past decade (Krasner, 1968; Franks, 1969; Neuringer and Michael, 1970; Ulrich, Stachnik, and Mabry, 1970). Most of the studies thus far reported have focused on the effectiveness of specific techniques on specific behaviors, often in research settings where no other treatment was available to patients. In this paper we describe the clinical use of these techniques in a comprehensive treatment program for severely disturbed adolescents in a state mental hospital. Operant conditioning was used in conjunction with psychoanalytically oriented psychotherapy, and practitioners of behavioral and psychoanalytic persuasions collaborated in structuring a 24-hour-per-

Reprinted by permission from the *Archives of General Psychiatry*, 25:515-521, 1971. Copyright 1971, American Medical Association.

day milieu program. More specifically, psychoanalysis provided us with a theory of the motivation of behavior and of the development and integration of personality and was thus helpful in deciding what behaviors to modify in what sequence and in evaluating the appropriateness of particular rewards and punishments. The psychoanalytic perspective also led us to emphasize the importance of "real-life" goals and rewards and the personal relevance of treatment to patients' verbalized and unverbalized needs and goals. Operant techniques were first introduced in order to overcome the apathy and behavioral disorganization that prevented many patients from becoming involved in an active treatment program, but were later used much more widely. In this paper we describe our uses of these techniques and present the hypothesis we have developed regarding conditions for successful treatment in our setting. We also address the issue of the compatibility of operant conditioning with psychoanalytically oriented insight therapy with severely disturbed adolescents.

DESCRIPTION OF THE ADOLESCENT SERVICE

SETTING

The Adolescent Service of Boston State Hospital was initiated in 1965 as a "participatory consultation" service (Kris and Schiff, 1969; Kelly, 1970; Schiff, unpublished), involved in every phase of the patient's treatment. It provides central daytime facilities for education and recreation and offers consultation to the primary caretakers of adolescents in the hospital's basic inpatient and outpatient services, who retain responsibility for treatment planning and decisionmaking.

The program at the Adolescent Service's central facilities include four schools (a high school, a remedial classroom, a vocational training program, and a class for the severely retarded), a library, an occupational therapy shop, a social lounge, and a variety of trips, games, and social activities. The Adolescent Service's programs operate seven days a week from 9 a.m. to 9 p.m. and thus provide the bulk of the daily experience of those involved with them.

PATIENTS

About 60 patients, aged 14 to 22, are involved in the treatment program at any one time. Although the full spectrum of major psychiatric problems occurring in adolescence are represented, the modal patient tends to be chronically ill. Approximately 50 percent at any one time are outpatients, but almost all are seen on an inpatient basis at some point in their treatment.

USE OF OPERANT CONDITIONING

Throughout the treatment program an emphasis is placed on the use of rewards that occur naturally in the patient's world outside the hospital and that are related to realistic, often long-term, goals rather than special rewards that are contrived within the hospital setting. We assume that the more similar our treatment program is to the contingencies in the real world, the more easily will patients be able to transfer what they have learned in the hospital to life outside. Thus, in the high school, patients receive a diploma through the Boston Public Schools which is indistinguishable from the one they would have earned if they had continued their education in the school at which they were registered before they came to the hospital. In the remedial school, where programmed materials, supplemented by tutoring, are used in sequence to teach arithmetic (Sullivan, 1968), reading (Science Research Associates, 1967; Buchanen, 1968), spelling (Buchanen, 1967), writing (Skinner and Krakower, 1968), and high school subjects (Performance Systems, Inc., 1968), students can see their progress at each step as they advance in preparation for the General Education Development Test for a high school equivalency certificate.

Another important guideline in selecting reinforcers has been their personal relevance to the patient. School materials are chosen to be inherently of interest to students of this age group. Similarly, patients play an important role in deciding what extracurricular activities are made available. Whenever attendance or enthusiasm fails in an activity, this is taken as a signal to reevaluate it and to change it or to discontinue it, if called for. At a weekly community meeting patients are encouraged to give suggestions for new activities as well as to make complaints about ones already in progress.

Nevertheless, because of the feelings of hopelessness, apathy, and fear of involvement that characterize the severely disturbed adolescent, these measures often, by themselves, are not sufficient to motivate the patients to participate actively in treatment. External incentives are often required to supplement the more natural reinforcers in order to overcome inertia and to involve patients in activities and personal relationships that may later become reinforcing in themselves. It was for this reason, for example, that a token economy was instituted in the Adolescent Service's milieu program.

In practice, treatment programs at home, on the ward, and at the Adolescent Service's central facilities are integrated, and programs for individual patients are decided upon in consultation with family members and hospital personnel serving all locations. For the purposes of exposition, however, the uses of operant techniques in each of these geographic areas will be discussed separately.

OPERANT CONDITIONING AT THE ADOLESCENT SERVICE'S CENTRAL FACILITIES

One of the most visible uses of operant conditioning at the Adolescent Service is the token economy. As we employ it, the token economy is a highly individualized system. Although there are many "standards" things for which all patients are charged or paid, most patients are on individualized programs in which special charges or payments are tailored to individual needs or problems. Patients are routinely paid for attendance and productivity in school and for participation in various extracurricular activities. The medium of exchange is "points," which may be redeemed at a penny per point for up to five dollars each week. In order to encourage saving and to teach delay of gratification, however, patients are not permitted to deplete their point balance to below 500 points by withdrawal of money. Patients can spend the balance of their points directly in a social lounge designed as a typical teenage hangout, with a soda fountain and grill. Points are used to buy food, e.g., pizza, hot dogs, hamburgers, cans of soda, ice cream, milkshakes, and, occasionally, complete meals, and to play the jukebox and various games, e.g., pinball, table tennis, and board games. A continual effort is made to find additional activities and goods that can be offered to back the point system. Special events during the past year for which patients paid points included parties, dances, and trips to local attractions, as well as several more ambitious expeditions, including a trip to Montreal, camping trips on Cape Cod, and mountain-climbing trips in New Hampshire.

Points are taken away from patients as punishment only for minor infractions of the rules, such as failing to pay for an item at the social lounge. Serious violations, however, (e.g., physical abuse of property, other patients, or staff) lead to automatic restriction from participation in all activities until the patient, with one of the Adolescent Service psychologists, has worked out a strategy for controlling his behavior and for undoing whatever damage he may have done. Although point fines and payment in points for repair or replacement of property are often imposed for these more serious infractions, they are not used alone because we have found, as others have (Krasner, 1968), that point fines alone are ineffective and that their use only stimulates unproductive struggles that may injure positive personal relationships.

All transactions take place through a credit-card system, rather than through the traditional medium of tangible tokens. This system has been described elsewhere in detail (Lehrer, Schiff, and Kris, 1970). One important effect of the point system that was not expected by some Adolescent Service staff members unfamiliar with the potential of token economies was the increase of communication between staff and patients that followed introduction of the system in our program. Discussion of points provided valuable structure to the weekly community meeting. These patients find it easier to talk about things that they are going to get or are required to pay than about less tangible, and often affectively charged, community issues. Such issues, it was found, could often be approached through discussions about the point system. Further, brief weekly individual meetings of the patient with his Adolescent Service nurse to evaluate his program through the concrete matter of his earning and spending often became important opportunities for personal exchange.

Several case examples of operant conditioning programs at the Adolescent Service central facilities will be offered here. Some of the interplay between these programs and a psychodynamic approach to pinpointing patients' problem areas is illustrated.

Case 1

Patient A, a compulsive point-earner, was known informally as the "Rockefeller" of the Adolescent Service since he amassed huge sums of points, rarely spent any, and *never* missed any opportunities to earn. This was an extremely obsessional psychotic boy who had previously done so poorly in school at another hospital and been made so anxious by it that he was referred to Boston State Hospital with the recommendation that he not attend school. In fact, he had responded well to the structure of the remedial school, had completed the sequence of material designed to bring his reading and mathematical skills to a sixth-grade level, and was beginning work on materials designed to prepare him for the high school equivalency certificate. His hoarding of points appeared to be helpful at first in increasing his self-esteem. Later, however, when it appeared that he never allowed himself to have fun, his hoarding was seen as another symptom. After he demonstrated his ability to succeed in school and in the Adolescent Service's point system a program was instituted to teach him to spend just for the fun of it. Initially, he was paid for playing games with other patients in the lounge. (Ordinarily patients must *pay* for the privilege.) He was required to play a specified minimum number of games in order to be paid any points for playing, and gradually this requirement was increased. Never before had the patient been observed to initiate games with other patients. Throughout the first few weeks of this program, however, he often invited other patients to play and regularly played more games than were required for him to earn points for playing. Then the program was changed so that he was no longer paid for playing games but was required to pay for playing. He was also now required to play a specified minimum number of games per week in order to earn *anything* for the week. His gameplaying behavior continued on a level well *above* the required minimum. He began to have fun.

Case 2

Patient B was a 15-year-old nonpsychotic, school-phobic patient who came from a broken home. His father had been severely alcoholic, had had a violent temper, and had been unable to take a role in the discipline of his children. His mother had attempted to enforce his going to school but his hypochondriacal symptoms and, eventually, his drinking kerosene, stabbing himself, and taking an overdose of aspirin, all in his battle to avoid school, led to his hospitalization on a stubborn child charge. His affect was angry and depressed, and, in an interview, he acknowledged strong feelings of having been abandoned by his parents and feelings of guilt over his violent outbursts. He was accident-prone and frequently got into various kinds of mischief. It was felt that he needed long-term treatment to reverse the dangerous, self-destructive path he was following. Major elements in the problem were thought to be his marked dependency and low self-esteem, intimately connected with inadequate development of self-discipline.

At the hospital he was provided with the strong controls he needed and was able to confide in a therapist and to attend school on a fairly regular basis. Occasionally his temper led him to violate some of the rules of deportment at the Adolescent Service, and this led to his restriction to the ward, but generally his behavior was entirely appropriate. Perfect school attendance was not required initially, to avoid premature confrontation. In the summer of his second year of hospitalization, however, the coordinator of special education of the Boston Public Schools, in reviewing the patient's school attendance, ruled that he must not miss any days of school during the summer session if he was to pass the ninth grade. The patient responded to this by dropping out of school and taking a job at a butcher shop without permission or approval. In view of the good relationship he now had with hospital personnel and in view of his increased self-esteem, it was felt that he was now ready for confrontation. He was required to leave his job and return to summer school.

A program was instituted whereby he was paid a bonus of 100 points for each perfect day of school. Any day on which he failed to come to school, either in the morning or in the afternoon, an attendant who had a good relationship with him was to be sent to look for him and to take him back to school. Whenever this was necessary, he was to be charged 100 points for "services rendered." On the first day of the program he frequently excused himself from the classroom, became nauseated, and fainted three times, behavior that, in milder form, had previously excused him from school. (This may be considered a typical example of the intensification of a previously reinforced response that often occurs during the early states of extinction [Notterman, 1970].) Limits were put on permission for him to leave the classroom and, within a week, he was attending regularly, paying attention, and making satisfactory academic progress. Although he was usually tardy and rarely earned his bonus, he needed to be brought by the attendant only on four occasions during the summer. He passed the ninth grade.

Case 3

Patient C, a 17-year-old boy with the diagnosis of autism, benefited demonstrably from the remedial school, which was organized as a programmed classroom, modeled after the CASE program at the National Training School for Boys in Washington, D.C. (Cohen, 1968). For years he could not function in the ordinary classroom. He was barely verbal, and he seemed completely unable to work independently on any prolonged task. He had been taught only on an individual tutorial basis. In the classroom, however, he was expected to do independent work. Although his subsequent course in school was stormy, he nevertheless made steady progress. One of the problems that interfered with his work was his tendency to give wrong answers deliberately. A teacher's attempts to correct his work and to tutor him generally led to an argument that resulted in both parties becoming angry and confused. This appeared to be a repetition of events at home, where his father would severely reprimand him for giving misinformation. He appeared to seek the confusion as a way of avoiding serious work on which he might be taken to task for his answers. A program combining reward with "timeout from reinforcement" (Ferster and Skinner, 1957) was used in order to modify this behavior. Whenever his errors appeared to be deliberate, his work was taken away from him and he was asked to sit in his seat without work or to leave the classroom until he was ready to work properly. During this time he could not earn any points. Also, since he liked to play with blocks, he was allowed to play with them for half an hour each time he correctly completed a specified minimum number of pages of work. Whenever he made an "honest" error in his work, he was not reprimanded but was shown the proper way to answer the problem. Appropriate materials were chosen so that he could learn while making a minimum of such mistakes. This program markedly reduced his tendency to make deliberate mistakes.

The patient's progress in the remedial classroom was dramatic. In arithmetic, where his work was initially evaluated in small units (by the page or by the individual problem), he successfully completed books on addition, subtraction, multiplication, and division and proceeded to fractions and decimals. He became able to work on this material independently for up to an hour at a time. In reading he began in a teacher-administered program taught in a small class and gradually advanced to books in which he was required to read independently and to retain several paragraphs at a time.

OPERANT CONDITIONING ON THE WARDS

We have already indicated that the ward staff are the primary treaters of adolescent inpatients at our hospital, and that they supervise and sponsor all the activities in the hospital in which patients engage, including those at the Adolescent Service. The ward is the one place in the hospital where violent and potentially violent behavior can be handled and is the place where patients feel safest when they are unsure of how well they can control themselves. Thus, patients ordinarily return to the ward voluntarily (and are encouraged to do so) when they get upset, and generally stay there until they feel more comfortable.

With the ward as a firm home base, the privilege of coming to the Adolescent Service can function as a strong and important reinforcer. Admission to the Adolescent Service's activities, however, is not unconditional. When a patient's behavior cannot be controlled at the Adolescent Service, he is excluded from its activities and is required to earn his way back by good behavior on his ward and by demonstrating his readiness to make proper use of the activities in which he chooses to engage. Only the physical security and 24-hour control available on a hospital ward can insure the effectiveness of a timeout program, for only on the ward can such powerful basic reinforcers as visiting privileges, grounds privileges, sleeping arrangements, or even the "privilege" of remaining out of a seclusion room be controlled and used systematically.

Case 4

The case of patient D illustrates how reinforcement contingencies on the ward were used, in conjunction with those in the remedial classroom, to treat a case of severe school phobia in a moderately retarded psychotic boy. The patient's experiences with school had been uniformly ones of complete failure. Eventually he sustained a series of losses that made him unable to tolerate the stress of school. These losses included his therapist, his ward administrator, and his nurse at the Adolescent Service who all left the hospital at about the same time. He stopped attending school and remained out for two months, making only two brief visits to school during this time. Numerous attempts at positive reinforcement met with failure. We supposed that this was related to the intense self-punitive attitude that characterized his depressive reaction to loss. To deal with this a program was implemented in which he was required to work for half an hour each day in the ward's occupational therapy shop in order to avoid having to spend the evening in a seclusion room. When he first learned of the program he appeared greatly relieved and he dramatically thanked us for proposing it. He attended occupational therapy faithfully every day and remained out of seclusion. After approximately one month he was also required to spend some time in the Adolescent Service's occupational therapy shop and, thereafter, some time in the classroom. Special programs were written for him to help him learn multiplication. His work was evaluated by a tutor after every arithmetic problem, and the patient was paid generously for his work. The seclusion provisions in the program were gradually eliminated. Within one month he was attending school for one and a half hours each day. The rest of the day was progressively filled with work assignments and other activities. Despite several severe stresses, including the admission of his mother to the hospital and several changes in ward administrator, he continued attending school regularly.

OPERANT CONDITIONING IN THE HOME

Parents are encouraged to join one or more of several groups conducted by the Adolescent Service soon after the patient's initial hospital contact. Some of these groups focus on orientation to the hospital, others on the experience of having a sick child and on gaining more personal insight. In addition there is a group called "Friends of the Adolescent Service" which plans social activities for the patients and hears invited speakers on topics relevant to their children's treatment. The general orientation has been to treat parents as co-workers in the treatment of their children.

A 10-week course in operant conditioning was offered to parents, irrespective of their participation in other groups. The parents of 15 patients volunteered to participate. Although there was reluctance on the part of some parents to see their children's problems as being treatable behavior problems (rather than problems of innate badness or physical illness), parents were nevertheless enthusiastic about receiving concrete help in handling their children's behavior at home. The course was modeled after ones given by Walder (1966) and by Patterson, Ray, and Shaw (1969) for parents of younger children. Parents met once weekly in a two-hour session. The first hour of each session consisted of a lecture on the basic principles of operant conditioning. Lecture topics included methods of observation, record-taking, schedules of reinforcement, extinction, punishment, shaping, and programming. The second hour consisted of individual meetings with a staff member in which the parents were trained and supervised in systematic observation of the behavior of their children and in the design of programs to modify it.

In the individual meetings, parents were first helped to isolate a behavioral problem that was important, that occurred frequently, and that was sufficiently well specified to be countable. It was thought that involvement in the course would be most helpful and appealing to the parents if they were given their initial choice of what behavior to work on. Thus, although the staff felt free to suggest important behaviors, the final choice was left to the parents. Choices included teaching new behaviors as well as eliminating "bad" ones. Frequently, both were done at once. After selecting a behavior, the parents were asked to take a baseline count on the frequency of occurrence of the target behaviors (or, in the case of behaviors not yet learned, to record the elements or approximations of the target behaviors that the patient was able to perform), and to record the antecedents and consequences of the behaviors. Considerable effort was invested in taking these preliminary steps with care. Only then was attention turned to modifying the behavior. The target behaviors chosen by parents included ones involving cleanliness and self-care (shaving, washing, care of hair), conversational abilities, getting up in the morning, doing chores at home, behaviors associated with independence (e.g., shopping, traveling by public transportation), talking to oneself, asking repetitive and annoying questions, bizarre gesturing, and aggressive behaviors. After the formal course was over, monthly follow-up meetings were held for one year in order to help parents continue working behaviorally with their children. Most of the parents were, in fact, able to modify significant behaviors in their children during the course. These led to important therapeutic advances and, often, to a "snowballing" of other, more global changes in the behavior of the patient and his family. Even in cases where parents were unable to carry out programs successfully with their children, they almost universally reported a new appreciation of the extent to which they punish their children for "bad" behavior, while ignoring good behavior. They saw the effectiveness of positive reinforcement and of teaching important behaviors in small steps. In several cases significant changes occurred in the *parents'* behavior, which were necessary in order to modify the behavior of their children, and which altered the general pattern of communication in the family.

Case 5

The mother of patient E chose to work on his talking to himself, which she saw as the hallmark of his chronic psychosis. When she observed the antecedents and consequences of this behavior, she noted that it tended to occur when he was not doing anything in particular and that one of the consequences of the behavior generally would be her nagging him to stop. This seemed to be a general pattern for the interaction between the patient and his mother. She would nag him about not doing the right things or about doing the wrong things, and generally she would overlook times when he did things on his own initiative. (Her capacity to face so squarely her own behavior was characteristic of parents in this group. The potential for relevant action offered by the course appeared to facilitate such insight.)

The effective program for eliminating his talking to himself involved his mother's counting the times he did it and taking him out to dinner at the end of each week in which he did not talk to himself for a specified number of evenings. She also established her own point system at home, and paid him in points for helpful things he did around the house without being asked (e.g., putting away his clothes and taking out the garbage). The points were exchangeable into gifts. In addition she made concerted attempts to engage him in conversation, especially about things he would read in the newspaper, as an incentive for him to spend time reading rather than talking to himself. After two months he stopped talking to himself and this behavior has not recurred for more than one year since then.

The parents of patient C (described above) decided initially to work on his repetitive questions. After observing the consequences of this behavior that usually occurred at home, they realized that they usually answered all of his questions and that eventually they became angry. The program consisted of their counting the number of times that he asked a question, and refusing to answer it after he repeated it four times. The patient became visibly upset when this program started and frequently asked whether his behavior was being counted. The repetitive questions disappeared within two weeks. He still tended to use language in a babyish way, however, generally with the effect of producing anger and confusion in his parents. Thus, it was decided to teach the family to talk together. The best site for this training seemed to be at the dinner table, where the patient and his parents were together every evening. Initially it was found that no communication ever took place at this time. Rather, the patient's mother would read a book while eating and his father would watch the news. The patient would receive attention only if he did something wrong. At first the program consisted of tape-recording the dinner table conversation and bringing the tape to the operant conditioning course for feedback. Some of these early conversations sounded as though the patient's father was giving him the "third degree" about school. The father asked pointed factual questions. The atmosphere was tense, and periodically the patient would give some wrong information, confuse the issues being discussed, and get his parents angry with him. It was suggested that the parents ignore instances of misinformation, that they bring more of their own daily experiences into the conversations, and that they expand on any topics that the patient brought up that were interesting. This program continued for about five months, during which his conversational ability markedly improved both at home and at the Adolescent Service, with a host of associated changes in social behaviors.

Several parents in the course were not successful in modifying their children's behavior. In three cases, violence on the patient's part required ward treatment to provide effective reinforcers and behavioral control. In another three cases, the parents could not see the relevance of the process to themselves (e.g., one mother was preoccupied with her marital difficulties and had no motivation to pursue the course), although one of these couples was later able to participate successfully in a conditioning program at home after subsequent events had demonstrated to them the importance of working on their child's behavior. In one instance a staff member's difficulty in setting limits with his patient made it impossible for him to help the parents, since no other approach was equally relevant in the case of this assaultive patient.

BEHAVIOR MODIFICATION AND PSYCHOTHERAPY

For the majority of our patients individual psychotherapy has been an important component of the treatment program. In our setting, with its wide range of diagnostic differences among patients and its considerable variation in aptitude, experience, and theoretical persuasion among therapists, psychotherapy is not closely definable as one kind of procedure. All versions share, however, the relative intimacy of private conversation, directed to an examination of the patient's personal experience, his hopes and fears, and, particularly, his feelings about the people close to him. No other setting offers the patient a comparable opportunity. For some patients psychotherapy becomes the central focus of treatment, while for others it appears never to achieve such intensity, although even in the latter case it may be of great importance to the patient. In this paper, however, we are not so much concerned with psychotherapy itself as with simultaneous use of psychotherapy and behavior modification techniques in the various forms described earlier.

In the past several years we have seen many cases in which behavior modification has facilitated psychotherapy but no cases in which the two have interfered with each other. In-

terference is, of course, often a matter of individual interpretation. Psychotherapists, ward administrators, and various
members of the Adolescent Service have often disagreed over
diagnosis or specific aspects of treatment planning, but these
disagreements have not as yet revealed areas of incompati-
bility between behavior modification and psychotherapy as
we have employed them.

The case of patient A (described above) illustrates how
involvement with the behavioral program in the Adolescent
Service enabled a seemingly unreachable patient to take advantage of psychotherapy. At the time of his admission he
was extremely anxious and, although he obsessively attempted to obey all the rules and to be approved of by everyone, he avoided close relationships with staff members and
with other patients. At times, his anxiety made it impossible
for him to carry on a conversation, for he could not concentrate on anything that someone else was saying. He adamantly
denied that he was a patient, and preferred to think of himself just as a student in the school. For these reasons, use of
psychotherapy, in our setting, at this time, would have been
ill-advised, and we made use of operant conditioning programs such as the one described earlier. After approximately
one year's involvement in the Adolescent Service, however,
during which he demonstrated, for the first time, that he
could succeed in school, he began to admit that he did, in
fact, have some problems, and he asked to have psychotherapy. During the approximately 10 months since therapy
began, the patient has been able to speak to this therapist
about his feelings of loneliness, his intense rage at people
who are even slightly critical of him (including his parents),
and his fear of becoming overtly psychotic again and becoming chronically hospitalized. He has markedly loosened up
during this period, his anxiety has diminished, and he has
begun, very tentatively, to express some of his anger and

depression more openly and to show a capacity for warmth and understanding both in his relationships with staff members and with other patients.

COMMENT

We have described the clinical use of operant conditioning for behavior modification in a comprehensive treatment program for a diverse population of disturbed adolescents. It will be evident to those familiar with inpatient treatment that proper administration (i.e., case-management by the patients' ward administrator) employs a similar behavioral frame of reference (Linn, 1959). For example, demands are regularly made on patients, requiring at least a minimal degree of behavioral organization, before the patient is allowed to leave the ward. Programs for adolescent inpatients have generally recognized, in addition, the need for developmentally relevant activities (e.g., school and recreation) as integral parts of hospital treatment (Beskind, 1962; Beckett, 1965; American Psychiatric Association, 1967; Schonfeld, 1967; Hartmann, Glasser, and Greenblatt, 1968). Our report has, therefore, been concerned less with these principles of treatment than with ways in which operant techniques can be used to systematize these aspects of treatment and apply them in various settings where treatment takes place.

Operant techniques and more traditional methods have been integrated into a consistent approach to treatment that has drawn from several bodies of psychiatric experience. A psychodynamic approach is taken to interviewing, to diagnosis, and to psychotherapy, and psychoanalysts and behaviorists cooperate in planning treatment programs. Choice of reinforcers and areas of reinforcement are influenced and directed by psychodynamic considerations. The decision to gratify patient A's need to hoard and, later, to challenge it, and the decision to avoid an early confrontation with patient

B but to insist upon one later are determined by assessments of many factors affecting their capacity to tolerate the new demands and to respond with benefit.

Operant techniques have been especially useful where other methods are least effective. Where words fail, these not necessarily verbal methods are powerful alternatives. Their emphasis on learning in a continuum of small, definable steps, with provision for recording of progress, their use of immediate, usually positive contingencies, and their attention to behavior and its consequences make them especially suitable for work with very sick adolescents, for whom action and nonverbal communication play such an important role. An indirect but nonetheless important aspect of operant techniques is inherent in their clarity and simplicity: They require that the goals of treatment be accurately specified. They can, therefore, be used to coordinate the efforts of a diverse staff scattered throughout a large hospital. As in every other aspect of treatment, however, proper diagnosis and timing are required in the use of operant conditioning. Further, these techniques do not obviate the need for personal investment in the patient nor is operant conditioning a substitute for the painful process of making life decisions. Also, patients develop deep emotional attachments to staff members who apply contingencies to their behavior, and the importance of these attachments must be considered in treatment planning.

The question is sometime raised: Does operant conditioning deal only with the surface, leaving the underlying problem untouched? The behaviorist argues that there is no "underlying" problem but that the behavior *is* the problem (Wolpe, 1958; Skinner, 1961). Neither the question nor the answer adequately represents our experience with operant techniques. Like the psychoanalytic approach to treatment (Freud, 1905a), operant techniques must *start* from the "surface," i.e., where problems are readily identifiable. In our experience, when we modify behaviors that most obviously interfere with a patient's academic and social adjustment and most directly contribute to his low self-esteem, we also often make the patient (e.g., patient A) more capable of fruitful self-examination. Similar observations have been made by others (Weitzman, 1967). Finally, as in the case of patient C, long-term sequential operant conditioning programs in various settings have, in fact, been found to deal effectively with the complexities of human behavior.

PART VI

Psychopharmacology

16

INTRODUCTION

Pharmacotherapy in Adolescent Psychiatry, by Michael G. Kalogerakis

Psychopharmacology has been spoken of as the "third revolution" in psychiatry, and has certainly profoundly affected the care of patients of all ages and clinical types over the past three decades. The treatment of adolescents has not escaped this trend, although the relatively clear guidelines that apply to adults on the one hand and to children on the other have been difficult to define for this transitional age group. Further, concerns about habituation and undesirable side effects have limited both research into and clinical application of drug treatment with adolescent patients.

In this chapter, written especially for this volume, Kalogerakis presents an up-to-date statement of current knowledge and practice in the treatment of adolescents with psychoactive medication. He spells out the pertinent cautions, limitations, and special phase-related considerations, but makes it clear that there are definite circumstances in which such treatment is not only useful, but clearly appropriate. He also emphasizes the fact that drug treatment must be only one element in a comprehensive program that involves psychological intervention, family support, and environmental management. He also points out areas of ignorance in which further research is urgently needed. His comprehensive sur-

421

vey of the existing literature is, in itself, a most valuable contribution.

16

Pharmacotherapy in Adolescent Psychiatry

Michael G. Kalogerakis, M.D.

The use of medication has an established place in the treatment of emotional disturbance in adolescence. Experienced clinicians familiar with a broad range of adolescent psychopathology attest to the usefulness of drugs in a variety of conditions. They tend not to make use of psychotropic agents as the preferred or initial treatment but use them when they are indicated.

This chapter summarizes the current state of the art in the pharmacotherapy of adolescent disorders. An effort has been made to be comprehensive and to keep in mind the practical problems faced by clinicians working in different settings. In addition to the purely clinical questions, relevant legal and ethical issues are considered.

PHARMACOTHERAPY IN PSYCHIATRY

As medical scientists pursue their research into the biochemical basis of mental illness, those working in clinical areas

First publication. The author is indebted for the writing of this chapter to the many who graciously shared their views and clinical experiences. In particular, Charles Popper of McLean Hospital in Belmont, Massachusetts, was most helpful.

have looked expectantly at their findings to see what they
might contain of value to the treatment of their patients. As
matters now stand, we still know far too little about how
psychotropic drugs work. Researchers believe that it is only
a matter of time before we solve the enigma of psychotic
illness and, in due course, discover the process by which
proven drugs have their effect. In the meantime, we must
content ourselves with empirical data, which, at least with
adult patients, are now substantial.

Extensive double-blind studies with adult patients have
demonstrated the effectiveness of specific psychotropic drugs
for particular clinical syndromes. Among the many general
principles derived from such studies which can be said to
apply to adolescents are the following:

1. Although careful diagnosis forms the basis for all
   therapeutic interventions, the prescription of psychotropic agents continues to be based primarily on
   the symptom picture, not on the diagnostic category
   per se.
2. Individual responses are highly variable, partially
   dependent on unknown factors, and often not predictable.
3. Within a given family of drugs, finding the most effective agent is generally a matter of trial and error.
4. The proper dosage is determined by titration, starting with a low dose and increasing it till the desired
   effect is obtained, then reducing the dose gradually
   until the smallest dose that still produces a therapeutic effect is reached.
5. The placebo effect, which is commonly observed, emphasizes the importance of psychological factors in
   the overall response of the patient.
6. As far as can be determined, drugs have no effect on

the underlying causes of the disorder, and are therefore not curative (as elsewhere in medicine); other therapeutic approaches (e.g., psychotherapy) which offer the possibility of definitive change must therefore be used in conjunction with medication for optimum results.

PHARMACOTHERAPY AND THE ADOLESCENT PATIENT

It is frequently said that pharmacotherapy as used with children is not applicable beyond puberty (Werry, 1978) and, further, that adolescents should be treated as adults since their reactions are basically similar. Though there is some truth to these assertions, neither is entirely correct, so that a psychopharmacology of adolescence is still sorely needed. Of the current standard works that address childhood psychopharmacology, only one (Wiener, 1977) attempts to deal with adolescents. As a result, much of what follows represents the impressions gathered over time by clinicians working independently, and is subject to change as empirical data accumulate and research specific to adolescence is reported.

It would appear that psychotropic agents are used far less commonly in adolescents than in adults and probably less frequently than in younger children. Furthermore, it is this writer's impression that over 80 percent of adolescents receiving prescribed psychoactive drugs either are or have been hospitalized. (This is certainly not the case among adults, who use hypnotics and anxiolytics such as diazepam in epidemic proportions.)

Several factors account for this restricted use. To begin with, the psychopathology of adolescence differs appreciably from that of other age groups. It is likely to be manifested in behavior disturbance rather than neurotic or psychotic symptomatology. Yet existing psychotropic substances are effective only against the latter. The major psychoses, although they may occur earlier, do not generally make their appearance until late adolescence and early adulthood, thus limiting the need for antipsychotic agents in the younger adolescent.

Many psychiatrists are reluctant to use medication with adolescents even when indicated, for fear they will encroach on normal growth and development. Reports that methylphenidate has had such an effect in younger children make the average adolescent psychiatrist wary, since he rarely has the depth of experience in the use of psychotropic drugs that many adult psychiatrists have.

Another source of reluctance is the awareness of the propensity many adolescents have to become drug-dependent. The drug abuse phenomenon remains quintessentially an expression of classical adolescent conflicts. Even the adolescent who has not abused drugs on the street must be considered vulnerable, so that few physicians are willing to risk introducing into a youngster's life medication that might later be misused.

In addition, one cannot always be certain that the adolescent is taking the medication as prescribed. Even the youth who is tacitly cooperative may secrete a phenothiazine tablet in his cheek, and spit it out moments later if he decides he doesn't want the drowsy effect that day. (Adolescents commonly have a low tolerance for side effects.) Needless to say, monitoring medication of an adolescent no longer in the hospital is virtually impossible, even when parents are thoroughly cooperative.

Finally, a number of psychodynamic considerations that lead to resistance may come into play. These have to do with the meanings that may be ascribed by the adolescent to the medication or to the act of being medicated. Most common are the following:

1. Medication changes his appearance (often true, as

with phenothiazines), and makes him look like a freak; this is especially important in the younger adolescent whose body-image concerns and dread of humiliation are intense.

2. Medication is a means of subduing him, rendering him passive and impotent, a plot on the part of the adult world to take away his autonomy.
3. Medication is poison.
4. Medication is magical and will cure him; he need not therefore do anything himself to get well.

Such fantasies are not necessarily observed only among psychotic youth, since they touch so directly on some of the most sensitive of normal adolescent concerns. They must be identified prior to prescribing medication and dealt with thoroughly, both to allay unnecessary anxiety and to insure maximum cooperation with the treatment.

A matter of considerable importance for the pharmacotherapy of children as well as adolescents, discussed by Klein, Gittelman, Quitkin, and Rifkin (1980), is involvement of the parents in the treatment. Thorough preparation of parents is essential when a youngster leaving the hospital must continue to receive medication. Since many adolescents cannot be relied on to take medication as prescribed, parents must be given detailed information about administration, dosage regulation, side effects, expected length of treatment, potential benefits, other needed treatment, and, commonly, the importance of maintaining contact with other observers such as schoolteachers. Failures in treatment are often the consequence of insufficient attention to such aspects of management and deny the adolescent patient our best effort.

General Principles of Drug Treatment

For all the foregoing reasons, the decision to use medication with an adolescent patient must be made after careful consideration of all appropriate alternatives. As is well known, many acute disturbances remit spontaneously. Except for emergency situations, therefore, a patient entering the hospital should not be started on medication until a fair trial without drugs fails to produce significant improvement. Such a period may vary from a few days to several weeks, depending on the nature of the disorder and the patient's course, but 10 days is an acceptable minimum. Such a drug-free period is essential to permit diagnostic evaluation of the patient in an unclouded field. Patients' medication prior to admission should be withdrawn gradually, with lithium the only exception.

An important part of every diagnostic evaluation is a careful history of drug treatment and drug abuse. What was prescribed and under what circumstances, what results were obtained, and what, if any, side effects were noted are critical pieces of information for the individual treatment plan. Unusual hypersensitivity and any truly allergic reactions (rare among psychotropic drugs) should of course be recorded. A history of abuse of mood-altering drugs peddled on the street provides invaluable clues to both biological responses of the individual adolescent to chemical agents and insights into the personality structure. Both should figure in any subsequent decision to medicate.

Parental attitudes and practices with regard to drug use are invariably transmitted consciously or unconsciously to children and should therefore be explored. Some otherwise adequately functioning families live in a veritable drug culture consisting of both medically prescribed and self-prescribed substances of all kinds. These practices are often closely guarded family secrets, rationalized in various ways to the children. Though this may lead to similar abuse in the latter, it may also create strong antipathy with subsequent inordinate resistance to needed medication. The unsuspecting physician seeking to medicate an adolescent in such families may run into impassioned and seemingly unreasonable refusal.

Of particular importance in the psychiatric examination of the adolescent is evidence of sensorial changes that suggest a toxic state. The possibility that such a state exists is an additional reason for not medicating a newly admitted patient until he is evaluated.

Differential diagnosis among psychotic or borderline states may lead to different choices of psychotropic agents. This applies particularly with regard to differentiating juvenile forms of manic-depressive illness from schizophrenia or other affective states (Feinstein, Feldman-Rotman, and Woolsey, 1980). It may also apply to the various conditions subsumed under the term "minimal brain dysfunction" (Wender, 1971).

The relevant information needed to arrive at a comprehensive diagnosis may require both a neurological evaluation and psychological testing. However, as Klein and his associates (1980) point out, these examinations are of little use in arriving at a decision with regard to choice of drug when pharmacotherapy is indicated. History and clinical (mental status) examination remain our best tools for this purpose.

In addition to the usual detailed observations of nursing staff, reports from schoolteachers and activities therapists, particularly in institutional settings where they may be trained by psychiatric staff, are invaluable for close monitoring of all psychotropic medication. The structure of a classroom places special demands on the adolescent, evoking behavior that might not be seen on the ward or at home. However, the reliability of school evaluations is extremely variable and totally dependent on the sensitivity of individual teachers and the quality of school-ward staff liaison.

The Psychotropic Agents and Their Uses

Any review of medication in current use must choose between a discussion organized around clinical syndromes and one that begins with the drugs themselves. The former is ideal but in this case impractical because of the continuing diagnostic confusion in adolescent psychiatry (DSM-III, 1978) and the degree to which specific drugs can be used in different conditions, a science still unfolding. This review therefore chooses the latter course, while acknowledging the deficiencies of the approach. No attempt is made to consider all drugs that may actually be in use. The reader is referred to the abundant literature in adult (Jarvik, 1978; Klein et al., 1980) and child (Wiener, 1977; Werry, 1978) psychopharmacology for discussions of the full spectrum of psychoactive agents.

STIMULANTS

It is perhaps appropriate to begin with this class of drugs since modern psychopharmacology may be said to have started with the use of stimulants in children (Bradley, 1937) well before the phenothiazines revolutionized hospital care of adult psychotics in the fifties. Cantwell (1979) states that the only definitely established indication for the use of stimulants is the hyperkinetic reaction of childhood (minimal brain dysfunction [MBD]) now officially known in DSM-III as Attention Deficit Disorder with Hyperactivity. Characterized in younger children by excessive motor activity, difficulty in sustaining attention, and impulsive behavior, there is evidence that it continues into adolescence and even adulthood with a modified clinical picture. Secondary symptoms may appear, especially antisocial behavior and learning disabilities, which may obscure the syndrome, although a careful history may reveal that it was present prepubertally in its classical form.

Mackay, Beck, and Taylor (1973), in a series of 10 cases of adolescents described as having minimal brain dysfunction, found, contrary to the then held belief, that they were not stimulated by methylphenidate but showed improvement in the capacity to learn, integrate, and remember. Two other studies involving delinquents found stimulants to be effective (Eisenberg, Lackman, and Molling, 1963; Maletsky, 1974). The latter compared two groups of adolescents, one placed on placebo, the other on dextroamphetamine, and found a significant difference in response, particularly in those youths who had been hyperactive in childhood.

Further study of adolescent populations is needed before definitive statements on the usefulness of stimulants in this age group can be made. For the time being, it is important to record that stimulants have demonstrated their value in childhood hyperkinesis, a 75 percent improvement rate being found for amphetamines, methylphenidate, and magnesium pemoline (Barkley, 1977). Cantwell (1979) recommends that thought be given to the use of stimulants for adolescents who manifest hyperactivity, conduct disturbance, or learning disability associated with difficulty in attention and impulsivity. Admittedly experimental at this point, such use is justified by the positive results with children and the absence of significant side effects. Of the latter, those seen include insomnia, anorexia, stomachaches, headaches, and moodiness, all short-term. One longer-term symptom, suppression of height and weight in prepubertal children, caused quite a furor in some circles a few years ago, but reestablishment of the normal growth rate is now known to occur after one to two years of medication, with no lasting effects on the final outcome.

It is impossible to recommend specific dosage schedules of stimulants because there is so much variability of response from one youngster to another. Starting low and titrating upward until a therapeutic response is achieved or side effects appear is the recommended procedure. Since stimulants are likely to be given on a long-term basis, drug holidays of one to two weeks every six months are advised to assess continuing therapeutic effect. Finally, although some authors minimize the risk of increased tolerance and drug-dependency, it is wise to remain alert to this danger when working with adolescents.

ANTIPSYCHOTICS (NEUROLEPTICS)

These are without doubt that drugs most commonly used with adolescents. In general, their use coincides with the first appearance of adult forms of schizophrenia, generally around 14 to 15 years of age. As elsewhere, our knowledge of how to use them is based largely on experience with adults, since there are no controlled studies involving adolescents reported in the literature.

The major groups of antipsychotics in current use are the phenothiazines, butyrophenones, and thioxanthenes. Since no clearcut advantages have been demonstrated for the last two, only the first will be considered here.

Of the phenothiazines, chlorpromazine is the most widely used and, in the experience of many clinicians, as effective as any other antipsychotic agent. What is important in selecting a drug is that the prescribing physician be familiar with it and that its effectiveness be determined empirically for each individual patient.

Indications

Neuroleptics should be reserved for the more severe psychiatric disturbances, with only rare exceptions. For the most part, this will coincide diagnostically with schizophrenic psychosis, although severe agitation unaccompanied by psychotic symptomatology, which has not remitted spontaneously after 10 days of hospitalization, also calls for a neuroleptic.

Toxic psychoses should be carefully ruled out, as must other psychotomimetic conditions such as encephalitis. Although phenothiazines may be given with good results in toxic states, establishing a diagnosis first and allowing time for spontaneous remission is essential. Manic-depressive illness does not respond well to phenothiazines and calls for the use of lithium (see p. 434).

Dosage

Initially, 50 to 100 mg orally per day of chlorpromazine, given preferably in three or four doses, should give an idea of therapeutic response. This can be raised until an adequate response is obtained and anticholinergics administered as side effects appear. On reviewing the literature on maintenance therapy, Davis (1975) emphasizes the consistent superiority of phenothiazine maintenance over placebo. He suggests that a first schizophrenic episode during adolescence may be treated with a short course of antipsychotic medication but that long-term maintenance be avoided since the relapse rate with this group is clearly lower than with others. Although the efficacy of depot neuroleptics (chiefly fluphenazine enanthate and fluphenazine decanoate) has been amply demonstrated with adults, Ayd (1975) advises against their use in "children" (age range uncertain) until additional studies support such use.

The intramuscular administration of chlorpromazine (25 to 50 mg) is occasionally necessary and is an effective means of achieving quick sedation of a violent, disturbed adolescent whose behavior threatens the safety of others or himself.

Side Effects

These may be significant with adolescents. In particular, akinesia and akathisia cause acute distress and lead to refusal of medication when uncontrolled (Van Putten, 1979). Titrating for the proper dose along with judicious use of anticholinergics should contain this problem in most adolescents. Trying other neuroleptics is recommended when this fails. Thioridazine is best avoided with male adolescents because of its potential for interfering with normal ejaculation. Tardive dyskinesia, the only toxic reaction which may be irreversible, is rare in adolescents, perhaps because few have been maintained on phenothiazines for very long periods.

LITHIUM

One of the more exciting developments in adolescent psychopharmacology has been the use of lithium for manic-depressive illness (MDI), now being diagnosed more frequently in the age group, and possibly for other emotional disturbances. It must be emphasized that at the present time our knowledge in this area is still limited and that lithium therapy is indicated for relatively few patients. As clinicians become more attuned to the possibility of bipolar illness in younger patients, we are certain to see a rise in the reported incidence of MDI and concomitant use of lithium. Carlson (1979) has aptly called our attention to the finding that one-fourth of bipolar patients admitted with mania to the National Institutes of Mental Health noted their first episode of illness before the age of 19. This author details three points that must be borne in mind in using lithium with adolescents: (1) The major use of lithium with adolescents is, as with adults, for the prevention and treatment of bipolar MDI. (2) History from both family and patient are essential, as is a systematic exploration of mood, cognition, and psychomotor and vegetative symptoms. (3) Lithium must be used in conjunction with other appropriate therapies.

Diagnostic Considerations

The use of lithium is perhaps the one area in the psychopharmacology of adolescence in which a specific diagnosis is of major importance. Since lithium works well in bipolar illness and other drugs do not, arriving at a diagnosis of MDI is an essential prerequisite to treatment. This should not mislead the reader into thinking that lithium should not be tried except for diagnosed MDI, however; it has been shown to be effective in some schizophrenics, and in depression, aggressive states, and so-called emotionally unstable personalities.

MDI rarely if ever appears in adolescents or children as the classical adult form described by Kraepelin. Yet it is apparent that precursors of the adult illness should be detectable as particular personality patterns or symptoms earlier in life. Several authors have attempted to tease out a syndrome which resembles bipolar affective disorder and has a positive response to lithium (Carlson and Strober, 1978; DeLong, 1978; Davis, 1979; Feinstein, Feldman-Rotman, and Woolsey, 1980). The following features have been emphasized:

1. Angry outbursts of a particular kind. These tend to be explosive, sudden, uncontrolled, lasting at least half an hour but often two to four hours ("affective storms" [Davis, 1979]). Some see these as transient psychotic states since the adolescent is out of touch with reality at the time and may show disorganized speech and delusional thinking. After the episode, the adolescent may recall having felt grandiose and may describe a continuing inner anger while nothing remains in evidence on the surface. Some (Feinstein, Feldman-Rotman, and Woolsey, 1980) note a very early appearance (as early as the first year of life) of affective extremes.

2. A family history of affective disturbance. Often this involves MDI proper, but unipolar depression, sui-

cide attempts, and other affective disturbances may be found (Youngerman and Canino, 1978).

3. A group of symptoms that might be called hypomanic and include hyperactivity, euphoria, distractibility, pressured speech, and hypersexuality. These have been variously noted and seem to vary partly in relationship to the age of the individual.

4. Absence of persistent psychosis. Most reporters agree that the psychotic symptomatology present in adult mania or bipolar depression is not seen during adolescence, although, as noted, transient psychotic states do occur.

5. A variety of other symptoms such as sleep disturbances, dysphoria, psychomotor retardation, concentration difficulties, guilt, suicidal ideation, and agitation—all of which are consistent with the depressive component of bipolar illness.

Treatment

Since the symptoms described are in general nonspecific and may occur in individuals who will neither go on to adult MDI or prove responsive to lithium, it is probably wise, after careful diagnostic evaluation and the usual medication-free period, to have a trial of phenothiazines before trying lithium. A careful medical history, with particular attention to cardiac or renal disease, and close medical monitoring, especially of thyroid function, are essential in lithium treatment. Carlson (1979) recommends an average daily dose of 900 mg with a range between 900 and 2700 mg. Side effects are minor, as in adults (chiefly gastrointestinal irritation), and are eliminated by reducing the dose. The response to lithium is often dramatic. In view of the familial nature of MDI, a positive response should lead to consideration of the drug for a disturbed parent who has not benefited from other medication.

The use of lithium for other disorders remains experimental and calls for controlled studies. Unfortunately, these are difficult to conduct on a ward with disturbed, volatile adolescents since staff tolerance of an unmedicated group is low and eligible patients are few. Also, ethical issues related to withholding potentially good treatment from adolescents in distress discourage many clinicians from such research.

ANTIDEPRESSANTS

The use of drugs for depression in children and adolescents is very restricted. This results from the simple clinical fact that endogenous depression as known in adults—the prime indication for the use of antidepressants—is very uncommon in younger individuals. Reactive and neurotic depressions are appropriately treated with psychotherapy.

Despite this generally cited principle, tricyclics (usually imipramine) have been used effectively in children for enuresis and conduct disorders with hyperactivity (see the excellent review by Rapoport and Mikkelsen, 1978), and are reported to be useful for adolescent depressions accompanied by specific vegetative symptoms. Workers at McLean Hospital in Belmont, Massachusetts, have evolved a different set of vegetative symptoms for younger adolescents (11 to 15 years) than are commonly cited for adults as indicators for use of tricyclics (Popper, personal communication). These include:

1. Excessive and unusually deep sleep. Such patients are hard to awaken and awake tired or sick, or angry and irritable. These symptoms disappear over the next two to six hours with the adolescent feeling more alert and energetic.
2. Inhibited sexual responsiveness. In males, there is a

decrease in the intensity and frequency of orgasm, spontaneous erection, and nocturnal emissions. In females, a diminution in sexual feelings and the intensity and frequency of orgasm is reported, with fewer sexual dreams. Also noted is an increase in premenstrual tension and irregularity of menses.

3. Psychomotor retardation may exist but is unlike that seen in adults: Movements are gentler, more effortful, speech may be faint, the ends of sentences trailing off. There is also less initiation of spontaneous speech.

4. Stomach aches are reported by about half the patients in this group.

The presence of the above in an adolescent who is otherwise depressed constitutes an indication for the use of antidepressants, at least after a trial of psychotherapy has failed to provide relief. Tricyclics should be used (not MAO inhibitors) in dosages that may have to exceed usual adult dosages, especially for the younger adolescent. Four to six weeks may be required for a therapeutic response, longer than for adults.

Side effects noted at McLean include tricyclic-induced seizures in brain-damaged youngsters (which are controlled by diphenylhydantoin) and "anger reactions," the previously withdrawn, depressed youngster becoming openly furious during the activation phase of the treatment. This development is often disturbing to parents who prefer the docile child they knew, and may cause them to withdraw permission for further treatment.

BENZODIAZEPINES

These are the major anxiolytic agents in current use. Diazepam is the only such agent approved for use with adolescents. Though effective, its use must be discouraged since it has been found to induce dependency and is too readily prescribed as an alternative to psychotherapy when the latter is the treatment of choice.

Are there instances when it may be appropriately used? In this writer's experience, carefully selected patients in psychotherapy who are suffering moderate to severe anxiety may benefit from a short course of treatment with diazepam. Care must be taken to exclude those who may be especially vulnerable to drug dependency such as known drug abusers or very dependent personalities. The patient and family must be prepared and the rationale for introducing diazepam explained. Once relief of handicapping anxiety is achieved (e.g., the patient is able to return to his studies), the drug should be withdrawn gradually, while psychotherapy is continued until treatment goals have been realized.

MISCELLANEOUS PSYCHOTROPIC AGENTS

Hypnotics. These should not be prescribed to adolescents. Difficulty in falling asleep must be treated as a psychological problem appropriately handled in psychotherapy. Occasional exceptions to this rule among institutionalized adolescents should be strictly limited to one or two nights at a time and only after nonchemical means have failed to provide relief. In such cases, chloral hydrate is the recommended drug in view of its effectiveness and low toxicity.

Sedatives. The barbiturates remain an important component in our armamentarium, although their use is confined largely to emergency situations. A short-acting barbiturate such as sodium amytal, given intramuscularly or intravenously, is the most effective and least intrusive agent for bringing a dangerously violent patient under control until other modalities of treatment can be brought into play (Kalogerakis, 1973). Chlorpromazine given intramuscularly may achieve a similar effect, although less rapidly.

Anti-convulsants. Tried experimentally for assorted disturbances other than epilepsy, diphenylhydantoin has failed to demonstrate its usefulness except for seizure disorders. It is likely that its use beyond epilepsy will continue and future studies may still reveal some additional uses. At the present time, however, this drug is not recommended for any adolescent emotional disorder uncomplicated by epilepsy.

LEGAL AND ETHICAL CONSIDERATIONS

The increasing involvement of the law in the practice of psychiatry, particularly institutional, has not failed to touch adolescents. Constitutional challenges to the physician's traditionally unquestioned authority to diagnose and prescribe have already forced changes in the way medicine is practiced. Although there are signs that this trend has gone about as far as it can go and that a return to more reasonable days is ahead, some principles have been established that will certainly endure.

Among these is the principle of informed consent. This has altered the course of much research and placed strictures on our freedom to use new drugs clinically. Where it concerns adolescents, it is wise (even when not mandated by law) to obtain the informed consent of parents and patient. It is without doubt good medical practice to involve both in the treatment plan as active participants from the start, as has been reflected throughout this chapter.

The right to treatment is another established principle, one that has already been addressed by the United States Supreme Court. It concerns us most when our research calls for setting up a control group which will receive placebo rather than a psychoactive substance. Although no law bars us from such a practice, in our clinical work we are often reluctant to withhold medication from patients in great distress. This has had an impact on research in adolescent pharmacotherapy and, in part, accounts for the scarcity of double-blind studies in this population.

Perhaps the most disruptive to traditional medical practice is the currently debated question of the right to *refuse* treatment. Originally confined to the use of lobotomy and ECT in voluntarily hospitalized patients, the dialogue has recently expanded (e.g., in Massachusetts) to include pharmacotherapy and behavior modification in all psychiatric patients. Whatever the outcome of this trend, it is clear that, for the foreseeable future, the law will be looking over the clinician's shoulders as he practices his art. In New York, a challenge to a state hospital's right to medicate patients on a unit for violent, disturbed delinquents over their objections led to the establishment of a working group of prominent psychiatrists to address the problem. A report by this group (Kalogerakis, 1978) set guidelines for the use of medication in institutionalized adolescents that were acceptable to legal and medical interests.

Summary

The use of psychotropic agents in adolescents presents problems not usually found in the psychopharmacological treatment of children or adults. Though pharmacotherapy remains a valuable component of our therapeutic armamentarium for adolescent disorders, it is useful primarily for a hospitalized population. Adolescent psychiatrists are advised to familiarize themselves thoroughly with a few proven drugs and to use them when specific indications are present. This is invariably most effective when done as part of a general treatment plan that includes simultaneous use of other modalities. Attention to the current legal and ethical questions attending the use of psychotropic drugs is essential.

PART VII

*The Treatment of Anorexia Nervosa:
Three Approaches*

17, 18, & 19

INTRODUCTION

Psychotherapy in Primary Anorexia Nervosa,
by Hilde Bruch

*The Role of the Family in the Treatment of
Anorexia Nervosa*, by Ronald Liebman,
Salvador Minuchin, and Lester Baker

*Treatment of Anorexia Nervosa with
Behavior Modification: Effectiveness of
Formula Feeding and Isolation*, by
Katherine A. Halmi, Pauline Powers,
and Sheila Cunningham

Preeminently a disorder of adolescence, anorexia nervosa remains, after decades of intensive study, a baffling and challenging illness. That its rarity is in reciprocal relationship to the amount of attention devoted to it in the psychiatric literature gives testimony to the difficulties it poses for the clinician. Recent reviews by Sours (1969), Bruch (1973), and others survey the field and the variety of theoretical and therapeutic approaches that have emerged from the wealth of studies devoted to the syndrome around the world.

There appears to be general agreement that classical psychoanalysis, and psychotherapy derived from it, have not proved particularly effective in reversing the malignant process of anorexia nervosa. In recent years, three treatment approaches have achieved prominence, each claiming substantial success where earlier methods have failed. Of the three, Bruch's is perhaps the closest to the traditional, since it is based on individual psychotherapy within the framework of a psychodynamic understanding of the patient's disorder. Bruch is explicit, however, in dismissing so-called "depth" interpretations; her focus is on the patient's cognitive distortions and problems of self-awareness, since she sees the disorder as derived from early "transactional" difficulties rather than from intrapsychic conflict. Her present paper is of particular interest in that it describes the treatment of that *rara avis*, a male anorectic.

A similar conception of etiology—that the anorectic's problem emerges out of pathological family interactions—leads Liebman, Minuchin, and Baker to a different therapeutic prescription. Rejecting what they call "linear" causal constructs, they favor a "contextual" or "ecological" view which leads them to direct their attention to the present, to the impact of those current family influences that shape the patient's symptom picture. They then attempt to alter these influences by means of family-centered techniques. These techniques are at times both innovative and, in the case of Minuchin's (Minuchin, Rosman, and Baker, 1978) own work, quite intrusive and directive. Their aim is to reduce the family's focus on eating as a vehicle for pathological interaction and to promote in the identified patient a greater sense of autonomy and self-direction. A similar approach is presented by Palazzoli (1978).

Halmi, Powers, and Cunningham operate from a rather different set of theoretical postulates—those of learning theory and behavior therapy. Conceiving of anorexia as a syndrome of learned maladaptation, they have sought to treat it with a regimen of behavior contingencies aimed at modifying the symptomatic behavior itself, through a planned series of reward/restriction steps predicated on weight gain. Bruch (1974) has challenged the long-range value of such an approach, but its proponents are impressed with their results, and modified behavioral measures have been incorporated into a number of more eclectic programs, including that of Liebman and his colleagues.

These three essays, then, offer a range of perspectives on the therapeutic approach to one of the most perplexing disorders in psychiatry. Current research on its biological substrate (see Vigersky, 1977) may provide leads for other kinds of treatment, but these papers seem to represent, at this time, the state of the art.

17

Psychotherapy in Primary Anorexia Nervosa

Hilde Bruch, M.D.

The literature on the value of psychotherapeutic intervention in anorexia nervosa is hopelessly inconclusive. This is due to the fact that authors frequently fail to differentiate between the genuine anorexia nervosa syndrome and emaciation associated with various psychological problems, and that only therapeutic models based on traditional psychoanalysis are considered.

Primary anorexia nervosa is characterized (1) by a relentless pursuit of thinness with body image disturbances of delusional proportions; (2) by a deficit in the accurate perception of bodily sensations, manifest as lack of hunger awareness and denial of fatigue; and (3) by an underlying, all-pervasive sense of ineffectiveness. This personality structure is conceived of as the outcome of childhood experiences lacking in appropriate confirming responses to child-initiated cues. These patients are singularly unresponsive to the traditional psychoanalytic therapy. A psychotherapeutic approach was formulated with the emphasis on correcting the deficits that

Reprinted by permission from the *Journal of Nervous and Mental Disease*, 150:51-67. Copyright 1971, The Williams & Wilkins Co., Baltimore.

have resulted from the faulty early transactional patterns. Interpretations are strictly avoided. Emphasis is on evoking awareness of feelings, thoughts, and impulses that originate in the patients themselves.

The treatment history of a young man who had been unsuccessfully in conventional psychiatric treatment for six and a half years, and who responded well to the new approach, will be used as an illustration. The change in the interaction with his family, and in his body awareness and self-concept, will be presented in detail.

Few conditions have been studied so thoroughly and with such contradictory approaches as the rare disease, anorexia nervosa. It represents a state of self-inflicted starvation, a refusal to eat with cachexia as the outstanding somatic symptom, frequently accompanied by constipation, amenorrhea, bradycardia, and dry, cool skin. Psychologically, the chief symptoms are denial of illness, relentless hyperactivity, and aggressive negativism against all treatment efforts.

The vivid descriptions of the early clinicians refer to a definite syndrome, which occurs chiefly, though not exclusively, in female patients around the time of puberty. Paradoxically, with increasing observations and study, the clinical picture of anorexia nervosa has become blurred and less well defined. Bliss and Branch (1960), failing to find in the literature a neat solution of differentiating it from other forms of undernutrition, decided to consider a loss of 25 pounds as a suitable definition of the condition, if the drop in weight was attributable to psychological causes. This definition is so overgeneral and colorless that it practically abolishes the concept of anorexia nervosa.

In recent years there has been increasing emphasis on differentiating between a syndrome of *genuine or primary anorexia nervosa*, and unspecific states of nervous malnutrition in connection with a variety of psychiatric problems. This has been expressed in a number of papers coming from different countries, by King (1963) in Australia, Crisp (1965a, b, c) in England, Thomä (1967) in Germany, and Palazzoli (1978) in Italy. My own studies, based on personal observation of 66 cases of self-starvation and severe weight loss in young persons, led to the same conclusions, namely, that differentiating between different types of psychologically determined emaciation is necessary for a meaningful understanding of the condition and appropriate therapeutic intervention (Bruch, 1962, 1965). Approximately two-thirds of the patients could be diagnosed as offering the primary picture.

In primary anorexia nervosa, pursuit of thinness is the motivating force; refusal of food is only the means of accomplishing this end. Three areas of disordered psychological functioning can be recognized. The first is a disturbance in the body image of delusional proportions. The truly pathognomic feature is a dramatic denial of illness, the absence of concern over the advanced emaciation, and the vigor and stubborness with which the often gruesome appearance is defended as normal, and not too thin. The weight loss may be just as severe in the unspecific forms of psychologically determined cachexia. In contrast to the primary group, these patients complain about their weight loss. Evaluation of the distorted body image is of importance in appraising treatment progress; without a change in self-awareness, gain in weight, which can be achieved in many ways, is apt to be only a temporary symptomatic improvement (Gottheil, Backup, and Cornelison, 1969).

The second outstanding characteristic is a disturbance of the accuracy of perception or cognitive interpretation of stimuli arising in the body. Awareness of hunger and appetite in the ordinary sense seems to be absent, and a patient's sullen statement, "I do not need to eat," is probably an accurate expression of what he feels and experiences most of the time.

The nutritional disorganization has two phases: failure of motivating desire, resulting in non-eating and weight loss, and uncontrollable impulses to gorge oneself, quite often without awareness of hunger or satiety, followed by self-induced vomiting.

Other manifestations of falsified awareness of bodily state are overactivity and denial of fatigue. Frequently, the overactivity appears long before the non-eating phase, and the drive for activity continues until the emaciation is far advanced. Instead of awareness of fatigue and weakness, there is a subjective feeling of not being tired and of wanting to do things. Failure of sexual functioning and absence of sexual feelings belong to the same area of perceptual and conceptual deficiency, as do sleeplessness, constipation, and urinary retention.

The third distinct psychological feature is a paralyzing sense of ineffectiveness, which pervades all thinking and activities. Anorexia nervosa patients experience themselves as acting only in response to the demands coming from other people or situations, and as not doing anything because they want to do it. While the two other characteristic features, the body image disturbance and the misperception of bodily states, are readily recognized, the third defect is camouflaged by these patients' enormous negativism and stubborn defiance. The paramount importance of this undifferentiated sense of helplessness was recognized during intensive psychotherapy and appeared rather surprising. It stands in striking contrast to the manifest aggressive and manipulative negativism, and the usual reports of a seemingly normal childhood characterized by excellent performance and few, if any, difficulties. Such patients impress one as exaggerated examples of the "accommodating" mode of integration of mental experiences, to use Piaget's concept, and, characteristically, the oppositional phase of early childhood has been absent. The development of anorexia nervosa may be conceived of as shouting an unrelenting "NO," which extends to every area of living, though most conspicuous with respect to food.

What is the background of this development of robot-like compliance during childhood and indiscriminate negativism at pubescence? In most cases the outer picture is that of devoted families who give excellent care to their children and many educational and other advantages and privileges. The mothers appear to be conscientious in their concept of motherhood, and the fathers stress success, outer appearances, fitness, and beauty. The parents are shocked and puzzled by the severity of a supposedly psychiatric illness in what they had conceived of as their happy homes. They are apt to deny any difficulties and focus only on the eating and weight loss. Detailed analysis reveals that the disturbing experiences are not related to one or another incident, but to an all-pervading attitude of doing for the child and superimposing the parents' concepts of his needs, with disregard of child-initiated signals. This deprives the child of a necessary learning experience, namely, the regular sequence of events of felt discomfort, signal, appropriate response, and felt satisfaction. Without such reciprocal and confirming responses to child-initiated cues, he will fail to develop a discriminate awareness of his needs and a sense of control over his impulses. He may even be lacking in the sense of ownership of his body. He will experience instead that he is not in control of his functions, with an overall lack of awareness of living his own life, and a conviction of the ineffectiveness of all his efforts and strivings.

When confronted with the task of independence and the need for a separate identity, such individuals may resort to rigid control over their bodies to establish a domain of self-

hood. Non-eating, the conspicuous feature of anorexia nervosa, is a very late step in this maldevelopment.

These considerations led to the formulation of a new psychotherapeutic approach to primary anorexia nervosa. These
patients, in my experience, are singularly unresponsive to
the traditional psychoanalytic approach, as has been pointed
out by Meyer and Weinroth (1957).

In view of the confusion about the differential diagnosis
of anorexia nervosa, the literature on suggestions for therapeutic intervention, and on treatment results, is hopelessly
inconclusive. Psychotherapy is referred to as useless (Kay and
Leigh, 1954), or, conversely, psychoanalysis is praised as the
only means of successful treatment (Thomä, 1967). Palazzoli
(1978), who formulated a concept of anorexia nervosa as a
condition in which the concrete use of the body serves as a
tool in an individual's struggle for an acceptable identity,
finds that a more pertinent understanding of the condition
was accompanied by increasingly better treatment results.

My own experiences go in the same direction. The essential
therapeutic task is conceived of as evoking awareness in such
patients that there are feelings and impulses that originate
in themselves, and that they can learn to recognize them.
Though a general statement needs to be made that the physician would not permit a patient to starve himself to death,
the eating function is not singled out for this investigation.
On the contrary, since most patients, by the time they come
for therapy, have been hounded with continuous exhorta-
tions to eat, or with questions of why they don't eat, it is safer
and more productive to clarify this sense of helplessness in
other areas.

In a later phase of treatment, these patients need help in
evaluating the appropriateness of their impulses and in judging the realistic possibilities of their plans and hopes. With
this new orientation, even patients who had been previously

resistant to all therapeutic efforts were able to abandon their sterile way of life and to progress to greater maturity.

CASE REPORT

I have chosen as illustration the case of a patient who offers in his own history a built-in control on the effectiveness of different psychotherapeutic models. Eric, as I shall call the patient, had begun to lose weight in the fall of 1952, when he was 12 years old. When he entered the New York State Psychiatric Institute six and a half years later, in March, 1959, he was 18½ years old, 59 inches tall, with a bone age of 13 years and a weight of only 40 pounds. He had been under continuous medical care and also in treatment with competent psychiatrists throughout this period. There had been several hospitalizations for diagnostic evaluations, or as a life-saving measure. His previous psychiatrists cooperated by giving reports on their treatment approaches.

Before going into details, I should like to give the important clinical data. There was agreement that Eric was an outgoing, bright, athletic, quite happy, somewhat tense child until age 12, in spite of some difficulties which when they occurred were considered "minor" and the importance of which could be understood only in retrospect. He had spent the summer of 1952 in camp, while his parents moved from a small city apartment to a home in the suburbs. He had objected to this and resented that they had moved while he was away. He was 56 inches tall and weighed 95 pounds when he came back from camp. He considered himself "too plump" and was concerned that he would not make friends in this new neighborhood. He found himself wanting to run and exercise uncontrollably. When he found exercising not effective in making him thinner, he began to eat less and less; his weight dropped from 91 pounds in September, 1952 to 57 pounds in May, 1953. After he had refused to eat anything for several days, he was admitted to the Babies Hospital for study and treatment. He was exceedingly resentful and gained only a few pounds in three weeks.

When 15 years old, he was admitted to the Rockefeller Institute for evaluation of his endocrine status. His height was 58¾ inches and his weight was 58 pounds. Bone age, according to roentgenogram of the knee, was 13 years. No evidence of endocrine abnormality was found except for delayed puberty and growth retardation, which were considered secondary to the malnutrition. Shortly thereafter, in the summer of 1956, he reached his highest weight during his illness, approximately 70 pounds. In 1957 he was on the psychiatric service for five months, and from December, 1958 to March, 1959 on the medical service of the Mt. Sinai Hospital for three months. On this second admission he weighed only 45 pounds and felt exhausted. Except for this period, he had felt alert and active during the whole period of his illness, and he had graduated from high school.

To anticipate results, improvement was marked and dramatic, after the first six months. He left the hospital in June, 1961, aged 20¾, 62 inches tall, and weighing 110 pounds. There was beginning pubertal development. An important landmark of his improvement was that during the second year he finally permitted a new endocrine evaluation. Treatment with depot testosterone, injected every three weeks, was begun on his 20th birthday when he weighed 94 pounds, nearly twice his admission weight, and was 60 inches tall, only one inch more than on admission. He has continued to do well on the outside and has kept in touch with his physician.

PREVIOUS PSYCHIATRIC APPROACHES

His first psychiatrist had found Eric exceedingly hostile and evasive, willing to go along only as long as "deeper issues" were avoided. He felt that the basic problem was Eric's struggle with his mother, an issue he would never face. He tried to show him how he was out to torture and destroy his mother through his symptoms and general attitude. He also saw the parents and was of particular help to the mother. He arranged for the various hospitalizations and the boarding school from which Eric graduated. Eric accused him later of having been in league with his parents and "against him."

His second psychiatrist, whose patient he became when at age 17 he was admitted to Mt. Sinai weighing only 45 pounds and in extremely poor physical condition, felt that the primary concern had been to keep him alive. He described his later approach as that of a sympathetic person who was "on his side." Interpretations were made regarding his eating habits and the self-destructive and suicidal aspects of his symptoms and his attempts to punish his parents with his bizarre eating and self-induced vomiting. Although the expression of unconscious material was not encouraged, certain fantasies were presented consistently (a frequent fantasy was one of being cut up and eaten) and it was pointed out to him how his thoughts interfered with his living, especially his eating. When there was no progress, he referred Eric to the New York State Psychiatric Institute.

His first physician there felt that further probing into underlying psychodynamics might not be useful and focused on his interpersonal difficulties, in particular, on his aggression and manipulative power struggle. When he discontinued treatment, he considered Eric a master of the technique of "divide and conquer." Eric had remained withdrawn, hostile, and suspicious of his therapist, but decided to sign out of the hospital when he learned that he had been assigned to another physician.

He had been admitted to the general service, where he did poorly. It was suspected that he vomited whatever food he ate. There were violent scenes about his being weighed, and often his weight was not taken. After two and a half months he weighed only 50½ pounds, and he was transferred to a small service with better supervision and nursing care. This had been avoided at the beginning because it was felt it would be discouraging for a new patient to meet another anorexic who had done poorly thus far and who received tube feeding twice a day. Eric correctly diagnosed this patient, a schizophrenic whose refusal to eat served as "atonement for his sins," as different from himself, as "weird," and he decided to eat—just enough to avoid tube feeding. With more effective supervision the vomiting stopped or occurred less often. There was increase in weight, to approximately 65 pounds in three and a half months, but no change in his attitude.

CHANGE IN THERAPEUTIC APPROACH

It was at this point that I accepted supervision of Eric's treatment. If the ideas which I had formulated about essential aspects of anorexia nervosa and the necessary modification of treatment had any validity, the longstanding illness of this young man, with extensive psychotherapy along traditional lines over many years, offered an opportunity for putting them to the test. I had used these ideas successfully in the treatment of private patients. By supervising residents, the element of my personality and experience was eliminated. In October, 1959, Dr. L. became Eric's therapist, and in October, 1960, Dr. M. took over. They were both in the beginning of their careers, with limited experience in psychotherapy, but with definite convictions about the positive value of psychoanalysis. They were about equal in intelligence and perceptiveness, yet quite different in their personalities. One factor of probable significance was the fact that Dr. L. was tall while Dr. M. was of about average height. Psychotherapeutic sessions were scheduled for three times a week, and twice a week during the last few months before discharge.

I saw Eric in several interviews during which his therapist was present. There were two joint conferences with his parents, one in May, 1960, and the other in March, 1961. These various conferences were recorded and the illustrations which I shall use here are taken from the transcript of these recordings.

The first task was familiarizing his new psychiatrist with the change in orientation. In many ways this approach is much simpler and less dramatic than the conventional model of psychotherapy in which the psychiatrist interprets on the basis of the knowledge he has acquired during his training what a patient's behavior means and indicates. It is important to avoid interpretations of this type; however correct or timely they may be, they represent to the patient the sad repetition of his lifelong experiences that someone else, not he himself, knows what he feels, thinks, or means. If there are things to be uncovered and interpreted, it is important that the patient make the discovery on his own and has a chance to say it first. The therapist has the privilege of agreeing, if it appears relevant.

The decisive, effective experience for such a patient is his becoming an active participant in the therapeutic process. He needs encouragement in becoming aware of impulses, thoughts, and feelings that originate within himself. Only in this way can he learn to discover his undeveloped and untapped resources and become alert and alive to what is going on within himself. These are necessary steps for his developing autonomy, initiative, and self-responsibility.

This approach makes new and unaccustomed demands on the patient, and he may find it difficult to switch gears if he has been in treatment before. He has usually used the previous experiences to express his rage and anger, and to blame others for his difficulties. In this new approach the emphasis is on his own role in the way he has lived his life, and on his assuming responsibility for a more effective self-discovery in therapy.

Such an open-ended, inquisitive approach also makes heavy demands on the therapist. His expertness is his faculty to listen. His self-awareness and perceptual apparatus must be realistic, his communication unambiguous. He should not suffer from doubts about his own intellectual abilities and professional competence, nor can he afford to be competitive with his patients. This approach implies a definite change in the therapist's concept of his role, and to make this change is not easy. It involves suspending one's knowledge and permitting a patient to express what he experiences without immediately explaining and labeling it. The current model of psychiatric training emphasizes early formulation of the underlying psychodynamic problems. Such early formulations may stand in the way of learning the truly relevant facts. A therapist who assumes that he understands the patient's problems is not quite so alert and curious in unraveling the unclear and confused periods. He may be tempted to superimpose his prematurely conceived notions on the patient.

In a previous paper (Bruch, 1963) I called this treatment approach "the constructive use of ignorance," using the word "ignorance" in the way a scientist might use it who, regardless of what discoveries have been made, is always ready to ask: "What is there that I do not know?" Patients respond well to this objective fact-finding attitude when they recognize that the therapist regards them truly as collaborators in the search for unknown factors and that the therapist does not have some secret knowledge which he holds back from them. In the patient who in previous treatment efforts has "resisted" any interpretation, or has become involved in endless intellectualizing arguments, a remarkable change takes place, often in a rather short time. Yet he can achieve the new goal, that of uncovering his own abilities, his resources, and his innate capacities for thinking, judging, and feeling, only in very small steps. For this he needs a relationship with a therapist who is warm and honest in his personal interest, and who, in his basic therapeutic attitude, reveals sincere respect for a human being struggling for his very existence in his thus far futile efforts to recognize something of value and significance within himself.

Several supervisory sessions were used to evaluate Eric's background history, his relations to his parents, and his behavior in the hospital and in psychotherapy, not from the angle of aggression and hostility, which were glaring and obvious, but in order to recognize the underlying lack of self-confidence, effectiveness, and competence, and the perceptual and conceptual deficits that had resulted in this misinterpretation of his place in life.

When a change in therapist became necessary, in October, 1960, Eric attended one of these briefing conferences with his new physician. He objected that he did not want to start "from scratch." When he recognized that he could not go back to "scratch," he took active part in formulating the problems that remained to be clarified. His understanding had advanced far enough that he could recognize, at ieast intellectually, that the therapeutic task was now a paradoxical one, namely, that he himself had to take active part in discovering errors in his thinking and deficits in his experiences. The more active he was in this process, the greater the chance of his making the necessary corrections.

Several conferences with the social worker were aimed at a reappraisal of the approach to the family. The mother was depressed, pessimistic, and hostile in her attitude toward her son, whom she described as "my supreme disappointment," and toward psychiatry, which had completely failed her family. She felt that she had been humiliated during Eric's previous hospitalizations by having been told that it had been her perfectionistic attitude that had caused his illness. She complained that nobody had asked about her husband; she felt that his terrible interest in appearance was as much to blame. The shift here, too, was away from pinpointing the one or other shortcoming to an effort to come to a new awareness of the subtle misunderstandings that had distorted their conscientious and devoted efforts at being good parents into something that had interfered with the development of their son. This same line was pursued in the joint family conferences, with avoidance of blame-fixing and emphasis on recognition of mutual misunderstandings or misinterpretations of well-meant efforts.

In therapy with Eric, interpretations of any one specific problem were avoided. Concrete situations in the present were used to help him recognize when and how he failed to exercise his basic right of being a person with feelings, wants, and needs of his own. It was essential not to get involved in his virtuosity of engaging other people in a struggle for power and control, and equally important to avoid vague permissiveness or inconsistent giving in.

The situation at the time of transfer offered an opportunity for his new physician to convey to Eric this different philosophy of treatment. Eric had signed out of the hospital and refused to see his doctor. Since he had gained some weight, he felt he was improving, had solved his problems, and did not need another therapist. His new physician went to see him on the ward but made no attempt to persuade him to stay. Within a few days Eric had to admit that he was in a trap, that he knew his parents did not want him home. Since he had no place to go, he was forced to withdraw his letter of signing out and to admit that he needed his doctor's help. In his customary way he argued this point from many different angles. Most acute was his concern about "losing face" on the ward. His doctor took the stand that this was an irrelevant point as compared to the important issue: the regard he owed himself and his chance of getting well. In many different ways it was conveyed to him that "there is only one thing that is important—you, your own life, and the way you value it." He acted as if he did not truly think of his own life as important, not rating it higher than what other people thought. If he did not value his life, then this needed to be recognized as an important sign of his illness. It did not matter whether his mother had been "wrong" in doing this or that, or whether his previous doctors had misunderstood him. Right now it was apparent that his problem was somewhere in this basic fact of his lacking self-regard. The leitmotif of the new treatment effort became that he had not only a right but also an obligation toward himself of which he did not seem to be aware. This was the one point where his doctor could be of help to him, namely, in finding out how it happened that he approached life with this tremendous error of not really respecting himself.

Needless to say, Eric continued to argue and complain, but this was now sidestepped with a consistent attitude of "this does not really matter—don't waste your time on it." It was acknowledged that there were many annoying routines in the functioning of a large hospital, that it was appropriate for him to feel discomfort about this, or to ask for changes if indicated, but that it had to be viewed in proportion to the real issues, namely, to use treatment time for understanding what had interfered with his own development, how to make up for this now, and the many additional deficits in his knowledge of life due to his long illness.

It is, of course, impossible to say whether this aspect had not been touched on by his previous psychiatrist. Eric's positive response suggests that this was the first time that he had heard this message, and that he experienced his doctor's interest not as intrusion but as benevolent support. He came to recognize his physician's basic attitude as one of respect but also that he, as a doctor, had the duty of insisting that everything be done for his patient's health until he himself could take care of it. He was eventually able to accept the need for a new physical checkup and endocrine treatment, something to which he had strenuously objected, when it was offered in terms of this orientation.

It so happened that about two months later he saw his first psychiatrist (who was teaching at the Institute). He became quite upset and told the psychiatrist that he had not understood his problem at all and that he should have sent him to this hospital immediately. This was the first place where he had had a physician who understood his problem and helped him come to the point of wanting to get better. Until then he had been so enraged at all doctors and treatment efforts that he had only wanted to get sicker.

Exploration of his developmental history did not reveal any startlingly new facts or events but helped him to gain a new picture of what had been going on. There was gradual improvement which could be recognized as change in many areas. I shall discuss here only a few aspects, his relationship to his family and to his own body and self-concept. Similarly, changes could have been illustrated in his dreams, in his ward behavior, and in his attitude toward his physician.

INTERACTION WITH FAMILY

When Eric came to the hospital, his relationship to his family, in particular to his mother, was one of bristling hostility. They had not seen each other alone for nearly two years because there was too much mutual hatred and accusation. The mother felt that "he fouled up our whole lives." She remembered only negative episodes of his having resisted every step. She was now resigned to his illness: "There is no hope for him, he will be a curse on us forever—and it has been going from bad to worse." The mere thought of taking him home was more than she could bear. Her resentment had been growing so that at times she had almost wished that he would die, though she recognized that his eccentric behavior was a sign of his sickness. She was exceedingly tense and complained that she could not sleep because she felt that she had "failed," and ruminated on the question, "Where have I gone wrong?" When Eric wanted to leave the hospital, there was no question of his coming home, because his family felt they could not stand it. They also were concerned as to how it would influence the life of their younger daughter and what her friends would say.

Eric was equally outspoken in his hatred of his mother and in his accusations of how she had ruined his life, always telling him what to do and never permitting him to do what he wanted. As he gained confidence in his new physician and the new approach to his problem, he spoke more and more freely about his family, chiefly about his mother, but also quite often about his father and younger sister. It puzzled him that she had been able to stand up against the pressure and that only he had become sick. It was the first indication of his being ready to reexamine his past development not in terms of his accusations against his mother but in terms of an effort to differentiate what she had done from what he had experienced. His therapist helped him in becoming more and more definite and detailed in talking about different episodes. He gradually learned to differentiate between occurrences that had been distressing because his mother had been neglectful or domineering, and others in which she had failed him because she did not know what he wanted. As he went into details, it became apparent to him that there had been many happenings that showed well-meaning intent and loving interest on her part but that had meant to him that she did not respect him. In the beginning it was for him more an intellectual interest in looking at things in a new way. As he became more objective in reviewing his life, he became at times quite anxious because he felt that he was no longer able to blame all his troubles and unhappiness on others and that he had to take responsibility for it. As he became more involved with the question of his own part in his illness, he began to change in his awareness of his body, as will be discussed later.

During the early months there was little contact with his parents. His father came to visit him, sometimes his sister. His first visit home was for Christmas Day, nine months after coming to the hospital and three months after beginning work with the second psychiatrist. When he came back, he reported in detail what he and his father had done and discussed, and how his sister had reacted, but he never mentioned his mother. He became angry when his attention was drawn to this, then admitted that she had been "hospitable" but not warm and that the only thing that had been good was that they had not bickered. He was still easily irritated and accused his doctor of "always looking for something." During January his mother went on a vacation in Florida. He was amused that she wrote to his sister, "Take care of Dad and Eric," but upset when she came back with a present. It was a cigarette lighter. She knew that he did not smoke and suggested, "You can light cigarettes for other people—it looks so gallant." He was enraged; that was the trouble with all her gifts, they were always something that she wanted him to do, never what he wanted. That's why gifts were disturbing to him: "I would rather have nothing, I cannot accept it with thanks—but I feel I have to use it. I can never throw anything away, only when it is old and I replace it with something new."

He went on to explain why he did not want gifts from her. There had always been a problem in relation to clothes. "As a child, mother always told me what to wear. I had to wear knickers because she had bought them but I hated them. I could not stop the clothes I had to wear, but I could stop the food. Oversupply makes me angry; I could never carry any extra paper in my looseleaf notebook."

After considerable improvement he requested to be transferred to the open service. He spoke to his mother on the phone. Instead of being pleased, she expressed skepticism. He had another outburst: "Maybe she is scared I will come home." It upset him that he could never please his mother. This was made the starting point of many discussions, that he did not live to please her but was entitled to pursue his own life. He began to recognize how much he had been in need of compliments from his mother and how he had always asked for compliments from her and how upset he had been when they were not forthcoming. He began to notice how much this had played a role in relation to all people, and could observe it in his relations on the ward, particularly to the nurses. When the head nurse one day noticed that he "looked happy," he was torn between pleasure that she had paid attention to him and indignation that she had dared to tell him how he felt. She was just like his mother, who had always done that.

A few weeks later, after a home visit, he felt for the first time "healthier" in his feelings about his parents. He felt they had had a good time, though no one had been very demonstrative. He was just satisfied being with them. "For the first time mother was *warm*. She brought me back to the hospital; she did not need to do so. It showed she cared." He was aware that he could accept her care now because he felt more independent, more of a self and a person.

By now he was actively interested in therapy, in particular, in the assessment of whether he could become an independent functioning person instead of remaining a helpless crea-

ture who was acted on by others and could assert himself
only by shouting "no." His obsessive wavering over small
decisions often became a starting point for clarifying underlying important issues. He discussed with many pros and cons
the question of going home for the Seder evening. The main
point of decision was whether he could go home alone, by
subway and bus, or whether he should phone his parents
when he reached the subway station so they could pick him
up by car. Eric hesitated because he did not feel he had the
right to impose upon them. If the situation had been reversed
and he was supposed to pick them up, he would do it without
hesitation. "I would be honored, because they are my parents
and I owe them something. I am their property—that's why
I owe them willingness to do things for them."

When the word "property" was singled out, he at first
wanted to dismiss it, that he had used the wrong expression,
that of course he was not their property. But then he took
it up in detail: "Everything I have and own comes from them.
I feel guilty that I have nothing to show for it. I keep taking
and taking from them. At least if I could produce, like my
sister, then they could be proud. That would be something
they would get from me, but all I do is take and take. Food,
money, sleep, everything I have is theirs. If I would say it
was mine, what would be the use, because I know it is not.
That's why I say everything is theirs, and I am theirs. As long
as I don't have to be responsible for making something out
of myself, what I am and do belongs to them. Only after I
have shown that I can make something out of myself, then
I can feel that I am myself and that things I have belong to
me."

He was aware that he was actually beyond this point, but
this basic conviction had dominated his life for such a long
time that it came out in this undisguised way. He went on to
speculate whether there had been a change in his feeling

about wanting to be himself as he grew older. Maybe it had been all right to take things and to think of himself as their property until he was eight or nine. But by the time he was 12 he needed to prove that he himself was "somebody." With his now nearly passionate interest in his own development it was rewarding to review his past history. This could be done in more objective terms because by this time the parents' relationship with the hospital had improved, and they were in good rapport with the social worker. It was learned that from age eight or nine onward Eric had been terribly concerned about his fitness and manliness. He had become a star athlete and would not only test the traditional biceps for strength but repeatedly examine the muscles of his thighs to see whether they were developed well enough. In his behavior at home the word "no" appeared more and more often, as if he were trying to prove himself as an independent individual.

A symptom that had aroused a certain degree of amusement began to acquire meaning in this context. Since the onset of his illness he had been unusually tight with money and exceedingly careful with all his possessions so that they would not wear out. He refused to own more than the minimum amount of shirts, pajamas, or other personal articles of clothing. If someone gave him a gift, he would reject it. It became apparent now that he felt that every possession made him more beholden to his parents, increasing his sense of responsibility or, conversely, his guilt at not fulfilling his obligations. In addition, he was so indecisive that he could not stand the strain of having to make a choice of what to use or wear.

He finally did go home for the holiday, and his father came to pick him up by car. To his great amazement his father seemed eager to do it and really enjoyed putting himself out for him. He felt there was real warmth, that they really cared for him. Even his mother did things just to make him feel more comfortable. During this weekend they had a meal in a restaurant and he was indignant when observing other parents and children together. He noticed that one father was called to the phone and had to go home because the baby was crying and the babysitter could not handle him. Eric was outraged: "That baby does not have the right to upset the family like this; of course, the baby doesn't know, but he still does not have the right to disturb them. Why should this newcomer break up this family?"

It was felt that there were glaring misconceptions underlying his reaction, and a joint family conference was planned to clarify what really had taken place in this family, how each member had tried to participate in a life together but how it had resulted in such serious misunderstandings. He was quite aware of the paradox of his reaction, that he now was so concerned over a baby interrupting a family meal when he had actually been this type of child himself in the most traumatic way. The question was how it had happened that from earliest childhood on he had felt an intruder and someone who was not doing his part of the bargain in return.

Though Eric felt so much better about his family, was touched by their solicitude when he came home, even felt something like homesickness—like calling home to tell his mother that he just wanted to talk to her—he strenuously objected to this conference. "Do I always have to repeat the things that made me sick? I will not go through that hell again." He agreed to come to the conference but not to talk. But then he worried, "I look like a dope for not cooperating. What will they think if I do not talk?" Though things were more relaxed, his mother, too, appeared reluctant to participate and was at first very defensive.

As to factual information, nothing new was learned, but by the end of this session the mother's defensive attitude had changed. For Eric it was the first time that he had listened seriously to what his parents had seen in him and hoped for him. In subsequent treatment sessions he took up to what extent his concern had remained focused on what his parents, particularly his mother, would think about him. He was equally concerned that she would think something was wrong when he did not talk as that she would be hurt or offended by what he did say.

Eric remained in the hospital and in intensive treatment for another year. During this time he regularly went home for holidays, gradually for whole weekends. When he finally felt ready to work, because he wanted to, not because someone else had suggested it or arranged it for him, he pointed out where his father had contacts. He asked for help in arranging an interview, without hesitating or even being quite aware of "taking from them," something he had so violently rejected in the past.

Finally it was felt that he was functioning with an adequate sense of self-reliance and appeared ready to leave the hospital. Another joint family conference took place in May, 1961, in which Eric participated as an equal. The general atmosphere was one of mutual pleasure in his progress and of hope for the future. The practical question was whether he should live at home. The parents had brought up the question of selling their home and moving into a new neighborhood to make things easier for Eric. This was examined from many angles, but in particular as to what extent this reflected a well-meaning attitude of devoted parents "anticipating problems," thereby depriving their son of the opportunity to work out his own solution. Both parents could see how much this had been the attitude toward their children. Finally, another problem of even greater importance was isolated, namely, the underlying assumption that there was something to be ashamed of, that Eric as well as his parents failed to take pride in the extraordinary effort he had made in working himself out of this serious illness. Eric openly admitted that he was ashamed and could accept that this was a problem to be worked out in further treatment. Something else became apparent as well, the extent to which anxiety and tension had been mutually infectious. Eric was particularly sensitive to and intolerant of any sign of anxiety in his mother, and he felt he had to fight back. The conference ended on a note of agreement, that his mother had the right to be anxious and that he had to lead his own life regardless of it. On the other hand, he was under no obligation to live his life according to her often exaggerated expectations.

A month later Eric was discharged. The family continued to live in the same neighborhood. Eric attended college and did well and found that he had become more tolerant of his mother's perfectionistic overconcern. He has since finished college and moved to a different city where he is working on his Ph.D. thesis.

CHANGING AWARENESS OF BODY AND SELF-CONCEPT

Anorexia nervosa is a disorder in which the body is used in a bizarre way to establish a sense of identity and selfhood. Anorexic patients suffer from delusional misconceptions about their appearance and needs. Corrective change in the body image is a prerequisite for lasting improvement (Bruch, 1962; Gottheil, Backup, and Cornelison, 1969).

Like other anorexics, Eric had violently denied that he was too skinny or that he needed to eat. In his struggles and fights he had often stressed: "It's my life. If I don't want to eat, why should my mother make a fuss over it"; or, "It's my life—I have the privilege to destroy it, but I have no interest in maintaining it." In the new approach, this disregard for his life and its value was focused on as the essence of his illness. Gradual changes in his concept about himself could be observed, and a few of them will be pointed out here.

His eating habits had been quite bizarre. There was angry refusal of food, often days of complete abstinence, but also, from the beginning, eating binges with subsequent vomiting. His former psychiatrists had pointed out that he did it to torture his mother, or that he would overeat to please her. He would make an issue of walking by her to go to the kitchen, make a lot of noise with the refrigerator to impress her, and then go to the bathroom and vomit. At one time it had been felt that he might do better with a neighbor who felt sympathetic toward him. There he would raid the freezer during the night, broil steaks, and then throw them up. At other times he would go on rigid starvation. Once when he was asked whether he had eaten his breakfast he answered sarcastically, "Of course, I ate my Cheerio."

He refused to discuss his eating habits, which he had maintained throughout his illness. When first admitted to the larger ward, he ate meals but did not gain weight. Efforts were made to weigh him weekly, but he made such scenes that for many weeks his weight was not taken. This point was the first he discussed, over several weeks, with his new physician. He was aware that his reaction to being weighed was abnormal—"like a phobia." He felt that the scale was his enemy, that it would give him away and reveal that there was something wrong with his body. In spite of his denial and fighting he admitted that he was no longer as unconcerned about his health as he acted. His fears had begun as "fear of the hospital" and then "fear of the tube," but now it was "the scale." Once when he had lost some weight he was terribly upset: "As if mother were here. When I lose, mother blows her head off." Or, "I feel I get evaluated by it and then I am panicky, of what they will say on rounds." Or, "If I gain, they are so proud—it is always somebody else's business."

Then he began to speak about his dreadful concern with what was "natural" for his body. Any special food, such as Sustagen or other protein products, impressed him as "unnatural." He was particularly afraid of endocrine treatment; it indicated both that there was something wrong with his body, or that he would be "forced" to change and to catch up too fast. The real fear was that he had permanently damaged his system.

In therapy the emphasis was on the extent to which this disowning of his own body had rendered him helpless in relation to others. Gradually he became aware of how much he had confused his own feelings and needs with his fear of other people's reactions. Everybody's concern had focused for so long on his weight that he could not truly accept that his progress was not rated in weight. A change began to occur after his visits home and when he had started to differentiate between his mother's overpowering good intentions and his violent and fearful reactions to them. As he improved, he spoke of working in the hospital. When a job was arranged for him, he set out to go to work but turned back. He was overpowered by fear that if he did something "extra" he no longer could be responsible for himself: "I am just managing now. I am afraid I might fail; maybe I'm capable but I do not want to rock the boat." He now often expressed unhappiness about his short size but the feeling of "wanting to stay the way I am" was stronger.

When his request to be transferred to the open floor was complied with, in February, 1960, there was a decided change. During the first week he gained five pounds and continued to gain, at a slower rate. His first reaction was fear of getting sick again; it had all started with his feeling too heavy. This was the most he had weighed since the onset of his illness and he worried: "I don't know whether to gain any more—how much more can I take." But he could also look at it with humor: "Me of all things to have to watch my weight!" He enjoyed being on the open ward and became more active in gym and showed interest in others. He expressed the feeling: "I am free—*I own my body*—I am not supervised anymore by nurses or by mother."

His greater optimism was expressed in his buying, with his own money, an electric shaver. He was aware how unusual this was in view of his enormous stinginess: "I will buy a shaver only when I am confident I can use it. This time I went ahead of time. I use it now to trim my hair while waiting—but there is a definite expectation that I will need it." His tightness with money pervaded all his actions and made for many difficulties, often of a humorous nature, with other patients.

His attitude toward his weight and eating underwent a complete change. He felt that even if he gained too much weight, he could no longer follow a diet: "I have controlled myself so long—now I want to enjoy food." When a soft diet was prescribed while extensive dental work was done that had become imperative after long neglect, he greatly resented it. Now that he had given up his starvation regime, he did not want to be left out: "Now if I lose weight it makes me feel sick, that I am losing something that is mine. If I cannot eat and they are serving something that I like, then I feel I am missing something. I was starved so long that now when I have a chance I do not want to miss anything anymore." Even if he now felt like not eating, he would still eat: "I would make myself do it." He also ate as a release: "It is a real pleasure—now I want to eat."

With this change in his attitude toward eating he began to express a feeling of responsibility for his body. If he had not been such a coward and so scared of pain, he would have gone to a dentist a long time ago. Now he made the decision that even though he was afraid of everything that was involved he would go through with it, and no longer let his teeth rot and decay. He also acknowledged that he was aware that he had mistreated his whole body in a similar way.

When collection of a 24-hour urine specimen was requested, he became alarmed that his body did not produce well enough; he seemed to notice that he passed less urine than on a similar test several years before. He also became concerned that the medical consultant was slow in making a decision. The effect on his growth of a protein-enriched diet was to be studied before endocrine treatment was instituted. Since the question of his vomiting after meals persisted, a nurse was assigned to watch his food intake in order to get a correct picture. This was explained to him. Now he was annoyed with himself for being angry: "I am angry when I see them watching. I won't eat when they watch me. Then I take it out on myself or I eat on the sly." He felt this was silly, that he was fighting fire with fire. Increasingly, he showed concern for his body instead of attacking it and even became angry with other patients who he felt did not care properly for their body: "My body was not my own. It was my parent's concern. By neglect I would get back at my mother. Now I am willing to treat my body well. I won't take it out on my body anymore. Now I know it is *my* body."

He could review his mother's concern with his health in a different light: "When I was a little kid she cared for me—she did things for me, mainly when I was sick. But now I know she helped me." He also recognized how his attitude toward his mother changed after anorexia nervosa developed. He particularly resented that she took him to doctors: "There was no warrant. She did not act the same way as when I had chicken pox. That was not my fault, but then they began to act as if it were all my fault. Now the warmth is coming back. She sees now that I am not hopeless, that something good is coming out of me. She sees me trying." During this time he needed extensive dental work, and also an eye checkup. He was touched that his father made arrangements for him to be seen by private physicians. This to him was proof that they really cared and saw something worthwhile in him.

His deficit in feeling differentiated from his parents, in particular from his mother, came up in many other ways. It had been rather puzzling that a boy as bright as he showed so little intellectual interest. It became apparent that his good school performance had also been something expected of him, and that he had been without true curiosity or eagerness to learn. Gradually he began to develop an interest in reading. He became aware to what extent he wanted things planned for him, how little he relied upon his own initiative. When choosing a book he would ruminate: "What would my mother say—shall I please my mother when I read or am I pleasing my self?" He recalled that his mother always had suggested what he should read and that he had never had the feeling that he was reading for his own enrichment.

He now accepted the need for endocrine treatment and began to pay attention to his bodily sensations. He talked about "feeling different," with no vocabulary to describe sexual feelings. Sex had never been discussed at home and during the years when other boys acquired knowledge of it he had been sick. There was constant amazement that his sister, who was dating at this time, was doing so well. He reacted with anger when his mother got interested in some "growth elixir."

With progressive improvement the need to consider the future became more imminent. He now clung to the idea that his short stature was an insurmountable obstacle, and became obsessively preoccupied with his size. He alternated between feeling guilty for having ruined his valuable body, and thinking of his body as the enemy who kept him from taking his role in the adult world. He would refer to himself as a teenage dwarf. It was not altogether undesirable that his first physician, who was very tall, left the service at this time, as Eric began to work with a new therapist. He again objected but now, in a common conference, treatment problems could be defined as including the problems of living in the adult world with a shorter than average stature.

His preoccupation with money became even more apparent, and he was finally willing to talk about it. He was aware that he was stingy and that hoarding money had been the very first sign of his illness. He would run errands for other patients for pay or would keep money for returned bottles, etc. He absolutely hated to lend or borrow money; it made him feel unclear as to what was his. He did not want any gifts, either; he considered himself unworthy for anybody to spend money on him. He had a dramatic reaction when a parallel was drawn between his attitude toward money and food. He recognized that he had tried to live as a closed system, as an island unto himself. Many episodes in his behavior on the ward showed to what extent he was afraid of being cheated, or felt that he was not treated as an equal, or feared that unjust impositions were made on him.

When endocrine treatment was finally instituted, on his twentieth birthday, he was eager for it, but also afraid that it would "hurt" his body. He anxiously watched for new sensations, particularly sexual feelings, and was disappointed when there were no immediate marked reactions. He needed support not to expect too much. His attitude became one of waiting, that he could not concern himself with anything new until he had grown. His failure in taking any initiative became more and more apparent. Though he had spent years accusing his parents for having done too many things for him, he now became increasingly aware that he was quite unable to start anything and was constantly trying to get directions about the simplest decisions. This was a difficult period for his new therapist because his repetitious complaining was a temptation to supply him with "motivation," thereby depriving him of the need to decide for himself.

As he began to note some effects of the endocrine treatment, growth of an inch, a change in the hairline, nocturnal erections, and beginning interest in girls, there was a gradual change. When he felt sure about his development, he decided that he wanted a job and used his father's connection to obtain a desirable position.

His behavior at work now showed how little understanding he had for other people's behavior or of what impressions he made on others. Now he could ask for help with his problems. It had been recognized before that he did not like to go to movies with other patients, even less to the theater, and avoided reading novels because he did not understand why people behaved the way they did. Simple situations were used to help him gain at least some outer knowledge of motivation and behavior.

His job involved contact with many different people, and he was excited about the new challenge and truly interested in the many problems that came up. When asked whether he had been scared, he eagerly denied it but then asked: "Why is my face so red and why are my hands so wet?" He needed help to identify the sensations that were associated with these somatic manifestations of anxiety. At work he had been indignant about being asked his age wherever he went. He was reluctant to accept the need for more adult clothing if he did not want to be mistaken for a 14-year-old kid in his t-shirt and dungarees. For a while his stinginess continued to interfere with the need to offer a more age-appropriate picture. When going to a movie, he would give an incorrect, younger age to get in on a child's ticket at half-price.

By the time he was ready to leave the hospital, he had

become a much more self-reliant person. He stood quite securely on an island of realistic awareness of his participation in his own life, not only in the most biological sense, but with greater awareness of his needs and sensations, vastly improved self-esteem and sense of effectiveness, and more discrimination and sensitivity in interpersonal relations.

COMMENT

Though this approach has been developed for the treatment of severe eating disorders, it is in no way specific to them alone. Anorexia nervosa, in spite of its rarity and unique manifest picture, is in its underlying structure not specific, but resembles other disorders of adolescence. The non-eating is a very late step in the overall development of the illness. Some adolescents in the same predicament will resort to overeating as a defense against their sense of "emptiness" and "nothingness"; some will alternate between phases of bulimia and anorexia. The great majority opts for other ways and means, not involving the eating function, in the search for selfhood.

One may call the struggle for a distinct identity, with awareness of control over one's functions, an essential task of adolescence. The fear of being influenced from without, of being empty and ineffective, can be recognized as the core issue in schizophrenics and in borderline cases, and in many others who are seeking deviant avenues toward self-differentiation.

This treatment approach has been used successfully in many other conditions characterized by "weak ego" or "diffused ego boundaries." It has been particularly useful in therapy of developmental obesity, borderline states, and schizophrenia (Bruch, 1966). Such patients are considered poor candidates for classical psychoanalysis. This approach represents a modification of the analytic process, with explicit and consistent emphasis on the patient's developing awareness of thoughts and impulses originating in himself. Through alert and consistent confirming or correcting responses to any self-initiated behavior, the patient will become able to participate actively in the therapeutic process and in the way he lives his life.

SUMMARY

For effective therapeutic intervention it is essential to differentiate between a specific anorexia nervosa syndrome and other psychiatric conditions associated with cachexia and self-starvation. In primary anorexia nervosa pursuit of thinness is the dominant issue. It appears as a late symptom in a life development that has been characterized by lack of self-initiated behavior due to a deficit of appropriate responses to child-initiated cues.

A therapeutic approach has been developed with emphasis on evoking awareness of impulses, thoughts, and feelings originating within the patient. Details have been presented from the progress of a patient who had been unsuccessfully in psychiatric treatment for seven years, with six months in the same hospital before the new therapeutic approach was instituted. Changes in the interaction within the family, and in body concept and self-awareness, were reported in detail to illustrate step-by-step development as treatment progressed.

18

The Role of the Family in the Treatment of Anorexia Nervosa

Ronald Liebman, M.D.,
Salvador Minuchin, M.D.,
and Lester Baker, M.D.

We have described in previous papers the importance of the family in the development and perpetuation of psychosomatic symptoms in children, and the effectiveness of structural family therapy in the treatment of anorexia nervosa, brittle diabetes, and intractable asthma (Baker and Barcai, 1970; Minuchin, 1970, 1971a; Liebman, Minuchin, and Baker, 1974a, b). Further, we have described a treatment program for anorexia nervosa which integrates operant reinforcement techniques within the context of structural family therapy.

Briefly, the integrated treatment program consists of the

Reprinted by permission from the *Journal of the American Academy of Child Psychiatry*, 13:263-274, 1974. New Haven: Yale University Press.

These studies were supported in part by USPHS Grant RR 240 and MH 21336.

The authors wish to thank Braulio Montalvo, of the Philadelphia Child Guidance Clinic, for his valuable assistance in the analysis of the family lunch session and in the organization and assigning of the family tasks. Also, Dr. B. Rosman and Ms. F. Hitchcock helped in the preparation of the final manuscript.

following steps: admission to the hospital for medical and neurological evaluation to rule out organic causes for the anorexia and weight loss; informal lunch sessions with the patient to assess the degree of negativism and anorexia; application of an operant reinforcement paradigm to initiate weight gain; family therapy lunch sessions to accelerate and reinforce weight gain; weekly outpatient family therapy to change the maladaptive patterns of family structure and functioning. Medications are not used. The average length of hospitalization is two to three weeks and results in significant weight gain and restoration of normal eating patterns. The duration of outpatient family therapy ranges from five to 12 months and is characterized by the lack of relapses following the cessation of therapy.

The purpose of this paper is to describe, in detail, the process of therapy of an anorectic girl and her family to illustrate the application of the principles of the above treatment program. In this case, an outpatient operant reinforcement paradigm is used within the context of the process of family therapy. There are other approaches to the outpatient family therapy of anorexia nervosa (Minuchin, 1970, 1974; Aponte and Hoffman, 1973; Combrinck-Graham, 1973) which do not utilize an operant reinforcement paradigm and have been successful. It is hoped that the detailed description of this case will be of practical value to help clinicians deal more effectively with a most frustrating, perplexing, and potentially fatal syndrome.

CASE EXAMPLE

Janet was a 14-year-old Jewish girl from an upper-middle-class professional family. When she was six, her mother died of breast cancer. As far as the father remembers, there was no anorexia or emaciation associated with the mother's death. The father and daughter lived with the father's parents for about two years, until the father remarried. The stepmother had two adopted children from her previous marriage, which ended when her first husband died. Thus, Janet's family is composed of her father, stepmother, a stepsister 10 months older, and a stepbrother one year younger. The father's work keeps him away from home two to three nights a week, leaving the mother responsible for settling most of the problems at home. The father relinquished these responsibilities to her, but criticized her for being incompetent and disorganized. A year before the onset of anorexia, the family's pediatrician recommended evaluation by a child psychiatrist because Janet was described as being emotionally immature, verbally and socially inhibited, and lacking in self-confidence. She was seen in individual psychotherapy for 10 months with some improvement. Occasionally, her parents were seen separately for counseling sessions. Four months after she stopped therapy, she began to diet because she thought her hips and thighs were too heavy, although she was not overweight. In four months she had gone from 112 pounds to 85 pounds. At this point, her parents telephoned the child psychiatrist, who arranged for hospitalization to evaluate the child's medical status, and to try to effect weight gain by separation from the family. Hospitalization revealed no medical causes for the anorexia, but all attempts to stimulate weight gain failed completely. A month later, Janet's weight had dropped to 72 pounds. At this point, she was referred to the authors at the Children's Hospital of Philadelphia.

Janet resembled a World War II concentration camp victim. Her emaciated skeletonlike appearance was repulsive. When the therapist first saw her, she was lying in bed, whining and continually wiping her mouth with tissue to avoid swallowing saliva because she feared that too much liquid could cause her to gain weight. She had all of the clinical characteristics described by Bruch (1973): disturbance of body image, misperception of internal physiological stimuli, a sense of ineffectiveness, and paradoxical hyperactivity.

Periodically, the therapist ate lunch with the patient. At these times, he told her that when he was hungry, his stomach hurt and he felt lightheaded. He said that it felt good to eat and be satiated. No attempt was made to get the patient to eat her lunch. The therapist asked her permission to eat some small part of her food, such as a piece of carrot or celery. Then he offered to share part of his lunch with her. This procedure enabled the therapist to ascertain the degree of negativism and anorexia manifested by the patient. It also provided an opportunity to relate to her around the issues of sharing and eating food, thus avoiding a power struggle over the act of eating. During the lunch sessions, information regarding the family and peer group and school relationships was obtained in an informal fashion.

On the second day of hospitalization, the pediatrician explained to Janet the details of the operant reinforcement paradigm which was put into effect on the third day by the pediatrician and his nursing staff under the supervision of the therapist.[1] The behavior paradigm made access to physical activity completely contingent on weight gain (Blinder, Freeman, and Stunkard, 1970). Janet was weighed every morning before breakfast. If she had gained less than half a pound compared to the previous morning's weight, she would not be allowed out of bed for any reason. If she had gained at least half a pound, she would be allowed to be out of bed to eat, watch television, have visitors, and use the

---

[1]The patients are hospitalized in the Clinical Research Center, which is a medical unit and in no way resembles a psychiatric hospital unit. When anorectics (as well as children with other psychosomatic illnesses) are treated, there is close collaboration between the family therapists and pediatricians. The nurses and other personnel are trained not to get into power struggles over the act of eating.

bathroom. She was also given a four- to six-hour period of unrestricted activity on the ward or in the hospital.

Janet was allowed to discuss the details of her menu with the pediatrician, nurses, and dietician. She could add or subtract certain foods as long as she ate a balanced diet at each meal. She could have three regular meals or five to six smaller ones. The goal was to give her an increased sense of autonomy and responsibility for her physical status.

For the first three days after the start of the inpatient behavior paradigm, Janet's weight stayed at 72 pounds. On the morning of the fourth day, she gained her first pound; nine days later she weighed 79 pounds. She then developed a viral gastroenteritis with nausea and vomiting which lasted for three days. On the morning of the sixteenth day, she weighed 76 pounds, a net gain of four pounds. That afternoon, the first family therapy lunch session was held.

The lunch session included the patient, her family, the pediatrician, and the psychiatrist. It was the first time that the family had met the psychiatrist and marked the beginning of the transition from the inpatient phase to the outpatient phase. It also demonstrated that the psychiatrist and the pediatrician worked together in a mutually supportive way with the common goal of helping the patient and her family.

The goals of the family therapy lunch session were: (1) to enable the patient to eat in the presence of her parents without the development of a power struggle, by preventing self-defeating intrusions from the parents; and (2) to redefine the presenting problem away from the family's myth that they were fine except for the presence of their medically sick child. This formulation had to be transformed into a recognition of the transactional conflicts which existed between the parents and Janet.

During the lunch session, the therapist engaged the parents on an affectual and verbal level to draw their attention away from Janet. In order to keep her in a conflict-free area, she was purposely avoided in the various discussions started by the therapist. The therapist told Janet that she could eat if she wanted to, or not eat if she didn't want to; then the therapist said that he was very hungry, and he immediately began to eat. Within a few minutes, the parents and the pediatrician began to eat their lunches spontaneously. At this point, the only person in the room who was not eating was Janet. Then the therapist asked Janet, and was granted, her permission to eat a small portion of her lunch, thus forcing her to compete with him for her lunch. Immediately thereafter, Janet began to eat and ate her entire lunch without any further difficulties. This was in marked contrast to what had been occurring at home during the six months prior to referral. Therefore, the family saw that change could occur, and were provided with a more optimistic and hopeful attitude.

At the end of the first family lunch session, the therapist stated that eating was no longer the problem in the family because Janet was able to eat her lunch. The pediatrician and therapist discussed Janet's status in the presence of the family, and agreed that she could go home when she reached 85 pounds.

On the morning of the first family lunch session, Janet had weighed 76 pounds. During the next six days, she gained 11.5 pounds, achieving the weight required for discharge. There were no episodes of bulimia. During this six-day period, she was allowed to eat in the hospital cafeteria, accompanied by family or nursing staff. She seemed happier and talked about leaving the hospital and returning to school. At the second family lunch session, seven days later, Janet was told that she could be discharged from the hospital. However, she stated that she was "not ready" to go home with her family. After all of the family members stated that they wanted her to return home and rejoin the family, she agreed to leave the hospital.

In the outpatient phase, the family psychiatrist assumed the primary responsibility, with the pediatrician functioning in a supportive-consultative way. This was the reverse of the system used during the inpatient phase. The general goals of the outpatient phase were: (1) to eliminate the symptom of refusing to eat and to stimulate progressive weight gain (this had top priority to prevent the family from concentrating on Janet's symptoms as a way of avoiding or detouring family conflicts); and (2) to elucidate and change the dysfunctional patterns in Janet's family which reinforced her symptoms.

The initial weight gain and family lunch sessions had started the process of changing Janet's role as the family's scapegoat.[2] This process was continued by the assignment of an outpatient operant reinforcement paradigm, which the parents enforced with the therapist's support. The behavior paradigm provided the parents with something concrete to do at home, decreasing their anxiety and previous feelings of helplessness in dealing with their sick child.

The outpatient paradigm was defined as an interpersonal process. The parents were told that it was their responsibility as parents to enforce the paradigm, and that if they worked together in a mutually supportive way, they would be successful. Janet was told that it was her responsibility to herself and to her parents to follow the paradigm. The family was told that Janet must gain a minimum of two pounds a week in order to maintain normal activities. If she gained less than two pounds, from Friday to Friday, she would not be allowed out of the house during the weekend, and she could not have

[2]This is referred to as disengagement: the process whereby family members are supported to function more competently and independently within the context of the family and with their respective peer groups.

friends come to the house. In addition, a member of the family had to stay at home with her. This produced a great deal of stress in the family system, causing the members of the family to join together to ensure that Janet ate. If she gained between two and two and a half pounds, she was allowed to be active on either Saturday or Sunday, but not both days. She was given the choice of days and the choice of activities. If she gained more than two and a half pounds in the preceding seven-day period, she was allowed to be active on Friday night, Saturday, and Sunday.

During the first two weeks following discharge, Janet tested her parents by gaining less than two pounds. The therapist supported the parents, who were able to enforce the behavior paradigm. By the third week, Janet had gained the required two pounds. She was told that she must weigh 112 pounds to go to summer camp with her siblings; she attained that weight by mid-June. Thus, she gained 25 pounds in the three months following discharge from the hospital.

Once weight gain was progressing in a gradual fashion, outpatient family therapy was concentrated upon family tasks to influence different subsystems of the family. These were directed toward expediting changes in the structure, organization, and functioning of the family and toward changing the quality of the interpersonal relationships in the family.

The following is a summary of some of the main points of the outpatient family therapy.

Janet's symptoms resulted from and were a manifestation of dysfunctional patterns in her family system. The parents were ineffective, disorganized, rigid, and incapable of resolving conflicts, finding solutions to problems, or dealing with stressful situations. Janet was emotionally close to her father and more distant from her mother, siblings, and peer group. The marital relationship was weak and inadequate, allowing Janet to be inappropriately involved in the parents' affairs. The family's pattern of functioning was characterized by constricting parental overprotectiveness, lack of privacy for individual members, denial of the existence of any problems except for the presence of Janet's symptoms, and a lack of resolution of spouse conflicts which remained submerged by the parents' concern for and total preoccupation with Janet. In this way, she detoured family conflicts, with the parents united around concern for their sick child. Therefore, her symptoms were reinforced within the context of the family. The first goal was to help Janet free herself from this position, and the first intervention was the assignment of the outpatient behavior paradigm. Defining the paradigm as a task for the parents to enforce separated Janet from the spouse subsystem and its conflicts.

Another important area for change was the relationship between the parents. The father and mother were given the task of discussing privately each evening any problems associated with the children or the behavior paradigm. These discussions were not to end until a plan of action had been organized. While the mother was given the responsibility of dealing directly with the children, the father's task was to coach her, but not to undermine or criticize her in any way. The therapist directed his major efforts to the father, supporting him to help his wife assume more of her maternal responsibilities in a competent fashion.

Two months after the beginning of outpatient therapy, the parents stated that eating was no longer a problem. The problem, as they now defined it, was Janet's poor interpersonal relationships, manifested by her lack of friends and outside interests. This indicated to the therapist that the family was ready for further changes.

With the older sister's permission, the parents were instructed to send Janet along to the parties and other activities the sister attended. The patient was told she must go and she did so, though initially with some reluctance. The parents were told to reward themselves for having become competent parents by planning to go out for a social evening alone, at least once each week. At the end of the third month of therapy, the parents went away for a weekend alone for the first time in their marriage. They also planned a two-week summer vacation during the time the children would be in camp. A closer relationship between the parents, within which their needs could be mutually satisfied, began to develop, freeing the children to develop relationships among themselves, in school and with their peer groups.

The children went to summer camp for July and August. Janet had an enjoyable summer, making many friends and volunteering for flood relief work in Pennsylvania. She developed obvious secondary sexual characteristics; she grew about two inches; her hair was stylishly longer; she was spontaneous and relaxed while she talked and joked with her siblings. In general, she appeared to be an attractive, confident teenager who seemed genuinely pleased with herself. She talked about the new school year, seeing her previous classmates, developing new friendships, and letting her hair grow longer.

After the summer vacation, therapy was resumed because the parents stated that more "work" needed to be done. However, the format was changed, the children and the parents coming to the clinic on different days in order to underline the disengagement process. Periodically, a family session was held to assess transactional patterns between the parents and the children. During one of the family sessions, the parents stated that they were more concerned about Janet's older sister, because they believed that Janet was stronger and demonstrated better judgment than her sister. Clearly, the role and status of the former patient in the family had changed.

Shortly after therapy was resumed, the therapist showed

the family a videotape of a previous session which demonstrated clearly how the mother had focused on some problem of the patient or her sister to decrease the peripheral position of her husband by stimulating his concern about the particular problem. This videotape, which was reviewed with the entire family in detail to point out the relevant transactional issues, served as a turning point. To reinforce further the disengagement process, the following tasks were put into effect: (1) the sisters were allowed to go on weekly unescorted shopping trips with their friends, and to use public transportation to keep those appointments with the therapist that did not involve the parents; (2) Janet was allowed to babysit for the neighbors and to go to the movies unescorted with her friends; (3) the brother was allowed to visit a friend in another part of the city to play baseball; and (4) the patient's older sister was allowed to begin dating.

The parents were supported in giving the children gradual increases in freedom and responsibility. The rationale was that the parents would be able to have more time and energy to satisfy themselves if their children were able to function in a more independent fashion. Instead of being concerned about the children, the parents could now concentrate on being concerned about each other. The remainder of the therapy dealt exclusively with resolving marital problems; the children were no longer seen. Therapy lasted 10 months.

At the time of the preparation of this paper, there has been an 18-month follow-up period, during which time Janet has continued without symptoms. Her eating patterns and weight are normal, and she appears to enjoy being physically attractive. She has done quite well academically, and she is very invested in age-appropriate peer group relationships and activities. The siblings have not manifested any significant problems, and the parents have been able to sustain the

marked improvements in their marital relationship and parental functions.

DISCUSSION AND CONCLUSIONS

In a clinical disorder in which there is a significant mortality
rate (five to 15 percent), the physician's top priority is to
ensure the survival of the patient. The behavior paradigm
and the family lunch sessions in the hospital begin the processes of weight gain and of disengaging the patient from the
arena of submerged parental conflicts. The outpatient behavior paradigm and the family tasks continue to support
weight gain and decrease the patient's role in detouring family conflicts. When used in the context of structural family
therapy, behavior modification paradigms are effective
methods of avoiding self-defeating power struggles. They
were used as a lever to start the therapeutic process moving.
However, the family interventions, such as the lunch sessions
and the family tasks, were vital to the outcome of therapy.

As a result of therapy, Janet's family was able to achieve
a new level of functioning in which the members were more
highly differentiated with more autonomy, freedom, responsibility, and spontaneity. The family system was more
flexible, with less rigidity of roles and more adaptive patterns
of communication and problem solving. As a result of
changes in family structure and functioning, conflicts could
be resolved and the need for detouring conflicts was eliminated. Then it was possible for Janet to move in the direction
of increased peer group activities and relationships. If the
structure of the family had not been changed, continuation
or reappearance of Janet's symptoms (or the appearance of
a new symptom bearer) might have occurred.

A review of the recent literature indicates that a combination of behavior therapy and chemotherapy has gained
popularity for the treatment of the acute cachectic phase of

anorexia nervosa (Dally and Sargant, 1960, 1966; Crisp, 1965a; Blinder, Freeman, and Stunkard, 1970; Stunkard, 1972). However, little has been reported about the clinical course of anorectics after they leave the hospital. It would appear that in many cases, improvement is not sustained after return to their environment. Blinder, Freeman, and Stunkard (1970), who were able to achieve an average weight gain of 3.9 to 4.8 pounds per week with three hospitalized patients, report that one of their patients committed suicide following discharge from the hospital, after a disturbing telephone conversation with her mother. Brady and Rieger (1974), reporting on 16 cases of anorexia (all of whom gained weight in the hospital), report two deaths, four rehospitalizations, and three patients with poor social adjustment at follow-up. Bruch (1973) reports that 30 of 50 cases of anorexia (for whom follow-up information is available) are leading restricted lives, are institutionalized, have died of anorexia, or are still anorectic.

From our combined experience with 20 cases, we believe that anorexia nervosa may best be approached with the therapeutic focus on the context of the patient's family. Direct involvement of the family early in the course of the acute cachectic phase may promote a rapid significant weight gain, facilitating return of the patient to the family and peer group in a comparatively short period of time (two to three weeks). Continued involvement of the family in ongoing outpatient therapy to change the structure and functioning of the family may make it possible for the family to prevent relapses and support the continued growth and development of its members.

19

Treatment of Anorexia Nervosa with Behavior Modification: Effectiveness of Formula Feeding and Isolation

Katherine A. Halmi, M.D.,
Pauline Powers, M.D.,
and Sheila Cunningham, R.N.

Anorexia nervosa, a disorder occurring predominantly in females and characterized by a refusal to eat, unusual food handling, a distorted attitude toward eating and body image associated with severe weight loss, amenorrhea, bradycardia, hypothermia, and exercising rituals or persistant overactivity, has been subjected to a variety of therapies, including hypnosis, psychoanalysis, family therapy (Thomä, 1967; Dally, 1969; Barcai, 1971), tube feeding, bed rest, electric convulsive therapy, chlorpromazine, subcoma doses of insulin, anabolic hormones, and prefrontal lobotomy (Dally and Sargant, 1960; Crisp, 1965a, b, c; Dally, 1969). The careless use of too inclusive, too general and vague criteria for the diagnosis of anorexia nervosa has made comparisons between various treatment programs difficult if not meaningless.

An effective therapy for this illness is crucial, since it is one

Reprinted by permission from the *Archives of General Psychiatry*, 32:93-96, 1975. Copyright 1975, American Medical Association.

of the few psychiatric disorders that can result in death. Follow-up studies of large numbers of anorexia nervosa patients have shown a mortality rate of 21.5 percent (Halmi, Brodland, and Rigas, 1975), 15 percent (Kay and Leigh, 1954; Dally and Sargant, 1960), and 17 percent (Seidensticker and Tzagournis, 1968; Theander, 1970). Also, increasing incidence of anorexia nervosa has been noted by Bruch (1970), Thomä (1967), Halmi (1974), and Duddle (1973).

Therapists using discriminating criteria for anorexia nervosa have recognized that classical psychotherapy with interpretations and stressing insight has not been effective with this illness (Groen and Feldman-Toledano, 1966; Rollins and Blackwell, 1968; Bruch, Chapter 17). Rather, Rollins and Blackwell (1968) have focused on interactions of the patient with her family and with others; Bruch (Chapter 17) places emphasis on "evoking awareness of feelings, thoughts, and impulses that originate in the patients themselves" (p. 450 above); and Groen and Feldman-Toledano (1966) state that a "superficial educative approach is preferable" (p. 680).

The most consistent published reports of successful treatment have described behavior modification, either with or without concomitant use of drugs. The behavior therapy has been that of operant conditioning with positive reinforcements, consisting of increased physical activity, visiting privileges, and social activities, contingent on weight gains (Hallsten, 1965; Lang, 1965; Leitenberg, Agras, and Thomson, 1968; Azerrod and Stafford, 1969; Blinder, Freeman, and Stunkard, 1970; Lobb and Schaefer, 1972; Bianco, 1972; Brady and Rieger, 1974). In addition to the above, some authors have concurrently used desensitization procedures (Hallsten, 1965; Lang, 1965; Leitenberg, Agras, and Thomson, 1968; Azerrod and Stafford, 1969; Brady and Rieger, 1974). It is impossible to evaluate the relationship of various drugs used in the above behavior modification programs to weight gains and general outcome.

A selective eating program in anorexia nervosa of taking in protein at the expense of carbohydrates or fats has been reported by Russell (1967) and Halmi and Fry (1974). With the hypothesis that taking away all food (thereby not allowing the patient to make a choice) and replacing it with a bland formula for a specified period would facilitate the patient's return to a normal eating pattern, a "Sustagen-like" formula was incorporated into the behavior modification program described below. Among the various reported cases of anorexia nervosa treated with behavior modification, only a few patients did not receive ataractic drugs concurrently. In order to gain an initial impression of the effects of behavior modification itself on weight gain in anorexia nervosa, we treated eight patients, meeting the rigorous criteria (slightly modified) of Feighner, Robins, and Guze (1972), with behavior therapy and no medications.

CLINICAL POPULATIONS AND METHODS

PATIENT SAMPLE

The following tabulation contains the criteria used to make the diagnosis of anorexia nervosa:

1. onset before 25 years of age;
2. anorexia with accompanying weight loss of at least 25 percent of original body weight;
3. a distorted, implacable attitude toward eating, food, or weight that overrides hunger, admonitions, reassurance, and threats; for example, (a) denial of illness, with a failure to recognize nutritional needs; (b) apparent enjoyment in losing weight, with over-manifestation that food refusal is pleasurable indulgence; (c) a desired body image of extreme thinness,

with overt evidence that it is rewarding to the patient
to achieve and maintain this state; (d) unusual hoarding or handling of food;

4. no known medical illness that could account for the
anorexia and weight loss;

5. no other known psychiatric disorder, with particular
reference to primary affective disorders, schizophrenia, obsessive-compulsive and phobic neuroses (It is
assumed that even though it may appear phobic or
obsessional, food refusal alone is not sufficient to
qualify for obsessive-compulsive or phobic disease.);

6. at least two of the following manifestations: (a) amenorrhea; (b) lanugo (persistence of downy pelage); (c)
bradycardia (persistent resting pulse rate of 60 beats
per minute or less); (d) periods of overactivity; (e)
episodes of bulimia (compulsive overeating); (f) vomiting (may be self-induced).

The patient sample, seven females and one male, is described in Table 1. (Details of case histories are available from
the senior author on request.) All patients in this study were
admitted and treated in the Clinical Research Center of the
University of Iowa General Hospitals, where they were also
part of comprehensive metabolic and hormonal study.

BEHAVIOR MODIFICATION PROGRAM

All eight patients were treated with the same operant conditioning program, with positive reinforcements of social activities, increased physical activities, and visiting privileges
contingent on weight gains. The patients were weighed each
morning under standardized conditions. After a three- to
five-day observation period, they were isolated and restricted
to their rooms. They were given a "Sustagen-like" formula,
diluted to 1 kcal/ml in six equal feedings as their only source

Table 1

Description of Anorexia Nervosa Patients During Hospitalization

Patient	Sex	Admission Age, yr.	Height, cm	Pretreatment Weight, kg	% Standard Weight*	Hospital Discharge Weight, kg	Total Weight Gain, kg	% Standard Weight	Weight Gain Per Week, kg
1	M	14	158	33.0	69	41.8	8.8	88	1.46
2	F	23	157.5	31.2	62	40	8.8	80	1.47
3	F	16	162	30.8	59	39.7	8.9	76	1.27
4	F	54	161.3	30	59	41.3	11.3	81	1.41
5	F	26	166	35.4	66	47	11.5	87	1.64
6	F	15	162.6	36.6	73	42.6	6.0	85	1.2
7	F	17	158	33.1	69	42	8.9	87	1.27
8	F	21	165	45.6	82	52	6.4	94	1.6

*For patients less than 18 years of age, Iowa Growth Charts used as reference for normal weight; for patients older than 18, normal weight references obtained from Metropolitan Life Insurance Company weight-height scales.

of nutrient for the first three weeks of treatment. Since a rapid weight gain can have serious medical complications (Dudrick, 1975), we instituted some control over the patients' rate of gaining weight by gradually increasing the total calories per day offered them. For the first week, the patient received 125 percent of the basal requirement, as determined by a nomogram (Mayo Clinic, 1951), to maintain the patient's weight measured on the first day of the treatment program. The second week the patient was offered 150 percent of baseline calories, and the third week 200 percent of baseline calories. The fourth week, the patient was given three meals of a regular diet, including a morning, afternoon, and evening snack. The meals were taken in the unit dining room, where the patient was given half an hour to complete each meal. The patient had to record all food she returned to the kitchen.

In order to earn increased privileges, the patient had to gain 0.5 kg (1.1 lb) per five-day period, with the exception of the first five days when she was required only to maintain her weight. If the patient did not gain weight at the end of five days, she received no advanced privileges. If she lost weight, she was tube fed until she attained the weight she had at the beginning of the five-day period.

For the first five days of the treatment program, the patients received no visitors, no phone calls, and no mail. A radio, but no television, and only hospital staff were allowed in their rooms. If a patient attained the appropriate weight, on the sixth day (or the beginning day of the next five-day period), she was allowed to make one phone call, receive her mail, have one visitor for one hour, and be out of her room one hour every day for the next five days. By the end of the next and each succeeding five-day period, the patient was required to gain 0.5 kg in order to have an additional visitor, or the same number of visitors for an additional hour, to receive her mail, to make additional phone calls, and to be out of her room each day for an additional hour. Phone calls, visitors, and mail were received only on the day privileges were earned. The patient chose which hours she spent out of her room, and while in her room could engage in any craft or reading of her choice. Each patient received from the staff some re-educative therapy with emphasis on her interactions with others.

The staff, relatives, and visitors were instructed not to discuss food and weight with the patients.

RESULTS

The average length of hospitalization for the eight patients was 6.25 weeks. Their average weight gain during hospitalization was 8.83 kg (19.4 lb). Weekly weight gain varied little among the patients with the average being 1.4 kg (3.1 lb) per week (see Table 1). At the conclusion of three weeks on the "Sustagen-like" formula, all patients eagerly ate the balanced meals presented to them. Only one patient, the male, had to be tube fed. He required six consecutive days of tube feeding during the "formula period." Only on rare occasions did the patients leave food on their trays, and then no particular type was left more frequently than another.

After discharge from the hospital, the patients were maintained on a behavior modification program. They were instructed as to the daily amount of calories necessary to maintain a weight within the normal range for their age and height. Individualized positive reinforcements such as new clothes and special activities were given by the family for a 0.5-kg (1.1-lb) weight gain per week until the patient reached normal weight range. If the patient had lost more than 1 kg (2.2 lb) at any follow-up visit, arrangements were made with the patient and relatives that she would be admitted to the psychiatric hospital for tube feeding. Cooperation from the parents or spouse was necessary for this agreement and was obtained as part of the "treatment plan" when the patient was admitted. Initial weekly follow-up visits were gradually decreased to less frequent checkups as the patients improved in weight and behavior.

Thus far none of the eight patients has required rehospitalization. The average number of months since their discharge is seven, and their average outpatient weight gain has been 4.2 kg (9.2 lb) (see Table 2).

An assessment was made at the last follow-up visit of the patients' general adjustment according to the following criteria: good—the patient is maintaining weight and functioning well at home, school, socially, and at work; adequate—the patient is maintaining weight but having minor behavioral problems; fair—the patient is maintaining weight but is functioning marginally in one or more important life areas (given above); and poor—the patient is not maintaining weight and is functioning marginally in important life areas.

All patients were maintaining their weight or gaining, and only one patient had substantial adjustment problems.

COMMENT

To date this is the largest number of reported anorexia nervosa patients successfully treated with behavior modification and without any type of drug therapy, to our knowledge. It must be recognized that any uncontrolled study, such as the present one, can never provide a definitive assessment of behavior therapy, regardless of the number of treatment successes obtained. However, before engaging in the time and expense of a controlled evaluation, it is desirable to have a substantial number of treatment successes under the therapeutic regimen in question. Short of a control group comparison, this study provides substantive additional evidence that behavior therapy is effective in producing weight gain

Table 2

Description of Anorexia Nervosa Patients at Follow-up

Patient	Mo Since Discharge at Last Follow-Up	Weight at Last Follow-up, kg	% Standard Weight*	Menstruation Returned	Adjustment at Last Follow-Up
1	6	47	99	NA†	Good
2	2	42	84	−	Good
3	13	47.6	92	+	Good
4	8	44	88	−	Fair
5	8	49	91	−	Adequate
6	12	47.6	95	−	Adequate
7	3	44.5	93	−	Adequate
8	6	61	111	+	Good

*For patients less than 18 years of age, Iowa Growth Charts used as reference for normal weight; for patients older than 18, normal weight references obtained from Metropolitan Life Insurance Company weight-height scales.
†Not applicable.

in anorexia nervosa. The slightly lower weekly weight gain of 1.4 kg (3.2 lb) compared to the 4.07 lb of Brady and Rieger's patients (Brady and Rieger, 1974) and the 4.7 lb of Dally and Sargant's anorectics (Dally and Sargant, 1966) might be explained by the initial calorie restriction in our program, and by the possible additive weight-gaining effect of the phenothiazines and tricyclic antidepressant drugs used in the other two studies, or both.

Because of redistribution of body fluids and changes occurring in body metabolism, we did not anticipate that the patients would have identical weight increases day after day. Giving positive reinforcements after an expected weight gain during a five-day interval allows for daily physiological variations to occur without penalizing the patient unjustly.

Since the anorectics have a selective eating pattern (Halmi, 1974) and since many have had a problem of being overweight prior to their illness (Halmi, 1974), providing them with a well-balanced diet of the appropriate number of calories to maintain a normal body weight a few weeks before hospital discharge may give the patient a necessary "eating-learning" experience.

Follow-up studies of anorectic patients who have received behavior therapy while hospitalized have shown that many need a continuing behavior modification program after discharge to maintain their weight (Crisp, 1965b; Dally and Sargant, 1966; Brady and Rieger, 1974).

Controlled, double-blind studies are needed for a more definitive assessment of the effectiveness of various drugs used to promote weight gain with behavior modification therapy. In addition, controlled studies are needed to determine what type of continuing therapy is most efficacious with the anorexia nervosa patients' behavioral and weight problems after hospitalization.

REFERENCES

Abend, S., Kachalsky, H., & Greenberg, H. R. (1968), Reactions of adolescents to short-term hospitalizations. *Amer. J. Psychiat.*, 124:949-954.

Ackerman, N. W. (1958), *The Psychodynamics of Family Life.* New York: Basic Books.

———(1966), *Treating the Troubled Family.* New York: Basic Books.

Aichhorn, A. (1925), *Wayward Youth.* New York: Viking, 1935.

———(1922-1948), *Delinquency and Child Guidance*, ed. O. Fleischmann, P. Kramer, & H. Ross. New York: International Universities Press, 1964.

Alt, H. (1960), *Residential Treatment of the Disturbed Child.* New York: International Universities Press.

American Psychiatric Association (1967), Summary of meetings of Council and Executive Committee. *Amer. J. Psychiat.*, 124:421-451.

Anthony, E. J. (1969), The reactions of adults to adolescents and their behavior. In: *The Psychology of Adolescence*, ed. A. H. Esman. New York: International Universities Press, 1975, pp. 467-493.

Aponte, H., & Hoffman, L. (1973), The open door: A structural approach to a family with an anorectic child. *Fam. Proc.*, 12:1-44.

Ariès, P. (1962), *Centuries of Childhood.* New York: Knopf.

Ayd, F. J., Jr. (1975), The depot fluphenazines: A reappraisal after 10 years' clinical experience. *Amer. J. Psychiat.*, 132:491-500.

Azerrod, J., & Stafford, R. (1969), Restoration of eating behavior in anorexia nervosa through operant conditioning and environmental manipulation. *Behav. Res. Ther.*, 7:165-171.

Baker, L., & Barcai, A. (1970), Psychosomatic aspects of diabetes mellitus. In: *Modern Trends in Psychosomatic Medicine*, Vol. 2, ed. O. W. Hill. New York: Appleton-Century-Crofts, pp. 105-123.

Barcai, A. (1971), Family therapy in the treatment of anorexia nervosa. *Amer. J. Psychiat.*, 128:286-290.

Barclay, L. E. (1969), A group approach to young unwed mothers. *Soc. Casework*, 50:379-384.

Barkley, R. (1977), A review of stimulant drug research with hyperactive children. *J. Child Psychol. & Psychiat.*, 18:137-165.

Barnard, J. E. (1970), Peer group instruction for primigravid adolescents. *Nursing Outlook*, 18:42-43.

Bartlett, D. (1975), The use of multiple family therapy groups with ado-

507

lescent drug addicts. In: *The Adolescent in Group and Family Therapy*, ed. M. Sugar. New York: Brunner/Mazel, pp. 262-282.

Bassin, A. (1968), Daytop Village. *Psychology Today*, 2(7):48-52.

Beckett, P. G. S. (1965), *Adolescents Out of Step: Their Treatment in a Psychiatric Hospital*. Detroit: Wayne State University Press.

Beels, C., & Ferber, A. (1969), Family therapy: A view. *Fam. Proc.* 8:280-332.

Begab, M. J. (1962), Recent developments in mental retardation and their implications for social group work. In: *Proceedings of the Institute for Social Group Work with the Mentally Retarded*, ed. M. Schreiber. New York: Association for the Help of Retarded Children, pp. 1-12.

Bell, N. W., & Vogel, E. F. (1960), The emotionally disturbed child as the family scapegoat. In: *The Family*, ed. N. W. Bell & E. F. Vogel. New York: Free Press.

Bellis, J. M., & Sklar, N. E. (1969), The challenge: Adjustment of retarded adolescents in a workshop. *J. Rehabil.*, 35:19-21.

Bender, L. (1947), Childhood schizophrenia: Clinical study of 100 schizophrenic children. *Amer. J. Orthopsychiat.*, 17:40-56.

———(1953), Childhood schizophrenia. *Psychiat. Quart.*, 27:663-681.

———(1956), Schizophrenia in childhood: Its recognition, description and treatment. *Amer. J. Orthopsychiat.*, 26:499-506.

Bergman, P., & Escalona, S. (1949), Unusual sensitivities in very young children. *The Psychoanalytic Study of the Child*, 3/4:333-352. New York: International Universities Press.

Berkovitz, I. H. (1972), On growing a group: Some thoughts on structure, process, and setting. In: *Adolescents Grow in Groups*, ed. I. H. Berkovitz. New York: Brunner/Mazel, pp. 6-28.

——— Chikahisa, P., Lee, M. L., & Murasaki, E. M. (1966), Psychosexual development of latency-age children and adolescents in group therapy in a residential setting. *Internat. J. Group Psychother.*, 16:344-356.

Bernfeld, S. (1923), Über eine typische Form der männlichen Pubertät. *Imago*, 9:169-188.

———(1929), Der soziale Ort und seine Bedeutung für Neurose, Verwahrlosung und Pädagogik. *Imago*, 15:299-312.

———(1938), Types of adolescence. *Psychoanal. Quart.*, 7:243-253.

Beskind, H. (1962), Psychiatric inpatient treatment of adolescents: A review of clinical experience. *Compr. Psychiat.*, 3:354-369.

Bettelheim, B. (1950), *Love Is Not Enough*. Glencoe, Ill.: Free Press.

Bianco, F. J. (1972), Rapid treatment of two cases of anorexia nervosa. *J. Behav. Ther. & Exper. Psychiat.*, 3:223-224.

Bigman, E. (1961), Group work with a group of severely retarded young adults. In: *Proceedings of the Institute for Social Group Work with the Mentally Retarded*, ed. M. Schreiber. New York: Association for the Help of Retarded Children, pp. 32-37.

Bion, W. R. (1961), *Experiences in Groups*. London: Tavistock.

Blaustein, F., & Wolff, H. (1972), Adolescent group: A "must" on a psychiatric unit—problems and results. In: *Adolescents Grow in Groups*, ed. I. H. Berkovitz. New York: Brunner/Mazel, pp. 181-191.

Bleuler, E. (1911), *Dementia Praecox, or The Group of Schizophrenias*. New York: International Universities Press, 1950.

Blinder, B. J., Freeman, D. M. A., & Stunkard, A. J. (1970), Behavior therapy of anorexia nervosa. *Amer. J. Psychiat.*, 126:1093-1098.

Bliss, E. L., & Branch, C. H. (1960), *Anorexia Nervosa*. New York: Hoeber.

Blom, G. E. (1972), A psychoanalytic viewpoint of behavior modification in clinical and educational settings. *J. Amer. Acad. Child Psychiat.*, 11:675-693.

Blos, P. (1941), *The Adolescent Personality*. New York: Appleton-Century-Crofts.

———(1962), *On Adolescence: A Psychoanalytic Interpretation*. New York: Free Press.

———(1970), *The Young Adolescent: Clinical Studies*. New York: Free Press.

———(1979a), *The Adolescent Passage*. New York: International Universities Press.

———(1979b), Modifications in the classical psychoanalytic model of adolescence. In: *The Adolescent Passage*. New York: International Universities Press, pp. 473-497.

Borenzweig, H. (1970), Social group work in the field of mental retardation: A review of the literature. *Soc. Sci. Rev.*, 44:177-183.

Bornstein, B. (1949), The analysis of a phobic child: Some problems of theory and technique in child analysis. *The Psychoanalytic Study of the Child*, 3/4:181-226. New York: International Universities Press.

Borowitz, G. (1973), The capacity to masturbate alone in adolescence. *Adolesc. Psychiat.*, 2:130-143.

Bowen, M. (1966), The use of family theory in clinical practice. *Comp. Psychiat.*, 7:345-374.

Bowlby, J. (1960a), Grief and mourning in infancy and early childhood. *The Psychoanalytic Study of the Child*, 15:9-52. New York: International Universities Press.

———(1960b), Separation anxiety. *Internat. J. Psycho-Anal.*, 41:89-113.

———(1961), Processes of mourning. *Internat. J. Psycho-Anal.*, 42:317-340.

———(1962), Childhood bereavement and psychiatric illness. In: *Aspects of Psychiatric Research*, ed. D. Richter et al. London: Oxford.

Brackelmanns, W. E., & Berkovitz, I. H. (1972), Younger adolescents in group psychotherapy: A reparative superego experience. In: *Adolescents Grow in Groups*, ed. I. H. Berkovitz. New York: Brunner/Mazel, pp. 37-48.

Bradley, C. (1937), The behavior of children receiving benzedrine. *Amer. J. Orthopsychiat.*, 94:577-585.

Brady, J. P., & Rieger, W. (1974), Behavioral treatment of anorexia ner-
    vosa. In: *Applications of Behavior Modification*, ed. T. Thompson & W.
    S. Dockens. New York: Academic Press, pp. 45-63.
Braverman, S. (1966), The informal peer group as an adjunct to treatment
    of the adolescent. *Soc. Casework*, 47:152-157.
Breuer, J., & Freud, S. (1893-1895), *Studies on Hysteria. Standard Edition*,
    2. London: Hogarth Press, 1955.
Brown, S. L. (1964), Clinical impression of the impact of family group
    interviewing on child and adolescent psychiatric practice. *J. Amer. Acad.
    Child Psychiat.*, 3:688-696.
————(1969), Diagnosis, clinical management and family interviewing. In:
    Science and Psychoanalysis, Vol. 14, ed. J. Masserman. New York: Grune
    & Stratton, pp. 188-193.
————(1970), Family for adolescents. *Psychiatric Opinion*, 7:6, 8-15.
Bruch, H. (1962), Perceptual and conceptual disturbances in anorexia
    nervosa. *Psychosom. Med.*, 24:187-194.
————(1963), Effectiveness in psychotherapy of the constructive use of
    ignorance. *Psychiat. Quart.*, 37:332-339.
————(1965), Anorexia nervosa and its differential diagnosis. *J. Nerv. Ment.
    Dis.*, 141:555-566.
————(1966), Psychotherapy with schizophrenics. *Arch. Gen. Psychiat.*,
    14:346-351.
————(1970), Changing approaches to anorexia nervosa. *Internat. Psychiat.
    Clin.*, 7:3-24.
————(1973), *Eating Disorders*. New York: Basic Books.
————(1974), Perils of behavior modification in treatment of anorexia
    nervosa. *JAMA*, 230:1419-1422.
Buchanen, C. (1967), *Spelling*, Books 1-6. Palo Alto, Cal.: Behavioral Re-
    search Laboratories.
————(1968), *Programmed Reading for Adults*, Books 1-8. New York:
    McGraw-Hill.
Buxbaum, E. (1945), Transference and group formation in children and
    adolescents. *The Psychoanalytic Study of the Child*, 1:351-365. New York:
    International Universities Press.
Cantwell, D. P. (1979), Use of stimulant medication with psychiatrically
    disordered adolescents. In: *Adolescent Psychiatry*, Vol. 7, ed. S. C. Fein-
    stein & P. L. Giovacchini. Chicago: University of Chicago Press, pp.
    375-388.
Carlson, G.A. (1979), Lithium carbonate use in adolescents: Clinical in-
    dications and management. In: *Adolescent Psychiatry*, Vol. 7, ed. S.C.
    Feinstein & P.L. Giovocchini. Chicago: University of Chicago Press.
———— & Strober, M. (1978), Bipolar manic-depressive illness in early
    adolescence. *J. Amer. Acad. Child Psychiat.*, 17:138-153.

Carroll, E. J. (1954), Acting out and ego development. *Psychoanal. Quart.*, 23:521-528.

Carter, W. W. (1968), Group counseling for adolescent foster children. *Children*, 15:22-27.

Caruth, E., & Ekstein, R. (1966), Interpretations within the metaphor: Further considerations. *J. Amer. Acad. Child Psychiat.*, 5:35-45.

Casriel, D. (1963), *So Fair a House: The Story of Synanon.* Englewood, N.J.: Prentice-Hall.

Charney, I. W. (1963), Regression and reorganization in the "isolation treatment" of children: A clinical contribution to sensory deprivation research. *J. Child Psychol. & Psychiat.*, 4:47-60.

Cohen, H. (1968), Educational therapy: The design of learning environments. In: *Research in Psychotherapy*, Vol. 3, ed. J. Shlien. Washington, D.C.: American Psychological Association.

Combrinck-Graham, L. (1974), Structural family therapy in psychosomatic illness: Treatment of anorexia nervosa and asthma. *Clin. Pediat.*, 13:827-833.

Crisp, A. H. (1965a), Clinical and therapeutic aspects of anorexia nervosa: A study of 30 cases. *J. Psychosom. Res.*, 9:67-78.

———(1965b), Some aspects of the evaluation, presentation and follow-up of anorexia nervosa. *Proc. Royal Soc. Med.*, 58:814-820.

———(1965c), A treatment regimen for anorexia nervosa. *Brit. J. Psychiat.*, 112:505-512.

Dally, P.J. (1969), *Anorexia Nervosa.* New York: Grune & Stratton.

——— & Sargant, W. (1960), A new treatment of anorexia nervosa. *Brit. Med. J.*, 1:1770-1773.

——— & ——— (1966), Treatment and outcome of anorexia nervosa. *Brit. Med. J.*, 2:793-795.

Davis, J. M. (1975), Maintenance therapy in psychiatry. I. Schizophrenia. *Amer. J. Psychiat.*, 132:1237-1245.

Davis, R. E. (1979), Manic-depressive variant syndrome of childhood: A preliminary report. *Amer. J. Psychiat.*, 13:702-706.

DeLong, G. R. (1978), Lithium carbonate treatment of select behavior disorders in children suggesting manic depressive illness. *J. Pediat.*, 93:689-694.

Deutsch, H. (1942), Some forms of emotional disturbances and their relationship to schizophrenia. In: *Neuroses and Character Types.* New York: International Universities Press, 1965, pp. 262-281.

DSM-III [Diagnostic and Statistical Manual of Mental Disorders, 3rd Ed.] (1978), Washington, D.C.: American Psychiatric Association.

Duddle, M. (1973), An increase of anorexia nervosa in a university population. *Brit. J. Psychiat.*, 123:711-712.

Dudrick, S. J. (1975), Historical considerations of intravenous hyperalimentation. In: *Intravenous Nutrition in High-Risk Infants*, ed. R. W. Winters & E. G. Hasselmeyer. New York: Wiley, pp. 7-31.

Easson, W. M. (1969), *The Severely Disturbed Adolescent: Inpatient, Residential, and Hospital Treatment*. New York: International Universities Press.

Eckermann, J. P. (1836), *Gespräche mit Goethe in den letzten Jahren seines Lebens*, ed. H. H. Houben. Leipzig: Brockhaus, 1910.

Edelson, M. (1970a), *Sociotherapy and Psychotherapy*. Chicago: University of Chicago Press.

———(1970b), *The Practice of Sociotherapy: A Case Study*. New Haven: Yale University Press.

Eisenberg, L., Lackman, R., & Molling, P. A. (1963), A psychopharmacologic experiment in a training school for delinquent boys: Methods, problems and findings. *Amer. J. Orthopsychiat.*, 33:431-447.

Eissler, K. (1949), A biographical outline of August Aichhorn. In: *Searchlights on Delinquency*, ed. K. R. Eissler. New York: International Universities Press, pp. ix-xiii.

———(1953), The effect of the structure of the ego on psychoanalytic technique. *J. Amer. Psychoanal. Assn.*, 1:104-143.

———(1969), Irreverent remarks about the present and the future of psychoanalysis. *Internat. J. Psycho-Anal.*, 50:461-471.

Ekstein, R. (1954), The space child's time machine: On "reconstruction" in the psychotherapeutic treatment of a schizophrenic child. *Amer. J. Orthopsychiat.*, 24:492-506.

———(1956), A clinical note on the therapeutic use of a quasi-religious experience. *J. Amer. Psychoanal. Assn.*, 4:304-313.

——— & Friedman, S. W. (1956), A technical problem in the beginning phase of treatment of a borderline psychotic child. In: *Case Studies in Childhood Emotional Disabilities*, Vol. 2, ed. G. Gardner. New York: American Orthopsychiatric Association, pp. 353-363.

——— & Wallerstein, J. (1956), Observations on the psychology of borderline and psychotic children. *The Psychoanalytic Study of the Child*, 11:303-311. New York: International Universities Press.

——— & Wright, D. (1952), The space child. *Bull. Menn. Clin.*, 16:211-223.

Elias, A. (1968), Group treatment program for juvenile delinquents. *Child Welfare*, 47:281-290.

Erikson, E. H. (1940), Studies in the interpretation of play. I. Clinical observation of play disruption in young children. *Genet. Psychol. Mon.*, 22:557-671.

———(1959), *Identity and the Life Cycle*. [*Psychological Issues*, Monogr. 1.] New York: International Universities Press.

Esman, A. H. (1982), Fathers and adolescent sons. In: *Father and Child*, ed. S. Cath, A. Gurwitt, & J. M. Ross. Boston: Little Brown.

Evans, J. (1966), Analytic group therapy with delinquents. *Adolescence*, 1:180-196.

Fairbairn, W. R. D. (1954), *An Object-Relations Theory of the Personality*. New York: Basic Books.

Federn, P. (1926-1952), *Ego Psychology and the Psychoses*, ed. E. Weiss. New York: Basic Books, 1952.

Feighner, J. P., Robins, E., & Guze, S. B. (1972), Diagnostic criteria for use in psychiatric research. *Arch. Gen. Psychiat.*, 26:57-63.

Feinstein, S. C., Feldman-Rotman, S., & Woolsey, A. B. (1980), Diagnostic aspects of manic-depressive illness in children and adolescents. In: *Essentials of Human Development and Child and Adolescent Psychiatry*, ed. M. Shafii & S. Shafii. Chicago: University of Chicago Press.

Fenichel, O. (1945), Neurotic acting out. *Psychoanal Rev.*, 32:197-206.

Ferenczi, S. (1924), *Thalassa: A Theory of Genitality*. New York: Psychoanalytic Quarterly, Inc., 1938.

Ferster, C., & Skinner, B. F. (1957), *Schedules of Reinforcement*. New York: Appleton-Century-Crofts.

Fine, R., & Dawson, J. (1964), A therapy program for the mildly retarded adolescent. *Amer. J. Ment. Def.*, 69:23-30.

Fliess, R. (1961), *Ego and Body Ego: Contributions to Their Psychoanalytic Psychology*. New York: Schulte.

Fraiberg, S. (1961), Homosexual conflicts. In: *Adolescents*, ed. S. Lorand & H. I. Schneer. New York: Hoeber, pp. 78-112.

Franklin, G. H., & Nottage, W. (1969), Psychoanalytic treatment of severely disturbed juvenile delinquents in a therapy group. *Internat. J. Group Psychother.*, 19:165-175.

Franks, C. M. (1969), *Behavior Therapy: Appraisal and Status*. New York: Appleton-Century-Crofts.

Freud, A. (1926), *Introduction to the Technique of Child Analysis*. New York & Washington, D.C.: Nervous and Mental Disease Publishing Company, 1928. [Reissued in revised translation as "Four lectures on child analysis," *The Writings of Anna Freud*, 1:1-69. New York: International Universities Press, 1974.]

———(1927), The theory of children's analysis. In: *The Psycho-Analytical Treatment of Children*. London: Imago, pp. 55-64. [Reissued in revised translation as "The theory of child analysis," *The Writings of Anna Freud*, 1:162-175. New York: International Universities Press, 1974.]

———(1931), *Introduction to Psycho-Analysis for Teachers: Four Lectures*. London: Allen & Unwin. [Reissued in revised translation as "Four lectures on psychoanalysis for teachers and parents," *The Writings of Anna Freud*, 1:71-133. New York: International Universities Press, 1974.]

———(1936), *The Ego and the Mechanisms of Defense*. *The Writings of Anna Freud*, 2. New York: International Universities Press, Rev. Ed., 1966.

———(1945), Indications for child analysis. *The Psychoanalytic Study of the*

Child. 1:127-149. New York: International Universities Press. [Reprinted in *The Writings of Anna Freud*, 4:3-38. New York: International Universities Press, 1968.]

————(1946), *The Psycho-Analytical Treatment of Children.* London: Imago.

————(1952), Studies in passivity. *The Writings of Anna Freud*, 4:245-259. New York: International Universities Press, 1968.

————(1958), Adolescence. *The Psychoanalytic Study of the Child*, 13:255-278. New York: International Universities Press. [Reprinted in *The Writings of Anna Freud*, 5:136-166. New York: International Universities Press, 1969.]

————(1962), Assessment of childhood disturbances. *The Psychoanalytic Study of the Child*, 17:149-158. New York: International Universities Press.

Freud, S. (1900), *The Interpretation of Dreams. Standard Edition*, 4 & 5. London: Hogarth Press, 1953.

————(1904), On psychotherapy. *Standard Edition*, 7:255-268. London: Hogarth Press, 1953.

————(1905a), Fragment of an analysis of a case of hysteria. *Standard Edition*, 7:1-122. London: Hogarth Press, 1953.

————(1905b), Three essays on the theory of sexuality. *Standard Edition*, 7:123-243. London: Hogarth Press, 1953.

————(1906), Psycho-analysis and the establishment of the facts in legal proceedings. *Standard Edition*, 9:97-114. London: Hogarth Press, 1959.

————(1909), Analysis of a phobia in a five-year-old boy. *Standard Edition*, 10:1-149. London: Hogarth Press, 1955.

————(1911), Formulations on the two principles of mental functioning. *Standard Edition*, 12:213-226. London: Hogarth Press, 1958.

————(1912), Contributions to a discussion on masturbation. *Standard Edition*, 12:239-254. London: Hogarth Press, 1958.

————(1914), On narcissism: An introduction. *Standard Edition*, 14:67-104. London: Hogarth Press, 1957.

————(1919), A child is being beaten. *Standard Edition*, 17:175-204. London: Hogarth Press, 1955.

————(1920), Beyond the pleasure principle. *Standard Edition*, 18:1-64. London: Hogarth Press, 1955.

————(1922), Some neurotic mechanisms in jealousy, paranoia and homosexuality. *Standard Edition*, 18:221-234. London: Hogarth Press, 1955.

————(1923), The infantile genital organization (an interpolation into the theory of sexuality). *Standard Edition*, 19:139-145. London: Hogarth Press, 1961.

————(1925a), Negation. *Standard Edition*, 19:233-239. London: Hogarth Press, 1961.

————(1925b), Die Verneinung. *Gesammelte Schriften*, 11:3-7. Leipzig, Vienna, Zurich: Internationaler psychoanalytischer Verlag, 1928.

————(1927), Fetishism. *Standard Edition*, 21:147-158. London: Hogarth Press, 1961.

————(1931), Female sexuality. *Standard Edition*, 21:221-243. London: Hogarth Press, 1961.

————(1933), *New Introductory Lectures on Psycho-Analysis. Standard Edition*, 22:1-182. London: Hogarth Press, 1964.

————(1937), Analysis terminable and interminable. *Standard Edition*, 23:209-253. London: Hogarth Press, 1964.

————(1938), An outline of psycho-analysis. *Standard Edition*, 23:139-207. London: Hogarth Press, 1964.

————(1940), Splitting of the ego in the process of defence. *Standard Edition*, 23:271-278. London: Hogarth Press, 1964.

Fried, E. (1956), Ego emancipation of adolescents through group psychotherapy. *Internat. J. Group Psychother.*, 5:358-373.

Friedman, A. S., Boszormenyi-Nagy, I., Jungreis, J. E., Lincoln, G., Mitchell, H. E., Sonne, J. C., Speck, R. Z., & Spizack, G. (1965), *Psychotherapy for the Whole Family*. New York: Springer.

Friedman, M., Glasser, M., Laufer, E., Laufer, M., & Wohl, M. (1972), Attempted suicide and self-mutilation in adolescence. *Internat. J. Psycho-Anal.*, 53:179-184.

Giovacchini, P. (1979), *Treatment of Primitive Mental States*. New York: Jason Aronson.

Gitelson, M. (1948), Character synthesis: The psychotherapeutic problem of adolescence. *Amer. J. Orthopsychiat.*, 18:422-431.

Glasser, W. (1965), *Reality Therapy*. New York: Harper & Row.

Glatt, M. M. (1967), Group therapy with young drug addicts—the addicts' point of view. *Nursing Times*, 63:519-521.

Glenn, J. (1978), Freud's adolescent patients: Katherina, Dora, and the "homosexual woman." In: *Freud and His Patients*, ed. M. Kanzer & J. Glenn. New York: Jason Aronson, pp. 23-47.

Gottheil, E., Backup, C. E., & Cornelison, F. S. (1969), Denial and self-image confrontation in a case of anorexia nervosa. *J. Nerv. Ment. Dis.*, 148:238-250.

Gralnick, A. (1966), Psychoanalysis and the treatment of adolescents in a private hospital. In: *Science and Psychoanalysis*, ed. J. H. Masserman. New York: Grune & Stratton.

Greenacre, P. (1952a), *Trauma, Growth and Personality*, 2nd Ed. New York: International Universities Press, 1969.

————(1952b), General problems of acting out. In: *Trauma, Growth and Personality*, 2nd Ed., New York: International Universities Press, 1969, pp. 224-236.

————(1953), Certain relationships between fetishism and the faulty development of the body image. *The Psychoanalytic Study of the Child*, 8:79-98. New York: International Universities Press.

———(1954), Problems of infantile neurosis: A discussion. *The Psychoanalytic Study of the Child*, 9:18-24, 37-40.

———(1955), Further considerations regarding fetishism. *The Psychoanalytic Study of the Child*, 10:187-194.

Greenson, R. R. (1950), The mother tongue and the mother. In: *Explorations in Psychoanalysis*. New York: International Universities Press, 1978, pp. 31-43.

Groen, J. J., & Feldman-Toledano, Z. (1966), Educative treatment of patients and parents in anorexia nervosa. *Brit. J. Psychiat.*, 112:671-681.

Grold, L. J. (1972), The value of a "youth group" to hospitalized adolescents. In: *Adolescents Grow in Groups*. ed. I. H. Berkovitz. New York: Brunner/Mazel, pp. 192-196.

Guntrip, H. (1961), *Personality Structure and Human Interaction*. New York: International Universities Press.

Haley, J. (1962), Whither family therapy. *Fam. Proc.*, 1:69-100.

———(1971), Family therapy. *Internat. J. Psychiat.*, 9:233-242.

——— & Hoffman, L. (1967), An interview with Carl A. Whitaker. In: *Techniques of Family Therapy*, ed. J. Haley & L. Hoffman. New York: Basic Books, pp. 265-360.

Hallsten, E. A. (1965), Adolescent anorexia nervosa treated by desensitization. *Behav. Res. Ther.*, 3:87-91.

Halmi, K. A. (1974), Anorexia nervosa: Demographic and clinical features in 94 cases. *Psychosom. Med.*, 36:18-26.

——— Brodland, G., & Rigas, C. (1975), A follow-up study of 79 patients with anorexia nervosa: An evaluation of prognostic factors and diagnostic criteria. In: *Life History Research in Psychopathology*, Vol. 4. Minneapolis: University of Minnesota Press, pp. 290-300.

——— & Fry, M. (1974), Serum lipids in anorexia nervosa. *Biol. Psychiat.*, 8:159-167.

Hammar, S. L., Campbell, V., & Woolley, J. (1971), Treating adolescent obesity. *Clin. Pediat.*, 10:46-52.

Harley, M. (1961a), Masturbation conflicts: In: *Adolescents*, ed. S. Lorand & H. I. Schneer. New York: Hoeber, pp. 51-77.

———(1961b), Some observations on the relationship between genitality and structural development at adolescence. *J. Amer. Psychoanal. Assn.*, 9:434-460.

Hartmann, E. L., Glasser, B. A., & Greenblatt, M. (1968), *Adolescents in a Mental Hospital*. New York: Grune & Stratton.

Hartmann, H. (1950), Comments on the psychoanalytic theory of the ego. In: *Essays on Ego Psychology*. New York: International Universities Press, 1964, pp. 113-141.

———(1954), Problems of infantile neurosis: A discussion. In: *Essays on*

Ego Psychology. New York: International Universities Press, 1964, pp. 207-214.

Heacock, D. R. (1966), Modifications of the standard techniques for out-patient group psychotherapy with delinquent boys. *J. Nat. Med. Assn.,* 58:41-47.

Hendrickson, W. J. (1969), Training in adolescent psychiatry: The role of experience with in-patients. Presented at the Conference on Training in Adolescent Psychiatry, University of Chicago, November.

——— Holmes, D. J., & Waggoner, R. W. (1959), Psychotherapy with hospitalized adolescents. *Amer. J. Psychiat.,* 116:527-532.

Hobbs, N. (1963), Strategies for the development of clinical psychology. *American Psychological Association, Division of Clinical Psychology Newsletter,* 16(2):3-5.

———(1966), Helping disturbed children: Psychological and ecological strategies. *Amer. Psychol.,* 21:1105-1115.

Holmes, D. J. (1964), *The Adolescent in Psychotherapy.* Boston: Little, Brown.

Honig, W. E. (1966), *Operant Behavior: Areas of Research and Application.* New York: Appleton-Century-Crofts.

Inhelder, B., & Piaget, J. (1958), *The Growth of Logical Thinking from Childhood to Adolescence.* New York: Basic Books.

Jackson, D. (1959), Family interaction, family homeostasis and implications for therapy. In: *Individual and Family Dynamics,* ed. J. Masserman. New York: Grune & Stratton, pp. 122-141.

Jacobs, M. A., & Christ, J. (1967), Structuring and limit setting as techniques in the group treatment of adolescent delinquents. *Commun. Ment. Health J.,* 3:237-244.

Jacobson, E. (1964), *The Self and the Object World.* New York: International Universities Press.

James, S. L., Osborn, F., & Oetting, E. R. (1967), The treatment of delinquent girls: The adolescent self-concept group. *Comm. Ment. Health J.,* 3:377-381.

Jarvik, M. E., Ed. (1978), *Psychopharmacology in the Practice of Medicine.* New York: Appleton-Century-Crofts.

Jokl, R. (1950), Psychic determinism and preservation of sublimation in classical psychoanalytic procedure. *Bull. Menn. Clin.,* 14:207-219.

Jones, E. (1922), Some problems of adolescence. In: *Papers on Psycho-Analysis,* 5th Ed., New York: William Wood, 1948, pp. 389-406.

Josselyn, I. (1952), *The Adolescent and His World.* New York: Family Service Association of America.

———(1972), Adolescent group therapy: Why, when, and a caution. In: *Adolescents Grow in Groups,* ed. I. H. Berkovitz. New York: Brunner/Mazel, pp. 1-5.

Kalogerakis, M. G. (1973), Therapy of assaultive psychiatric patients. In:

Current Psychiatric Therapies. Vol. 13, ed. J. H. Masserman. New York: Grune & Stratton, pp. 207-214.

—— Ed. (1978), *Pharmacotherapy for Institutionalized Adolescents.* New York: New York State Office of Mental Health.

Kanner, L. (1943), Autistic disturbances of affective contact. *Nervous Child,* 2:217-250.

——(1949), Problems of nosology and dynamics of early infantile autism. *Amer. J. Orthopsychiat.,* 19:416-426.

Katan, A. (1937), The role of "displacement" in agoraphobia. *Internat. J. Psycho-Anal.,* 32:41-50, 1951.

Kaufmann, P. N., & Deutsch, A. L. (1967), Group therapy for pregnant unwed adolescents in the prenatal clinic of a general hospital. *Internat. J. Group Psychother.,* 17:309-320.

Kay, D. W. K., & Leigh, D. (1954), The natural history, treatment and prognosis of anorexia nervosa, based on a study of 38 patients. *J. Ment. Sci.,* 100:411-429.

Kelly, M. J. (1970), Comprehensive long term treatment of a schizophrenic adolescent. *Psychiatric Opinion,* 7:36-41.

Kernberg, O. F. (1966), Structural derivatives of object relationships. *Internat. J. Psycho-Anal.,* 47:236-253.

——(1968), Some effects of social pressure on the psychiatrist as a clinician. *Bull. Menn. Clin.,* 32:144-159.

——(1975), *Borderline Conditions and Pathological Narcissism.* New York: Jason Aronson.

King, A. (1963), Primary and secondary anorexia nervosa syndromes. *Brit. J. Psychiat.,* 109:470-479.

Klein, D. F., Gittelman, R., Quitkin, F., & Rifkin, A. (1980), *Diagnosis and Drug Treatment of Psychiatric Disorders: Adults and Children,* 2nd Ed. Baltimore: Williams and Wilkins.

Klein, H., & Erlich, H. S. (1970), Is hospital democracy possible? Problems encountered in the therapeutic community as it reflects the community-at-large. *Ment. Health & Soc.,* 1:34-48.

—— & ——(1975), Some dynamic and transactional aspects of family therapy with psychotic patients. *Psychother. Psychosom.,* 26:148-155.

—— & ——(1976), Some psychoanalytic structural aspects of family function and growth: In: *Adolescent Psychiatry,* Vol. 6, ed. S. Feinstein & P. Giovacchini. Chicago: University of Chicago Press, 1978, pp. 171-194.

Klein, M. (1950), *The Psycho-Analysis of Children.* London: Hogarth Press.

——(1961), *Narrative of a Child Analysis.* New York: Basic Books.

Kohut, H. (1977), *The Restoration of the Self.* New York: International Universities Press.

Kraft, I. (1968), An overview of group therapy with adolescents. *Internat. J. Group Psychother.,* 18:461-480.

Kramer, C. H. (1970), *Psychoanalytically Oriented Family Therapy: Ten Year Evolution in a Private Child Psychiatry Practice*. Chicago: Family Institute of Chicago (unpublished).

Krasner, L. (1968), Assessment of token economy programmes in psychiatric hospitals. In: *CIBA Foundation Symposium: The Role of Learning in Psychotherapy*. London: J. & A. Churchill, Ltd., pp. 155-173.

Kris, A. O., & Schiff, L. F. (1969), An adolescent consultation service in a state mental hospital: Maintaining a treatment motivation. *Seminars in Psychiatry*, 1:15-23.

Kogerer, H. (1934), *Psychotherapie*. Vienna: Maudrich.

Kubie, L. S. (1968), Pitfalls of community psychiatry. *Arch. Gen. Psychiat.*, 18:257-266.

Lang, P. (1965), Behavior therapy with a case of nervous anorexia. In: *Case Studies in Behavior Modification*, ed. L. P. Ullman & L. Krasner. New York: Holt, Rinehart & Winston, pp. 217-221.

Laufer, M. (1965), Assessment of adolescent disturbances. *The Psychoanalytic Study of the Child*, 20:99-123. New York: International Universities Press.

———(1968), The body image, the function of masturbation, and adolescence: Problems of the ownership of the body. *The Psychoanalytic Study of the Child*, 23:114-137. New York: International Universities Press.

———(1973), Studies of psychopathology in adolescence. In: *Adolescent Psychiatry*, Vol. 2, ed. S. C. Feinstein & P. L. Giovacchini. New York: Basic Books, pp. 56-69.

———(1974), The analysis of an adolescent at risk. In: *The Analyst and the Adolescent at Work*, ed. M. Harley. New York: Quadrangle Books, pp. 269-296.

———(1978), The nature of adolescent pathology and the analytic process. *The Psychoanalytic Study of the Child*, 33:307-322. New Haven: Yale University Press.

Lazarus, A. (1971), *Behavior Treatment and Psychoanalysis*. New York: McGraw-Hill.

Lehrer, P., Schiff, L., & Kris, A. (1970), The use of credit cards in a token economy. *J. Applied Behav. Anal.*, 3:289-291.

Leitenberg, H., Agras, W. S., & Thomson, L. E. (1968), A sequential analysis of the effect of selective positive reinforcement in modifying anorexia nervosa. *Behav. Res. Ther.*, 6:211-218.

Leonard, M. (1966), Fathers and daughters. *Internat. J. Psycho-Anal.*, 47:325-334.

Levitt, L. (1968), Rehabilitation of narcotics addicts among lower-class teenagers. *Amer. J. Orthopsychiat.*, 38:56-62.

Lidz, T., Fleck, S., & Cornelison, A. A. (1965), *Schizophrenia and the Family*. New York: International Universities Press.

Liebman, R., Minuchin, S., & Baker, L. (1974a), An integrated treatment program for anorexia nervosa. *Amer. J. Psychiat.*, 131:432-436.

—— —— & ——(1974b), The use of structured family therapy in the treatment of intractable asthma. *Amer. J. Psychiat.*, 131:535-540.

Linn, L. (1959), Hospital psychiatry. In: *American Handbook of Psychiatry*, Vol. 2, ed. S. Arieti. New York: Basic Books, pp. 1829-1839.

Lobb, L. G., & Schaefer, H. H. (1972), Successful treatment of anorexia nervosa through isolation. *Psychol. Rep.*, 30:245-246.

Loewenstein, R. M. (1958), Remarks on some variations in psycho-analytic technique. *Internat. J. Psycho-Anal.*, 39:202-210, 240-242.

Mack, J. E., & Barnum, M. C. (1966), Group activity and group discussion in the treatment of hospitalized psychiatric patients, *Internat. J. Group Psychother.*, 16:452-462.

Mackay, M. C., Beck, L., & Taylor, R. (1973), Methylphenidate for adolescents with minimal brain dysfunction. *N.Y. J. Med.*, 73:550-554.

MacLennan, B. W. (1967), The group as reinforcer of reality: A positive approach in the treatment of adolescents. *Amer. J. Orthopsychiat.*, (Digest Issue), 37:272-273.

—— & Felsenfeld, N. (1968), *Group Counseling and Psychotherapy with Adolescents*. New York: Columbia University Press.

Maletsky, B. (1974), D-Amphetamine and delinquency: Hyperkinesis persisting? *Dis. Nerv. Syst.*, 35:543-547.

Malmquist, C. (1978), *Handbook of Adolescence*. New York: Jason Aronson.

Masterson, J. F. (1967), *The Psychiatric Dilemma of Adolescence*. Boston: Little, Brown.

——(1968), The psychiatric significance of adolescent turmoil. *Amer. J. Psychiat.*, 124:1549-1554.

——(1972), *Treatment of the Borderline Adolescent: A Developmental Approach*. New York: Wiley.

——(1978), The borderline adolescent: An object relations view. In: *Adolescent Psychiatry*, Vol. 6, ed. S. C. Feinstein & P. L. Giovacchini. Chicago: University of Chicago Press, pp. 344-359.

—— & Rinsley, D. B. (1975), The borderline syndrome: The role of the mother in the genesis and psychic structure of the borderline personality. *Internat. J. Psycho-Anal.*, 56:163-177.

Mayo Clinic (1951), The Bootby and Berkson food nomogram. *Postgrad. Med.*, 9:109.

Menninger, W. C. (1936), Psychiatric hospital treatment designed to meet unconscious needs. *Amer. J. Psychiat.*, 93:347-360.

——(1937), Psychoanalytic principles applied to the treatment of hospitalized patients. *Bull. Menn. Clin.*, 1:35-43.

——(1939), Psychoanalytic principles in psychiatric hospital therapy. *Southern Med. J.*, 32:348-354.

Meyer, B. C., & Weinroth, L. A. (1957), Observations on psychological aspects of anorexia nervosa. *Psychosom. Med.*, 19:398.

Miezio, S. (1967), Group therapy with mentally retarded adolescents in institutional settings. *Internat. J. Group Psychother.*, 17:321-327.

Miller, D. H. (1957), The treatment of adolescents in an adolescent hospital. *Bull. Menn. Clin.*, 21:189-199.

———(1974), *Adolescence: Psychology, Psychopathology and Psychotherapy*. New York: Jason Aronson.

——— & Feinstein, S. (1980), Psychoses in adolescence. In: *Basic Handbook of Child Psychiatry*, ed. J. Noshpitz. New York: Basic Books, pp. 708-722.

Minuchin, S. (1970), The use of an ecological framework in the treatment of a child. In: *The Child in His Family*, ed. E. J. Anthony & C. Koupernik. New York: Wiley, pp. 41-57.

———(1971a), Anorexia nervosa: Interactions around the family table. Presented at the Institute for Juvenile Research, Chicago.

———(1971b), Re-conceptualization of adolescent dynamics from the family point of view. In: *Teaching and Learning Adolescent Psychiatry*, ed. D. Offer & J. D. Masterson. Springfield, Ill.: Charles C Thomas, pp. 87-108.

———(1974), *Families and Family Therapy: A Structural Approach*. Cambridge, Mass.: Harvard University Press.

——— Rosman, B., & Baker, L. (1978), *Psychosomatic Families*. Cambridge, Mass.: Harvard University Press.

Mishler, E. G., & Waxler, N. E. Eds. (1966), *Family Processes and Schizophrenia*. New York: Science House.

Moadel, Y. (1970), Adolescent group psychotherapy in a hospital setting. *Amer. J. Psychoanal.*, 30:68-72.

Mordock, J. B., Ellis, M. H., & Greenstone, J. L. (1969), The effects of group and individual therapy on sociometric choice of disturbed institutionalized adolescents. *Internat. J. Group Psychother.*, 19:510-517.

Moreno, J. L. (1964), *Psychodrama*, 3rd Ed. Beacon, N.Y.: Beacon House, Inc.

Mowrer, O. H. (1963a), *The New Group Therapy*. Princeton, N.J.: Van Nostrand.

———(1963b), Payment or repayment? The problem of private practice. *Amer. Psychol.*, 18:577-580.

Neuringer, C., & Michael, J. L. (1970), *Behavior Modification in Clinical Psychology*. New York: Appleton-Century-Crofts.

Notterman, J. M. (1970), *Behavior: A Systematic Approach*. New York: Random House.

Nunberg, H. (1947), *Problems of Bisexuality as Reflected in Circumcision*. London: Imago.

Offer, D. (1969), *The Psychological World of the Teen-Ager*. New York: Basic Books.

O'Shea, C. (1972), "Two gray cats learn how it is" in a group of black teenagers. In: *Adolescents Grow in Groups*. ed. I. H. Berkovitz. New York: Brunner/Mazel, pp. 134-148.

Palazzoli, M. S. (1978), *Self-Starvation*. New York: Jason Aronson.

Pankratz, L. D., & Buchan, L. G. (1966), Techniques of the warm-up in psychodrama with the retarded. *Mental Retardation*, 4:12-15.

Pascal, G. R., Cottrell, T. B., & Baugh, J. R. (1967), A methodological note in the use of videotape in group psychotherapy with juvenile delinquents. *Internat. J. Group Psychother.*, 17:248-251.

Patterson, G. R., Ray, R. S., & Shaw, D. A. (1969), *Direct Intervention in Families of Deviant Children*, Vol. 8, No. 9, Oregon Institute Research Bulletin.

Paul, N. L., & Grosser, G. H. (1965), Operational mourning and its role in conjoint family therapy. *Comm. Ment. Health J.*, 1:339-345.

Peck, H. B., & Bellsmith, V. (1954), *Treatment of the Delinquent Adolescent—Group and Individual Therapy with Parent and Child*. New York: Family Service Association of America.

Performance Systems, Inc. (1968), *Advanced General Education Program*. Washington, D.C.: Office of Economic Opportunity.

Persons, R. W. (1966), Psychological and behavioral change in delinquents following psychotherapy. *J. Clin. Psychol.*, 22:337-340.

———(1967), Relationship between psychotherapy with institutionalized boys and subsequent community adjustment. *J. Consult. Psychol.*, 31:137-141.

——— & Pepinsky, H. B. (1966), Convergence in psychotherapy with delinquent boys. *J. Counsel. Psychol.*, 13:329-334.

Pottharst, K. E., & Gabriel, M. (1972), The peer group as a treatment tool in a probation department girls' residential treatment center. In: *Adolescents Grow in Groups*, ed. I. H. Berkovitz. New York: Brunner/Mazel, pp. 225-232.

Powdermaker, F. B., & Frank, J. D. (1953), *Group Psychotherapy: Studies in Methodology of Research and Therapy*. Cambridge, Mass.: Harvard University Press.

Rachman, A. W. (1969), Talking it out rather than fighting it out: Prevention of a delinquent gang war by group therapy intervention. *Internat. J. Group Psychother.*, 19:518-521.

Rachman, S. (1959), The treatment of anxiety and phobic reactions by systematic desensitization psychotherapy. *J. Abnorm. Soc. Psychol.*, 58:259-263.

Rado, S. (1956), *Psychoanalysis of Behavior*, Vol. 1. New York: Grune & Stratton.

————(1962), *Psychoanalysis of Behavior*, Vol. 2. New York: Grune & Stratton.

Rafel, S., & Stockhammer, R. (1961), The impact of a community group work agency in serving a retardate and his family. In: *Proceedings of the Institute for Social Group Work with the Mentally Retarded*, ed. M. Schreiber. New York: Association for the Help of Retarded Children, pp. 24-29.

Rapaport, D. (1953), Some metapsychological considerations concerning activity and passivity. In: *The Collected Papers of David Rapaport*, ed. M. M. Gill. New York: Basic Books, 1967, pp. 530-568.

Rapoport, J. L., & Mikkelsen, E. J. (1978), Antidepressants. In: *Pediatric Psychopharmacology*, ed. J. S. Werry. New York: Brunner/Mazel, pp. 208-223.

Redl, F. (1966), *When We Deal with Children*. New York: Free Press.

———— & Wineman, D. (1951), *Children Who Hate*. Glencoe, Ill.: Free Press.

———— & ————(1952), *Controls from Within*. Glencoe, Ill.: Free Press.

———— & ————(1957), *The Aggressive Child*. Glencoe, Ill.: Free Press.

Reich, W. (1932), Der masochistische Charakter. *Internat. Z. für Psychoanal.*, 18:303-351.

Riegel, B. (1968), Group meetings with adolescents in child welfare. *Child Welfare*, 47:417-427.

Rinsley, D. B. (1963), Psychiatric hospital treatment with special reference to children. *Arch. Gen. Psychiat.*, 9:489-496.

————(1965), Intensive psychiatric hospital treatment of adolescents: An object-relations view. *Psychiat. Quart.*, 39:405-429.

————(1967a), The adolescent in residential treatment: Some critical reflections. *Adolescents*, 2:83-95.

————(1967b), Intensive residential treatment of the adolescent. *Psychiat. Quart.*, 41:134-143.

————(1968), Economic aspects of object relations. *Internat. J. Psycho-Anal.*, 49:38-48.

————(1972), Group therapy within the wider residential context. In: *Adolescents Grow in Groups*. ed. I. H. Berkovitz. New York: Brunner/Mazel, pp. 233-242.

———— & Hall, D. D. (1962), Psychiatric hospital treatment of adolescents: Parental resistances as expressed in casework metaphor. *Arch. Gen. Psychiat.*, 7:286-294.

———— & Inge, G. P. III (1961), Psychiatric hospital treatment of adolescents: Verbal and nonverbal resistance to treatment. *Bull Menn. Clin.*, 25:249-263.

Rollins, N., & Blackwell, A. (1968), The treatment of anorexia nervosa in children and adolescents: Stage I. *J. Child Psychol. & Psychiat.*, 9:81-91.

Root, N. N. (1957), A neurosis in adolescence. *The Psychoanalytic Study of the Child*, 12:320-334. New York: International Universities Press.

Rosen, H. G., & Rosen, S. (1969), Group therapy as an instrument to develop a concept of self-worth in the adolescent and young adult mentally retarded. *Mental Retardation*, 7:52-55.

Rotman, C. B., & Golburgh, S. J. (1967), Group counseling mentally retarded adolescents. *Mental Retardation*, 5:13-16.

Russell, G. F. M. (1967), The nutritional disorder in anorexia nervosa. *J. Psychosom. Res.*, 11:141.

Schonfeld, W. (1967), The adolescent in contemporary American psychiatry. *Arch. Gen. Psychiat.*, 16:713-719.

Schulman, I. (1956), Delinquents. In: *The Fields of Group Psychotherapy*, ed. S. R. Slavson. New York: International University Press, pp. 196-214.

Schween, P. H., & Gralnick, A. (1965), Factors affecting family therapy in the hospital setting. *Compr. Psychiat.*, 7:424-431.

Schwing, G. (1954), *A Way to the Soul of the Mentally Ill*. New York: International Universities Press.

Science Research Associates (1967), *Job Corps Graded Reading Program*. Washington, D.C.: Office of Economic Opportunity.

Sechehaye, M. (1951), *Symbolic Realization*. New York: International Universities Press.

———(1956), *A New Psychotherapy in Schizophrenia*. New York: Grune & Stratton.

Seidensticker, J. F., & Tzagournis, M. (1968), Anorexia nervosa—clinical features and long-term follow-up. *J. Chronic Dis.*, 21:361-367.

Shapiro, E. (1978), The psychodynamics and developmental psychology of the borderline patient: A review of the literature. *Amer. J. Psychiat.*, 135:1305-1315.

Shapiro, R. L. (1963), Adolescence and the psychology of the ego. *Psychiatry.*, 26:77-87.

———(1966), Identity and ego autonomy in adolescence. In: *Science and Psychoanalysis*, ed. J. Masserman. New York: Grune & Stratton, pp. 16-23.

———(1967), The origin of adolescent disturbances in the family: Some considerations in therapy and implications for therapy. In: *Family Therapy and Disturbed Families*, ed. G. H. Zuk & I. Boszormenyi-Nagy. New York: Science and Behavior Books, pp. 221-238.

Shelly, J. A., & Bassin, A. (1965), Daytop Lodge—a new treatment approach for drug addicts. *Corrective Psychiatry and Journal of Social Therapy*, 11:186-195.

Simmel, E. (1929), Psycho-analytic treatment in a sanitarium. *Internat. J. Psycho-Anal.*, 10:70-89.

Skinner, B. F. (1961), *Cumulative Record*. New York: Appleton-Century-Crofts.

————— & Krakower, S. (1968), *Handwriting with Write and See*, Books 1-6. Chicago: Lyons & Carnahan.

Slagle, P. A., & Silver, D. S. (1972), "Turning on" the turned off: Active techniques with depressed drug users in a country free clinic. In: *Adolescents Grow in Groups*, ed. I. H. Berkovitz. New York: Brunner/Mazel, pp. 108-121.

Slavson, S. R. (1945), *An Introduction to Group Therapy*. New York: International Universities Press.

Sours, J. (1969), Anorexia nervosa: Nosology, diagnosis, developmental patterns and power-control dynamics. In: *Adolescence: Psychosocial Perspectives*, ed. G. Caplan & S. Lebovici. New York: Basic Books, pp. 185-212.

Spiegel, L. A. (1951), A review of contributions to a psychoanalytic theory of adolescence. *The Psychoanalytic Study of the Child*, 6:375-393. New York: International Universities Press.

—————(1954), Acting out and defensive instinctual gratification. *J. Amer. Psychoanal. Assn.*, 2:107-119.

Stanley, E. J., Glaser, H. H., Levin, D. G., Adams, P. A., & Coley, I. L. (1968), The treatment of adolescent obesity: Is it worthwhile? *Amer. J. Orthopsychiat.* (Digest Issue), 38:207.

Stanton, A. H., & Schwartz, M. S. (1954), *The Mental Hospital*. New York: Basic Books.

Stebbins, D. B. (1972), "Playing it by ear," in answering the needs of a group of black teen-agers. In: *Adolescents Grow in Groups*. ed. I. H. Berkovitz. New York: Brunner/Mazel, pp. 126-133.

Sterba, R. (1951), A case of brief psychotherapy by Sigmund Freud. *Psychoanal. Rev.*, 38:75-80.

Sternlicht, M. (1966), Treatment approaches to delinquent retardates. *Internat. J. Group Psychother.*, 16:91-93.

Stewart, W. A. (1963), An inquiry into the concept of working through. *J. Amer. Psychoanal. Assn.*, 11:474-499.

Stranahan, M., Schwartzman, C., & Atkin, E. (1957), Group treatment for emotionally disturbed and potentially delinquent boys and girls. *Amer. J. Orthopsychiat.*, 27:518-527.

Stunkard, A. (1972), New therapies for the eating disorders. *Arch. Gen. Psychiat.*, 26:391-398.

Sugar, M. (1972), Psychotherapy with the adolescent in self-selected peer groups. In: *Adolescents Grow in Groups*, ed. I. H. Berkovitz. New York: Brunner/Mazel, pp. 80-94.

—————(1975), Defusing a high school critical mass. In: *The Adolescent in Group and Family Therapy*, ed. M. Sugar. New York: Brunner/Mazel, pp. 118-141.

Sullivan, H. S. (1953), *The Interpersonal Theory of Psychiatry*. New York: Norton.

Sullivan, M. (1968), *Programmed Math*, Books 1-15. New York: McGraw-Hill.

Szasz, T. S. (1965), *The Ethics of Psychoanalysis: The Theory and Method of Autonomous Psychotherapy*. New York: Basic Books.

Taylor, A. J. (1967), An evaluation of group psychotherapy in a girl's borstal. *Internat. J. Group Psychother.*, 17:168-177.

Teicher, J. D. (1966), Group psychotherapy with adolescents. *Cal. Med.*, 105:18-21.

Theander, S. (1970), Anorexia nervosa. *Acta Psychiat. Scand.*, 214:29-31.

Thomä, H. (1967), *Anorexia Nervosa*. New York: International Universities Press.

Truax, C. B. (1971), Degree of negative transference occurring in group psychotherapy and client outcome in juvenile delinquents. *J. Clin. Psychol.*, 12:132-136.

Ulrich, R., Stachnik, T., & Mabry, J. (1970), *Control of Human Behavior: From Cure to Prevention*, Vol. 2. New York: Scott Foresman.

Van Putten, T. (1979), Antipsychotic drugs in adolescence. In: *Adolescent Psychiatry*, Vol. 7, ed. S. C. Feinstein & P. L. Giovacchini. Chicago: University of Chicago Press, pp. 389-401.

Vigersky, R. (1977), *Anorexia Nervosa*. New York: Raven.

Wachtel, P. (1977), *Psychoanalysis and Behavior Therapy*. New York: Basic Books.

Walder, L. O. (1966), Teaching parents to modify the behaviors of their autistic children. Presented to the American Psychological Association convention, New York.

Wallerstein, R. S. (1968), The challenge of the community mental health movement to psychoanalysis. *Amer. J. Psychiat.*, 124:1049-1056.

Walter, B. (1947), *Theme and Variations*. New York: Knopf.

Weitzman, B. (1967), Behavior therapy and psychotherapy. *Psychol. Rev.*, 74:300-317.

Wender, P. (1971), *Minimal Brain Dysfunction in Children*. New York: John Wiley & Sons.

Werry, J. S. (1978), *Pediatric Psychopharmacology*. New York: Brunner/Mazel.

——— & Wollersheim, J. (1967), Behavior therapy with children: A broad overview. *J. Amer. Acad. Child Psychiat.*, 6:346-370.

Whitaker, C. (1968), Interview. In: *Techniques of Family Therapy*, ed. J. Haley & L. Hoffman. New York: Basic Books, pp. 265-360.

Wiener, J. M. (1977), *Psychopharmacology in Childhood and Adolescence*. New York: Basic Books.

Williams, F. S. (1967a), Family therapy: A critical assessment. *Amer. J. Orthopsychiat.*, 37:912-919.

———(1967b), Family interviews for diagnostic evaluations in child psychiatry. Presented to the American Orthopsychiatric Association, New York.

————(1968), Family therapy. In: *Modern Psychoanalysis*, ed. J. Marmor. New York: Basic Books, pp. 387-406.

————(1970), Alienation of youth as reflected in the hippie movement. *J. Amer. Acad. Child Psychiat.*, 9:251-263.

Winnicott, D. W. (1965), Adolescence: Struggling through the doldrums. In: *The Family and Individual Development*. New York: Basic Books, pp. 79-87.

Wolk, R. L., & Reid, R. (1964), A study of group psychotherapy results with youthful offenders in detention. *Group Psychotherapy & Psychodrama*, 17:56-60.

Wolpe, J. (1958), *Psychotherapy by Reciprocal Inhibition*. Palo Alto, Cal.: Stanford University Press.

Wynne, L. C. (1965), Some indications and contraindications for exploration of family therapy. In: *Intensive Family Therapy*, ed. I. Boszormenyi-Nagy & J. L. Framo. New York: Harper & Row, pp. 289-322.

Yalom, I. D. (1970), *The Theory and Practice of Group Psychotherapy*. New York: Basic Books.

Youngerman, J., & Canino, I. (1978), Lithium carbonate use in children and adolescents: A survey of the literature. *Arch. Gen. Psychiat.*, 35:216-224.

Zellermayer, I. (1975), Reflections on adolescence. *Israel Annals Psychiat.*, 12:261-274.

Zentner, E. B., & Aponte, H. J. (1970), The amorphous family nexus. *Psychiat. Quart.*, 44:91-113.

Zinner, R., & Shapiro, R. (1972), Projective identification as a mode of perception and behavior in families of adolescents. *Internat. J. Psycho-Anal.*, 53:523-529.

NAME INDEX

SUBJECT INDEX